KEY TOPICS IN

OTOLARYNGOLOGY AND HEAD AND NECK SURGERY

The KEY TOPICS Series

Advisors:

T.M. Craft *Royal United Hospital, Bath, UK*
C.S. Garrard *Intensive Therapy Unit, John Radcliffe Hospital, Oxford, UK*
P.M. Upton *Sir Humphry Davy Department of Anaesthesia, Bristol Royal Infirmary, Bristol, UK*

Key Topics in Anaesthesia

Key Topics in Obstetrics and Gynaecology

Key Topics in Accident and Emergency Medicine

Key Topics in Paediatrics

Key Topics in Orthopaedic Surgery

Key Topics in Otolaryngology and Head and Neck Surgery

Forthcoming titles include:

Key Topics in General Surgery

Key Topics in Ophthalmology

KEY TOPICS IN
OTOLARYNGOLOGY AND HEAD AND NECK SURGERY

N.J. ROLAND
FRCS

*Senior Registrar and Lecturer in Otolaryngology
and Head and Neck Surgery,
Royal Liverpool University Hospital, Liverpool, UK*

R.D.R. McRAE
FRCS

*Senior Registrar in Otolaryngology
and Head and Neck Surgery,
Royal Liverpool University Hospital, Liverpool, UK*

A.W. McCOMBE
MD, FRCS

*Senior Registrar and Lecturer in Otolaryngology
and Head and Neck Surgery,
Bristol Royal Infirmary, Bristol, UK*

Consultant Editor
A.S. JONES
MD, FRCS

*Professor of Otolaryngology and Head and Neck Surgery,
University of Liverpool, UK*

βIOS
SCIENTIFIC
PUBLISHERS

First published 1995

A CIP catalogue record for this book is available from the British Library.

ISBN 1 872748 68 6

BIOS Scientific Publishers Ltd
9 Newtec Place, Magdalen Road, Oxford OX4 1RE
Tel. +44 (0)1865 726286. Fax. +44 (0)1865 246823

DISTRIBUTORS

Australia and New Zealand
    DA Information Services
    648 Whitehorse Road, Mitcham
    Victoria 3132

Singapore and South East Asia
    Toppan Company (S) PTE Ltd
    38 Liu Fang Road, Jurong
    Singapore 2262

India
    Viva Books Private Limited
    4346/4C Ansari Road
    New Delhi 110002

USA and Canada
    Books International Inc.
    PO Box 605, Herndon VA 22070

Typeset by Chandos Electronic Publishing, Stanton Harcourt, UK.
Printed by Redwood Books, Trowbridge, UK.

CONTENTS

[a] Contributed by J. Sutherland (FRCA), Registrar in Anaesthetics, Bristol Royal Infirmary, Bristol, UK.

[b] Contributed by T.H. Lesser (MS, FRCS), Consultant in Otoneurology, Walton Hospital, Liverpool, UK.

[c] Contributed by A. Leach (FRCA), Consultant in Anaesthesia, Royal Liverpool University Hospital, Liverpool, UK.

[d] Contributed by J.H. Rogers (FRCS), Consultant in Otolaryngology, Alder Hey Children's Hospital, Liverpool, UK.

[e] Contributed by J. Kabala (FRCR), Consultant Radiologist, Bristol Royal Infirmary, Bristol, UK.

[f] Contributed by M. Pringle (FRCS (ORL)), Senior Registrar in Otolaryngology and Head and Neck Surgery, The Royal Devon and Exeter Hospital, Exeter, UK.

[g] Contributed by P. Young (BSc (Hons), MCSLT), Senior Speech Therapist, Royal Liverpool University Hospital, Liverpool, UK.

ABBREVIATIONS

AIDS	Acquired immunodeficiency syndrome
AJC	American Joint Committee
ARC	AIDS-related complex
ASA	American Society of Anesthesiologists
ASOM	acute suppurative otitis media
BAHA	bone-anchored hearing aid
BEHA	behind-the-ear hearing aid
BERA	brainstem electrical response audiometry
BIPP	bismuth iodoform paraffin paste
BKB	Bench, Koval and Bamford
BW	body-worn
c-ANCA	cytoplasmic anti-neutrophil cytoplasmic antibody
CHOP	cyclophosphamide, hydroxydaunorubicin, oncovine, prednisolone
CPAP	continuous positive airway pressure
CROS	contralateral routing of signal
CSF	cerebrospinal fluid
CSOM	chronic suppurative otitis media
CT	computerized tomography
DPOAE	distortion-product otoacoustic emission
DSF	delayed speech feedback
EAM	external auditory meatus
EBV	Epstein–Barr virus
ECG	electrocardiogram
ECochG	echocochleography
EEG	electroencephalogram
EEMG	evoked electromyography
ELISA	enzyme-linked immunosorbent assay
EMG	electromyogram
EMLA	eutectic mixture of local anaesthetic
ENG	electronystagmography
EPS	exomphthalmos-producing substance
ERA	evoked response audiometry
ESR	erythrocyte sedimentation rate
EUA	examination under anaesthetic
FBC	full blood count
FESS	functional endoscopic sinus surgery
FNA	fine-needle aspiration
FNAC	fine-needle aspiration cytology
FTA	fluorescent treponemal antibody test
HIB	*Haemophilus influenzae* type B
HIV	human immunodeficiency virus
HL	hearing level

HPL	half-peak level
HPLE	half-peak level elevation
HPV	human papillomavirus
IHC	inner hair cell
IR	intrinsic rhinitis
KTP	potassium titanyl phosphate
LA	local anaesthetic
MEN	multiple endocrine neoplasia
MRI	magnetic resonance imaging
MSGC	minor salivary gland carcinoma
NCEPOD	National Confidential Enquiry into Perioperative Deaths
Nd-YAG	neodymium–yttrium aluminium garnet
NF2	neurofibromatosis type 2
NHL	non-Hodgkin's lymphoma
NIHL	noise-induced hearing loss
NOHL	non-organic hearing loss
NPC	nasopharyngeal carcinoma
OAE	otoacoustic emission
ODS	optimum discrimination score
OHC	outer hair cell
OM	occipitomental
OME	otitis media with effusion
OPG	orthopantogram
OSA	obstructive sleep apnoea
p-ANCA	perinuclear anti-neutrophil cytoplasmic antibody
PE	pharyngo-oesophageal
PHN	postherpetic neuralgia
PLF	perilymph fistula
PORP	partial ossicular replacement prosthesis
PRIST	plasma radioimmunosorbent test
PTA	pure tone audiometry
PTS	permanent threshold shift
RAST	radioallergosorbent test
SCC	squamous cell carcinoma
SL	sound level
SMR	submucosal resection
SNHL	sensorineural hearing loss
SOAE	spontaneous otoacoustic emission
SPL	sound pressure level
SRT	speech reception threshold
STIR	short tau inversion recovery
SVR	surgical voice restoration
TENS	transcutaneous electrical nerve stimulation
TEOAE	transient evoked otoacoustic emission
TFT	thyroid function tests

TGN	trigeminal nerve
TMJ	temporomandibular joint
TORP	total ossicular replacement prosthesis
TPHA	treponema pallidum haemagglutination antigen
TSH	thyroid-stimulating hormone
TSI	thyroid-stimulating immunoglobulin
TTS	temporary threshold shift
UICC	International Union Against Cancer
UPPP	uvulopharyngopalatoplasty
URTI	upper respiratory tract infection
VMA	vanillylmandelic acid
WG	Wegener's granulomatosis

PREFACE

Otolaryngology encompasses a broad range of supraspecialties in a rapidly changing discipline. Many weighty texts exist which give exhaustive coverage of the subject, but they risk hiding the wood from the trees. Common problems occur commonly. This is as true for postgraduate examinations as it is for clinical practice. Certain 'key topics' tend to present themselves far more frequently than others. The aim of this book is to give a succinct overview of the key topics in otolaryngology and head and neck surgery in a comprehensible, easy to read text.

Basic information is contained in some topics (e.g. Examination of the ear, nose and throat), and symptom-orientated approach is used in others (e.g. Epistaxis, Foreign bodies, Otalgia, Otorrhoea). Topics on specific commonly seen diseases (e.g. Acute sinusitis, Otitis media with effusion, Otitis externa) are also included. We feel that this makes the book an ideal introduction to the specialty for medical students, and an accessible source of reference for general practitioners and junior doctors cross-covering ENT surgery when they are on call.

The text is up-to-date and provides sufficient detail to be used as a valuable revision aid to those studying for post-graduate examinations in otolaryngology and head and neck surgery. Scrutiny of past papers and discussion with candidates reveals that there are certain key areas which tend to be repeated. We have endeavoured to cover these areas using a common framework for each topic. It is hoped that this will engender an approach which, when adopted, will be of use to the candidate considering questions in areas not discussed in the book. Other material which does not lend itself to this format (e.g. anaesthesia, cochlear implants, lasers in ENT, speech therapy) is also included as we feel that it is of sufficient importance.

A text of this size cannot pretend to be comprehensive and this one does not set out to be so. Anatomy is only described in the context of a particular clinical topic and only the principles of surgical technique are covered when deemed appropriate. Clarity and brevity have been our aim. We suggest the book be used early in the revision process before turning to the more major texts. The reader is encouraged to refer to the articles and texts which are recommended for further reading at the end of each topic. We feel that *Key Topics in Otolaryngology and Head and Neck Surgery* will be of particular value in those heady days just before examination for which we wish you every success!

N.J. Roland
R.D.R. McRae
A.W. McCombe

ACOUSTIC NEUROMA

Acoustic neuroma represents 8% of all intracranial tumours and 80% of cerebellopontine angle tumours. They arise from Schwann (neurolemmal) cells. The commonest nerve of origin is the superior vestibular nerve, followed by the inferior vestibular and then, rarely, the cochlear nerve. Many surgeons prefer therefore the term vestibular schwannoma to acoustic neuroma.

Pathology

As the medial portions of the cranial nerves are covered with glial stroma, acoustic neuromas are situated lateral to the porus, originating within the internal auditory meatus. The sexes are equally affected and, whatever the time of onset and rate of progression, the presentation is most often between the ages of 40 and 60. The majority of these tumours are unilateral, and the small proportion that are bilateral (5%) are seen in multiple neurofibromatosis type 2 (NF2). This is a genetic disease due to an aberration on the long arm of chromosome 22.

Macroscopically the tumour appears as a firm yellowish encapsulated mass with the nerve splayed out on its surface. Histologically the tumour consists of packed sheaves of connective tissue cells (fasciculated) or may be composed of a disorderly loose network of cells with intercellular vacuoles and cysts (reticular pattern). In the latter type, haemorrhage can occur, leading to a sudden increase in size and therefore marked symptoms such as acute vertigo or sudden deafness.

Clinical features

Clinically, two phases can be recognized: an *otological phase* in which a small intracanalicular tumour compresses only structures in the meatus; and a *neurological phase* as the tumour expands medially into the cerebellopontine angle.

1. Otological symptoms. Unilateral deafness of less than 10 years' duration, often associated with tinnitus, is the usual presenting symptom. Vertigo is an unusual complaint as compensation for vestibular nerve damage usually keeps pace with the slow rate of neural destruction.

2. Trigeminal nerve symptoms. Facial pain, numbness and paraesthesiae may all occur.

3. Headache. Discomfort and dull aching around the ear and mastoid area are probably caused by posterior fossa dura irritation due to the enlarging tumour.

4. Late symptoms. Like most motor nerves, the facial nerve is resistant to pressure deformity and symptoms of facial weakness or hemifacial spasm are uncommon. Ataxia and unsteadiness develop with progressive brain stem displacement and cerebellar involvement. Diplopia due to pressure on the VIth cranial nerve, and hoarseness with dysphagia due to involvement of the IXth and Xth nerves is rare.

5. Terminal symptoms. The raised CSF pressure causes failing vision due to papilloedema, headache and eventually coma.

In the otological phase, general examination will reveal no abnormalities. The patient may have a unilateral neural hearing loss. Later the patient may have evidence of ataxia. Loss of the corneal reflex is an early sign of trigeminal nerve impairment. Nystagmus when present may be of the vestibular or cerebellar type. Facial nerve impairment is usually of the sensory element and can be elicited as a lack of taste on electrogustometry or loss of lacrimation on Schirmer's test. Slight facial weakness may show as a delay in the blink reflex. Neurological signs of the other cranial nerve palsies will eventually become apparent.

Investigations

1. Audiometry. A unilateral or asymmetrical sensorineural hearing loss can usually be demonstrated by a *pure tone audiogram.* The hearing loss is classically a neural lesion with no loudness recruitment, abnormally rapid adaptation and disproportionately poor speech discrimination. *Stapedial reflex decay* can be measured using impedance audiometry, and this gives a low-false negative rate of around 5%. *Brainstem electric response audiometry* has only a 3% false-negative rate and, where it is available, is undoubtedly the audiological investigation of choice. It demonstrates a retrocochlear lesion by an increased latency between N1 and N5 waves. If the pure tone threshold hearing loss is greater than 70 dB, the accuracy of audiometric testing is poor.

2. Vestibular investigations. Caloric responses are usually reduced in or absent from the affected side, but there is no abnormality in some patients with small tumours.

3. Radiological investigations. Computerized tomography (CT) scanning with high definition and enhancement techniques will accurately diagnose and delineate most tumours, but the most accurate means of identifying small intracanalicular tumours is *magnetic resonance* (MRI) scanning with gadolinium enhancement.

Differential diagnosis of a tumour at the cerebellopontine angle

1. Acoustic neuromas (constitute 80% of cerebellopontine angle tumours).

2. Meningioma.

3. Neuroma of the VIIth nerve.

4. Congenital cholesteatoma.

5. Aneurysm of the basilar or vertebral arteries.

6. Cholesterol granuloma of the petrous apex.

7. Cerebellar tumour.

Management

The ideal management is a single stage total removal of the lesion, with preservation of all neural function and with minimal morbidity and mortality. However, this ideal is not always possible. Each case must be assessed on its own merits, with careful consideration of the age and general condition of the patient and the size, site and rate of growth of the lesion.

Removal of acoustic neuroma is associated most commonly with injury to the VIIth and VIIIth cranial nerves. Cerebrospinal fluid leak (often from the Eustachian tube) and meningitis are also relatively common. The morbidity and mortality from both tumour growth and its operative removal increase with large tumours. A small tumour can be extracted from the meatus with negligible hazard and preservation of the facial nerve. Early diagnosis and removal of these tumours should therefore be the rule. Small, slow-growing tumours in elderly patients can be watched by carrying out CT or MRI scanning at regular intervals to gauge the rate of expansion. Stereotactic radiosurgery has been applied to the tumour margin to control growth. This technique is limited in current practice to patients unable or unwilling to undergo surgery.

There are three approaches to the cerebellopontine angle and the choice depends on the position and size of the tumour and preoperative assessment by the otoneurologist and neurosurgeon.

1. *Middle fossa route.* This gives a limited access and is used for only very small intrameatal tumours. Hearing and the facial nerve can be preserved.

2. *Translabyrinthine approach.* This allows removal of intrameatal tumours that do not extend for more than a few millimetres into the cerebellopontine angle. The facial nerve can be preserved but all hearing is lost. The approach tends to be used for patients with a severe sensorineural hearing loss.

3. *Suboccipital approach.* This is needed for large tumours. The patient's hearing and facial nerve can be preserved, so this approach is also used for small tumours when there is good hearing.

Further reading

Chandler CL, Ramsden RT. Acoustic schwannoma. *British Journal of Hospital Medicine,* 1993; **49**(5): 3–16; 335–43.
Kveton JF. Evaluation and management of acoustic neuroma. *Current Opinion in Otolaryngology and Head and Neck Surgery*, 1993; **1**: 53–63.
Ludman H. Tumours of the inner ear. In: Ludman H (ed.) *Mawson's Diseases of the Ear*, 5th edn. London: Edward Arnold, 1988; 648–62.

Related topics of interest

Evoked response audiometry (p. 85)
Radiology in ENT (p. 259)
Tinnitus (p. 313)
Vertigo (p. 334)
Vestibular function tests (p. 338)

ACUTE SINUSITIS

Acute inflammation of one or all the sinuses may occur (pansinusitis). The maxillary sinus is clinically the most commonly affected, followed by the ethmoid, frontal and sphenoid sinuses in that order.

Aetiology

1. *Acute infective rhinitis (common cold or influenza).*

2. *Dental extraction or infection.*

3. *Swimming and diving.*

4. *Fractures involving the sinuses.*

Predisposing factors

1. *Local.*

- Pre-existing rhinitis (allergic, vasomotor, rhinitis medicamentosa, etc.).
- Nasal polyps.
- Nasal foreign body.
- Upper respiratory tract infection (tonsillitis and adenoiditis).
- Nasal anatomical variations (septal deviation, abnormal uncinate process, middle turbinate or ethmoid bulla) narrow the infundibulum and predispose to its occlusion when there is intercurrent disease.
- Nasal tumour.

2. *General.*

- Debilitation.
- Immunocompromised host.
- Mucociliary disorders (e.g. Kartagener's syndrome).

Pathology

The majority of cases follow a viral upper respiratory tract infection which involves all of the respiratory epithelium including the paranasal sinuses. Such infections cause hyperaemia and oedema of the mucosa, which blocks the ostia. There will be cellular infiltration and an increase in mucus production.

The infection will also paralyse the cilia, leading to stasis of secretions predisposing to secondary bacterial infection. The usual causative organisms are *Streptococcus pneumoniae, Streptococcus pyogenes, Staphylococcus aureus* and *Haemophilus influenzae. Klebsiella pneumoniae, Escherichia coli* and *Streptococcus faecalis* may spread from a dental source. Acute fungal infections (for example mucormycosis and aspergillosis) are rare, but may develop in immunocompromised or elderly diabetic patients.

Clinical features

The symptoms usually occur several days after developing an upper respiratory tract infection. The patient will have pain over the infected sinus, nasal congestion, fullness in the face, malaise and possibly a pyrexia. The fullness in the face and pain may be exacerbated by bending forward or stooping down.

Specific features may indicate the sinus that is infected. Pain developing in the cheek or upper teeth indicates maxillary sinus involvement. Frontal sinusitis produces pain in the forehead and tenderness below the eyebrows. Ethmoid sinusitis may cause pain between the eyes accompanied by frontal headache. Sphenoid infection may produce retro-orbital pain, or pain anywhere across the vault.

Anterior rhinoscopy nasal mucosa and turbinates may show red oedematous. Posterior rhinoscopy may reveal pus in the middle meatus or sphenoethmoidal recess. It may also be possible to elicit tenderness over the infected sinus. Percussion over the upper teeth may elicit tenderness, suggesting a dental origin of maxillary sinusitis.

Differential diagnosis

1. *Migraine.*

2. *Dental pain.*

3. *Trigeminal neuralgia.*

4. *Temporal arteritis.*

5. *Herpes zoster.*

6. *Erysipelas.*

7. *Sinonasal tumour.*

Investigations

An elevated white cell count and erythrocyte sedimentation rate (ESR) will confirm an acute infection. Where possible pus from the nose should be cultured and blood cultures should be taken if there is systemic upset. Radiological investigation may show an opacity or fluid level. Standard radiographic views of the paranasal sinuses include:

- Occipitomental (maxillary sinus).
- Occipitofrontal (ethmoid and frontal sinus).
- Lateral (sphenoid sinus).

When there is doubt about the diagnosis, further confirmation can be obtained by a high-definition coronal CT scan, ideally using both soft-tissue and bone window settings.

Management

The aims of treatment are to resolve and limit the course of the acute infection, to prevent complications and to correct any precipitating factor.

1. Medical treatment. In the acute stages the patient should have:

- Bed rest and adequate simple analgesia (e.g. paracetamol).
- Broad-spectrum antibiotic (e.g. co-anoxyclav).
- A decongestant (e.g. pseudoephedrine or xylometazoline).

The patient should have a full 7-day course of the antibiotic. The decongestant may reduce nasal oedema, and hopefully open the natural ostia of the sinuses to allow free drainage. It can be given locally or systemically. The current practice of many rhinologists is to shrink the mucosal lining, and aid infundibular drainage, by placing a pledget of cocainized cotton wool into the middle meatus for 20 minutes.

2. Surgical treatment. Functional endoscopic sinus surgery (see p. 119) is now considered to be the treatment of choice, but the classical management is described as it is still used in many centres and is asked about in the examination. If acute sinusitis fails to respond to medical treatment within 24 hours or so then the patient needs an antral puncture and washout. This will not only treat any infection in the maxillary sinus but will also promote drainage from the other sinuses as the oedema in the middle meatus settles. Any pus obtained should be cultured. If the patient has suffered recurrent infections it may be appropriate to perform an intranasal antrostomy for better and longer-lasting drainage. Frontal sinusitis which does not respond to these measures requires trephining of the floor of the sinus via a small incision above the medial canthus. The ethmoid sinuses can be uncapped to promote drainage if they are specifically diseased and an anterior sphenoidotomy may be necessary for acute sphenoiditis.

Follow-up and aftercare

The patient should be reviewed 2 weeks after the resolution of the acute phase. Correction of any obvious precipitating factor (e.g. septoplasty for septal deviation) should be organized. It may be necessary to perform repeat antral washouts for some patients. Those surgeons who follow the philosophy of functional endoscopic sinus surgery claim that if definitive endoscopic sinus surgery is performed in the acute phase no further washout should be necessary.

Related topics of interest

ACUTE SUPPURATIVE OTITIS MEDIA

Definition

Otitis media is an inflammation of part or all of the mucosa of the middle-ear cleft, the collective term for the Eustachian tube, tympanic cavity, attic, aditus, antrum and mastoid air cells.

Classification

It may be classified as acute or chronic with the suffix suppurative or non-suppurative. A third category, 'specific otitis media', has been used to describe tuberculous and syphilitic otitis media which may present acutely or chronically, with or without suppuration. A fourth category, namely 'adhesive otitis media', has been used to describe tympanosclerosis (hyaline degeneration and calcification) and adhesion formation within the tympanic cavity but should more accurately be regarded as a sequel of otitis media.

Acute suppurative otitis media (ASOM)

Aetiology

This is a bacterial disease caused by pus-forming organisms, *Streptococcus pneumoniae* (40%), *Haemophilus influenzae* (30%) and *Branhamella (Moraxella) catarrhalis* (10%) being the most commonly implicated. It may occur as a primary or a secondary infection after a viral acute non-suppurative otitis media. Bacteria enter the middle-ear cleft via the Eustachian tube, a perforated tympanic membrane or may more rarely be blood-borne. Infants have a short, wide more horizontally placed Eustachian tube, allowing contamination from the regurgitation of feed and when actively vomiting. Teething increases the incidence of infection. Poor sanitation and hygiene, overcrowding and malnutrition are predisposing factors. Children aged 3–7 have the highest incidence, direct extension from a bacterial or secondary to a viral upper respiratory tract infection being the most common aetiological factor. Risk factors in all age groups are recurrent or chronic rhinosinusitis, adenoiditis, chest disease and Eustachian tube dysfunction. Causes of the latter are nasopharyngeal tumours, including adenoidal hypertrophy, abnormal Eustachian patency and cleft and submucous cleft palate. Pathogenic bacteria have been isolated from the nasopharynx in up to 97% of children with ASOM.

Clinical features

The two main symptoms are:

- *Pain*, which may increase rapidly in intensity to become deep and throbbing.
- *Deafness* initially described as a blocked ear and secondary to Eustachian tube dysfunction.

Deafness progresses as suppuration supervenes and both symptoms may rapidly improve if the tympanic membrane ruptures to produce a mucopurulent otorrhoea.

The initial event after infection is mucosal oedema, causing Eustachian tube occlusion and a dull tympanic membrane on examination. Hyperaemia rapidly follows and leashes of vessels may be seen running along or parallel to the malleus handle. Soon radial vessels are visible on the drumhead and a middle-ear effusion occurs. The drumhead takes on a full (i.e. opposite to retraction), red, angry appearance and pus may be seen bulging posteroinferiorly. Pressure necrosis of this region may cause the drumhead to rupture, allowing mucopus to drain into the external ear canal. Children are usually fretful with a high pyrexia (>39°C) and there may be signs of complications of ASOM.

Treatment

1. Rest in a warm, well-humidified room.

2. Antibiotics in an adequate dose administered until resolution. Amoxycillin will cover the most common pathogens provided the patient is not allergic to penicillin and the organisms are not resistant, the latter occurring in about 14% of cases and increasing. In these circumstances, gleaned from bacterial sensitivity studies or lack of clinical response, a β-lactamase-resistant antibiotic should be chosen, for example coamoxyclav. Oral medication is adequate in the absence of complications.

3. Systemic and topical decongestants have a theoretical adjuvant role although, as in glue ear trials, they have not been proven to be of significant value.

4. Conditions predisposing to ASOM should be treated on their own merit after resolution of the acute infection.

Complications

- *Mucositis may progress to an osteomyelitis*, namely acute mastoiditis, if the mastoid air cells are affected or acute petrositis should the petrous apex become involved. Gradenigo's syndrome, comprising signs of ASOM, in particular a discharging ear, an ipsilateral abducent nerve palsy causing paralysis of the external rectus and pain in the distribution of the ipsilateral trigeminal nerve, is a classical feature of petrositis. The cranial nerves are separated from the petrous apex only by a layer of dura so that an extradural abscess or pachymeningitis (meningitis extending to the dural layer) of this region from a generalized meningitis may also cause the combined cranial nerve signs.

- *Meningitis.*
- *Citelli's abscess* (a subperiosteal abscess which has spread through the medial aspect of the mastoid, into the digastric fossa) or *Bezold's abscess* (an abscess which has tracked inferiorly within the sheath of sternomastoid to form a fluctuant mass along its anterior border).
- *Extradural and subdural abscess.*
- *Cerebellar, temporal lobe and perisinus abscess.*
- *Lateral sinus thrombosis*, rarely extending in an antegrade direction to thrombose the internal jugular vein and in a retrograde direction causing a cavernous sinus thrombosis.
- *Otitic hydrocephalus.*
- *Lower motor neurone facial nerve paralysis.* This occurs usually in that group of patients with a congenital dehiscence of the horizontal portion of the facial nerve comprising 6% of the population.
- *Serous and suppurative labyrinthitis.*

Sequelae of ASOM

- *Non-suppurative middle-ear effusion.* This persists for over 30 days in 40% of children and for over 3 months in 10%.
- *High-tone sensorineural hearing loss*, perhaps secondary to bacterial toxins migrating across the round window.
- *Tympanic membrane perforation.*
- *Adhesions* between the tympanic membrane, ossicles and the medial wall of the middle ear.
- *Tympanosclerosis,* which may spread from the tympanic membrane to the ossicular chain, fixing the latter.
- *Erosion of the ossicular chain*, in particular the long process of the incus, especially following recurrent episodes of ASOM.
- Sequelae of ASOM complications.

Further reading

Haddad J Jr. Treatment of acute otitis media and its complications in paediatric otology. *Otolaryngologic Clinics of North America*, 1994; **6:** 431–41.

Pichichero ME. Assessing the treatment alternatives for acute otitis media. *Paediatric Infectious Diseases Journal*, 1994; **13:** 27–34.

Stutman HR, Arguedas AG. Comparison of cefprozil with other antibiotic regimes in the treatment of children with acute otitis media. *Clinical Infectious Diseases*, 1992; **14** (Suppl. 2): 204–8.

Related topics of interest

ADENOIDS

The adenoids are a mass of lymphoid tissue found at the junction of the roof and posterior wall of the nasopharynx. They are a normal structure with a function in the production of antibodies (IgA, IgG and IgM). The size of the adenoids varies, but in general they attain their maximum size between the ages of 3 and 8 years and then regress.

Pathology

Inflammation due to acute viral and bacterial infections results in hyperplasia with enlargement and multiplication of the lymphoid follicles. Most of the pathological effects related to the adenoids are due to this increase in size. The symptoms caused by hypertrophy result not from the actual size of the lymphoid mass, but from the relative disproportion in size between the adenoids and the cavity of the nasopharynx. The effect of the enlargement is to produce obstruction of the nasal airways and possibly obstruction of the Eustachian tubes.

Clinical features

1. Nasal obstruction leads to mouth breathing, snoring and hyponasal speech. Infants may have difficulty in feeding because they have to stop sucking intermittently to take a breath. Nasal discharge and postnasal drip or catarrh may develop as a result of secondary chronic rhinitis and sinusitis. Besides snoring, some children may suffer from episodes of sleep apnoea. The child with the characteristic adenoid facies appearance (an open lip posture, prominent upper incisors, a short upper lip, a thin nose and a hypoplastic maxilla with a high arched palate) is rarely seen.

2. Eustachian tube obstruction may result in earache and deafness due to recurrent bouts of acute otitis media and otitis media with effusion (glue ear).

The clinical features of adenoid hypertrophy are not always clear cut, and unfortunately the parents' history is not always reliable. Symptoms are frequently wrongly attributed to enlarged adenoids. In some children examination of the nasopharynx with a postnasal mirror will identify large adenoids, but in many children it is impossible to assess the adenoids in this way

Investigations

The only reliable means of assessing the size of the adenoid is examination under general anaesthetic, but some preoperative investigations may suggest enlargement. The most useful investigation is a lateral soft-tissue radiograph. This will give a measure of the absolute size of the adenoids and an assessment of their proportion in relation to the size of the airway. This is not always accurate and some children will still need an examination of the postnasal space under general anaesthetic. If enlarged adenoids are present then they can then be curetted.

Indications for adenoidectomy

Generally speaking, an adenoidectomy is only indicated if troublesome symptoms can be attributed to abnormal adenoid hypertrophy. The evidence for their removal in otitis media with effusion and acute otitis media is debatable. Some studies have shown a benefit after adenoidectomy and others no effect in control of these diseases. The indications for adenoidectomy are as follows:

- Nasal obstruction.
- Otitis media with effusion (glue ear).
- Recurrent acute otitis media.
- Chronic rhinosinusitis.
- Sleep apnoea.

Contraindications for adenoidectomy

- Recent upper respiratory tract infection.
- An uncontrolled bleeding disorder.
- Cleft palate. The adenoids assist in closure of the nasopharynx from the oropharynx during speech and deglutition. They should never be removed in a child who has had a cleft palate repair or a congenitally short palate. All children who have a bifid uvula should have a submucous cleft excluded.

Complications of adenoidectomy

1. *Immediate.*

- Anaesthetic complications.
- Soft palate damage.
- Dislocation of the cervical spine.
- Reactionary haemorrhage.

2. *Intermediate.*

- Secondary haemorrhage.
- Subluxation of the atlanto-occipital joint (secondary to infection).

3. *Late.*

- Eustachian tube stenosis.
- Hypernasal speech (rhinolalia aperta).
- Persistence of symptoms.

The most serious complication is reactionary haemorrhage. This is treated in the same manner as post-tonsillectomy haemorrhage. The child should be returned to theatre and an attempt made to localize and diathermy the bleeding point. A postnasal pack should be inserted if necessary. Hypernasal speech can be a troublesome complication in some children. It often improves with time and speech therapy but may be sufficiently severe to require a pharyngoplasty to correct the problem. It is less likely to occur if children with palatal abnormalities are excluded from operation. Some surgeons advocate removal of the upper part of the adenoid mass leaving a lower ridge of adenoid tissue against which the defective palate may continue to make contact.

Follow-up and aftercare In view of the problems with accurate diagnosis and the potential long-term complications it is worthwhile reviewing adenoidectomy children in the outpatient clinic 6 months postoperatively.

Further reading

Hotaling AJ, Silva AB. Advances in adenotonsillar disease. *Current Opinion in Otolaryngology and Head and Neck Surgery*, 1993; **1**: 177–84.
Potsic WP. Assessment and treatment of adenotonsillar hypertrophy in children. *American Journal of Otolaryngology*, 1992; **13**: 259–64.

Related topics of interest

ALLERGIC RHINITIS

Allergic rhinitis is an IgE-mediated, type 1 hypersensitivity reaction in the mucous membranes of the nasal airways. The disease is very common, affecting approximately 30% of the Western population. It can be either seasonal (summer hayfever) or perennial (sometimes with seasonal exacerbations).

Aetiology

Allergy is a hypersensitivity reaction of tissues to certain substances called allergens. The commonest allergens are highly soluble proteins or glycoproteins with a molecular weight in the range of 10 000 – 40 000. Typical allergens include pollens, moulds, house dust mite (*Dermatophagoides pteronyssinus* and *D. forinae*) and animal epithelia.

Pathogenesis

Immunoglobulin E is formed by plasma cells which are regulated by T suppressor lymphocytes and T helper cells. In normal individuals this system maintains a constant function. In allergic patients the IgE T helper cells appear to promote overproduction at times of exposure to the allergen, or suppressor T cells may not be functioning correctly. The IgE antibody is composed of an Fc and an Fab portion. The Fc portion of IgE has an affinity for mast cells and basophils, which have receptors for the immunoglobulin on their cell membrane. The Fab portion of IgE is free to combine with an allergen. The allergen is thought to interact with two adjacent cell-bound IgE antibody molecules, so forming a cross-link composed of IgE–allergen–IgE. This triggers a chain of events with the synthesis and release of arachidonic acid metabolites (prostaglandin D, leukotrienes and other chemotactic factors) and initiates disruption of the mast cell with degranulation of lysosomes (releasing histamine, proteases and more chemotactic factors). The effect is that capillaries become more permeable, the ground substance viscosity is reduced by enzymes such as hyaluronidase, eosinophils infiltrate the tissues and oedema occurs. This produces the typical features of vascular congestion, oedema, rhinorrhoea and irritation.

Clinical features

Seasonal rhinitis usually occurs any time from early summer to early autumn depending on the specific allergen. The patient suffers from rhinorrhoea, nasal irritation and sneezing, associated with itchy and watering eyes. Some individuals (described as atopic) will have a strong family history of allergy or a previous history of eczema or asthma. Long-standing cases of perennial allergy may not display all these features, but they often have nasal obstruction due to hypertrophy of the inferior turbinates sometimes associated with hyposmia. Patients with perennial rhinitis are almost invariably allergic to house dust mite and typically have more than one allergy.

On examination the nasal mucosa classically appears moist, pale and swollen, and the turbinates hypertrophied. Sometimes the mucosa is red and the turbinates may have a blue hue to their appearance. Polyps may be present, but they are more often seen in intrinsic rhinitis.

Investigations

There are many investigations available, but clinically the most useful are the skin tests and plasma IgE measurements.

1. Skin tests. The epidermal prick test and the intradermal injection test use an allergen placed on the skin of the flexor aspect of the forearm. If the patient has an allergy to this then a wheal and flare will come up within 20 minutes. A negative control (carrier substance) and a histamine-containing solution (positive control) are used to ensure that the patient is not allergic to the carrier substance and does react in the normal fashion to histamine. A battery of common allergens (e.g. pollens, moulds, feathers, house dust mite, animal epithelia, etc.) are compared with the controls by the wheal they produce. Specific substances can be used depending on the history. If the patient is highly sensitive a widespread or even an anaphylactic reaction may result. Resuscitation equipment must always be available although the epidermal prick test is safe if properly performed. If an adverse reaction occurs, a tourniquet should be placed proximally to contain it and the patient given intravenous hydrocortisone, chlorpheniramine and adrenaline.

2. Blood tests. Total plasma IgE levels may be measured in the plasma radioimmunosorbent test (PRIST) and IgE to specific allergens in the radioallergosorbent test (RAST). These tests are more convenient, do not expose the patient to the risks of the skin tests and do not rely on the use of a specific allergen. However, they are more expensive and have no diagnostic superiority over skin tests. An eosinophilia may occur in an acute allergic reaction but is unusual in allergic rhinitis.

3. Nasal smears. An increase in eosinophils in a nasal smear indicates an allergic rhinitis but is not diagnostic.

4. Provocation tests. A drop of the suspected allergen squeezed into the nose may cause symptoms (rhinorrhoea, sneezing, etc.). The effect can be measured objectively by rhinomanometry.

Management

1. Avoidance of the precipitating allergen is obviously helpful, but not always possible.

2. Oral antihistamines which selectively block histamine receptors, cause minimal or no drowsiness and can be given once daily are now available (e.g. astemizole, terfenadine, oratidine, cetirizine). Some patients still prefer the older antihistamines which may cause drowsiness (e.g. chlorpheniramine and triprolidine) and they should be warned of this. Intranasal antihistamine sprays (e.g. azelastine hydrochloride) have the advantage of minimal absorption.

3. Topical steroid sprays and drops are now considered to be the cornerstone in the treatment of rhinitis. They are safe and effective. Crusting and bleeding are the main side-effects. Systemic absorption is negligible, as is the chance of promoting fungal infections. Examples include beclomethasone dipropionate, fluticasone propionate and budesonide.

4. Depot intramuscular injections of steroids (e.g. triamcinolone acetonide) should be reserved for when symptoms interfere with special events (e.g. school examinations). Oral steroids are even more rarely indicated.

5. Sodium cromoglycate stabilizes mast cell membranes and therefore prevents the release of the allergic response mediators. It has few side-effects, but needs to be used five to six times per day for adequate prophylaxis. It works in relatively few people but may be effective in children.

6. Desensitization involves a series of injections of small amounts of the proven allergens in a purified form, in the hope that blocking IgG antibodies will be produced. It is really only of use in patients who are sensitive to only one or two allergens, in particular pollen allergy. The main complication of this treatment is anaphylaxis, and for this reason its use in the UK has been discouraged. Resuscitation equipment must always be available where this therapy is performed, and in case of anaphylaxis there must be a supply of intravenous hydrocortisone, chlorpheniramine and adrenaline.

7. Surgical treatment has little role to play other than turbinate surgery when there are symptoms of nasal obstruction.

Follow-up and aftercare Most cases of allergic rhinitis can be managed by the patient's general practitioner. If the offending allergen is identified by any of the tests then the patient should be given general advice on avoidance. When there are any nasal abnormalities (e.g. deflected nasal septum or turbinate hypertrophy) or concomitant disease of the sinuses that complicate and exaggerate the symptoms of the rhinitis, they should be treated on their own merit.

Further reading

Norman PS. Allergic rhinitis. *Journal of Allergy and Clinical Immunology*, 1985; **75**: 531–45.
The cellular and clinical aspects of treating rhinitis with fluticasone propionate. *European Respiratory Review*, 1994; **4**: 245–73.

Related topics of interest

ANAESTHESIA – GENERAL

Approximately 5% of general anaesthetics given in the UK are for ENT procedures. The majority are elective procedures with an increasing proportion as day cases. One of the most important points is that successful surgery and anaesthesia depend on cooperation and understanding of the problems involved between the surgeon and the anaesthetist. There should be a high level of liaison and dialogue at all times.

Problems

Shared airway

1. Access. Operations on the nose and throat require the anaesthetist and surgeon to share the airway. Many otolaryngeal procedures require the trachea to be intubated to facilitate adequate ventilation, protect the airway from blood and debris and ensure surgical access. The tracheal tube should always be secured to prevent dislodgement, disconnection or kinking. The last is a particular risk during tonsillectomy when a gag is used and during procedures that involve instrumentation of the airway, e.g. endoscopy.

2. Bleeding in the airway.
(a) Preoperatively with epistaxis or post tonsillectomy haemorrhage. It must be assumed that blood has entered the stomach, and laryngoscopy may be difficult owing to blood clots and continued bleeding. Adequate resuscitation is essential before induction to prevent acute cardiovascular collapse. An experienced anaesthetist is required. Intubation may be performed following a rapid-sequence intravenous induction or a gaseous induction in the left lateral, head-down position. A rapid-sequence induction is preceded by preoxygenation and is performed with a predetermined dose of intravenous anaesthetic agent. Cricoid pressure is applied at induction to prevent regurgitation of gastric contents into the airway. Intravenous induction of anaesthesia causes more hypotension than a gaseous induction, however anaesthetists are more familiar with intubating in a supine position rather than in the left lateral position.
(b) Intraoperatively. Blood loss may be reduced by smooth induction of anaesthesia and the avoidance of coughing or straining and thus venous congestion. Patients with local infection or allergy-related disorder have increased

airway sensitivity and may require deep anaesthesia or neuromuscular blockade to avoid this. General anaesthesia with deliberate hypotension may minimize intraoperative blood loss.

(c) Postoperatively. If blood is present in the airway, the patient is extubated, after pharyngeal suction, in the left lateral, head-down position.

3. *Laser surgery.* This risks an airway fire after ignition of the tracheal tube or the fresh gas mixture. The tracheal tube should be flexometallic, wrapped in aluminium foil or laserproof. The tracheal tube cuff is filled with saline or preformed with foam. If airway fire occurs, the surgery must be discontinued and ventilation stopped until the fire is extinguished with a pre-filled syringe of saline. The tracheal tube should then be replaced, the patient ventilated with 100% oxygen, a bronchoscopy performed, steroids commenced and antibiotics and prolonged ventilatory support provided as necessary.

Induced hypotension

This can reduce blood loss during head and neck operations. It may result in cerebral or myocardial ischaemia and renal or hepatic hypoperfusion. It is contraindicated in patients with coexisting hypertension, ischaemic heart disease, previous cerebrovascular accident, pregnancy, anaemia, hypovolaemia or impaired renal or hepatic function.

Techniques of inducing hypotension include:

- The prevention of anxiety-related tachycardia by good premedication.
- The avoidance of hypertension during laryngoscopy and intubation.
- Controlled ventilation without positive end-expiratory pressure.
- Volatile agent-induced vasodilatation.
- The use of head-up positioning to encourage venous drainage from the operative site.

Specific drugs used to induce hypotension include:

- *d*-Tubocurare, which is a muscle relaxant that releases histamine and blocks sympathetic ganglia.
- Sodium nitroprusside, which directly dilates arterioles and venules.
- Glyceryl trinitrate, which dilates capacitance vessels.
- Trimetaphan, which releases histamine, blocks ganglia and directly reduces peripheral vascular resistance.

- Labetolol, which reduces arteriolar tone and heart rate (useful in preventing the reflex tachycardia seen in response to hypotension).

Large-bore intravenous access and an arterial cannula to facilitate direct blood pressure monitoring are required if profound hypotension is to be induced, but this is rarely, if ever, warranted in ENT surgery.

Nitrous oxide (N_2O)

This has been in use for 120 years as a general anaesthetic. It is 35 times more soluble in blood than nitrogen, and thus diffuses into air-containing spaces such as the middle ear, leading to an increase in pressure. This is maximal after 40 minutes of anaesthesia and is implicated in the adverse positioning of grafts, altered appearance of the tympanic membrane and postoperative nausea and vomiting. Nitrous oxide may be excluded by substituting air or by total intravenous anaesthesia. It has been suggested that packing the middle ear during surgery reduces the clinical significance of nitrous oxide-induced pressure changes.

Anaesthetic management

The following investigations are generally required:

- FBC
  Females of menstrual age.
  All patients over 60.
  Before major operations.
  After significant blood loss.
- U&E
  All patients over 60.
  Patients with diabetes, renal or hepatic impairment, hypertension, or on medications such as diuretics and antihypertensives.
- ECG
  All patients over 60.
- Chest radiography
  All patients over 60.

These guidelines are modified according to each individual patient's signs and symptoms. Treatment of medical conditions should be optimized preoperatively. Patients require steroid cover if they have received steroids in the past 12 months, or antibiotic prophylaxis if valvular heart disease is present.

Premedication

Premedication may be used to reduce anxiety and decrease the incidence of nausea and vomiting. A benzodiazepine with an antiemetic is a suitable combination, although patients with a compromised airway should not be sedated. Oral sedative agents are often used in children who also require EMLA (eutectic mixture of local anaesthetic – lignocaine 2.5% with prilocaine 2.5%). EMLA cream is applied to potential venepuncture sites under an occlusive dressing. Anticholinergics may be given as an antisialogogue, glycopyrolate being the best as it causes less tachycardia and does not cross the blood–brain barrier thus avoiding confusion. They are not given if hypotension is required as the resulting tachycardia antagonizes this effect.

Specific procedures

1. Myringotomy. Intubation is not required; the effects of N_2O should be considered. A laryngeal mask airway may be used.

2. Nasal operations. Injection of local anaesthetic with a vasoconstrictor may induce arrhythmias, especially if halothane is used, as this sensitizes the myocardium to catecholamines.

3. Upper airway obstruction. An experienced anaesthetist is required to perform either a gaseous induction or an awake intubation. The findings at indirect laryngoscopy should be available. The latter agent is now rarely used in the UK.

4. Microlaryngoscopy. The cords are sprayed with lignocaine 10% to prevent laryngospasm.

5. Tracheostomy. Once dissection to the trachea is achieved, 100% oxygen is given and oropharyngeal suction performed prior to opening the trachea. The endotracheal tube is then withdrawn to just above the tracheotomy and the tracheostomy tube is inserted.

6. Laryngectomy. Preoperative radiotherapy may result in tissue scarring and a difficult intubation. The tumour itself may also make intubation difficult. Proceed as for tracheostomy, except when the trachea is cut the endotracheal tube may be replaced initially by a modified tracheal tube to facilitate surgical access. The tracheostomy tube is used only at the end of the procedure.

7. Pharyngolaryngo-oesophagectomy. Traction on the mediastinum may produce arrhythmias. Damage to the pleura may result in a pneumothorax.

Further reading

Craft TM, Upton PM. *Key Topics in Anaesthesia,* 2nd edn. Oxford: BIOS Scientific
  Publishers, 1995.
MacRae WR. ENT and ophthalmology. In: Nimmo WS, Smith G (eds) *Anaesthesia*, Vol. 1.
  Oxford: Blackwell Scientific Publications, 1989; 522–37.

Related topics of interest

Anaesthesia – local (p. 25)
Hypopharyngeal carcinoma (p. 133)
Laryngeal carcinoma (p. 148)
Paediatric airway problems (p. 234)
Stridor and stertor (p. 301)
Tracheostomy (p. 323)

ANAESTHESIA – LOCAL

Local anaesthetic (LA) agents produce a reversible block in the transmission of peripheral nerve impulses. With the exception of benzocaine, they act from the interior of the axon, on the sodium channels, to prevent the influx of sodium ions. Removal by the blood, diffusion, metabolism or dilution reduces tissue concentration of the LA allowing it to diffuse out of the axon, thereby restoring nerve function.

All LA agents consist of a benzene ring and an amine group with either an ester or amide linkage. They are weak bases and the degree of ionization depends on the individual drug's pK_a and the surrounding pH. At a low pH, e.g. in infected tissue, more of the drug remains in the ionized form, preventing it from diffusing across the axonal membrane and therefore reducing efficacy.

Problems

1. *Toxicity.* This depends on the total dose and blood flow to the area. In ENT surgery, toxicity most commonly results from direct intravascular injection or rapid absorption via mucous membranes. Systemic effects include:

- CNS: Lightheadedness, perioral paraesthesia, slurred speech, tinnitus, facial twitching, convulsions and coma.
- CVS: Bradycardia, hypotension and cardiac arrest.
- RS: An initial increase in respiratory rate followed by respiratory depression, hypoxia and respiratory arrest.

Treatment depends on the severity of the reaction. Prior to a LA block an IV cannula should be inserted. If toxicity is suspected the injection of LA is stopped and 100% O_2 given. CPR may be required. Bupivacaine has a long duration of action on the myocardial cell membrane, necessitating prolonged cardiac massage.

2. *Allergic reactions.* These are more common with esters, e.g cocaine, than with amides. Cardiopulmonary collapse requires ventilation with 100% oxygen, IV fluids and adrenaline 1:10 000 in 1-ml aliquots. Bronchodilators may be required.

Specific agents

1. *Cocaine.* An ester hydrolysed by plasma cholinesterases. It is a vasoconstrictor, potentiates catecholamine activity and sensitizes the myocardium to adrenaline. It is available as a 20% paste or a 4–20% solution and is used topically to facilitate nasal surgery. Max dose 1.5 mg/kg or total 100 mg in a fit adult. Duration of action 30–60 minutes.

2. *Lignocaine.* An amide metabolized in the liver. It is available in injectable form as 0.5–2%, sprays as 4% or 10%

and ointments of 2–5%. It is a mild vasodilator and is often given with a vasopressor, e.g. adrenaline 1:200 000.

Max dose: 3 mg/kg or 7 mg/kg with adrenaline.

Duration of action: (when infiltrated) 90 minutes without adrenaline.

3. Prilocaine. An amide with no vasodilating effect and lower systemic toxicity. Metabolism to *o*-toluidine may cause methaemoglobinaemia.

Max dose: 5 mg/kg or 7 mg/kg with adrenaline.

Duration of action: 140 minutes.

4. Bupivacaine. A vasodilating amide with a long duration, useful for postoperative analgesia. At toxic levels cardiac events, especially ventricular fibrillation, may precede neurological events.

Max dose: 2 mg/kg or 3 mg/kg with adrenaline.

Duration of action: 240 minutes without adrenaline.

Vasopressors

Combined with a LA agent these reduce the risk of systemic toxicity and intraoperative bleeding and prolong the duration of action. Vasopressors are contraindicated in patients with ischaemic heart disease, hypertension or thyrotoxicosis and in those on monoamine oxidase inhibitors. Halothane, a volatile anaesthetic agent, sensitizes the myocardium to adrenaline and this should not be used in the presence of high inspired concentrations. Vasopressors must also be avoided in areas supplied by end arteries. Felypressin is less toxic than adrenaline, but has a slower onset of action.

Local anaesthetic uses

1. Nose. LA used on its own or combined with general anaesthesia.

(a) Modified Moffet's technique. The nasal cavities are sprayed with LA and the patient placed supine with the head extended over the end of the trolley. A 2-ml volume of 5% cocaine is applied to each nasal cavity using a specially angulated cannula. After 10 minutes the nose is pinched and any remaining solution removed.

(b) Nasal pack. After applying LA to the nasal cavity, ribbon gauze soaked in LA is packed into the nose and left for 10 minutes. After removal of the pack, two wool applicators soaked in LA are applied, one to the region of the sphenopalatine foramen and the other to the anterior end of the cribriform plate.

Additional anaesthesia may be supplied by anterior ethmoidal or maxillary nerve blocks or by infiltration of the columella.

2. *Pharynx, larynx and trachea.* LA is used for direct laryngoscopy or awake intubation. The oropharynx is anaesthetized by spraying or nebulizing 4% lignocaine, or using a benzocaine lozenge. When using a fibreoptic bronchoscope LA is sprayed as the scope is advanced. Alternatively, the following blocks may be used:

(a) Superior laryngeal nerve:
- Krause's method – a swab soaked in 4% lignocaine is held, by Krause's forceps, in each piriform fossa for 1 minute.
- Percutaneous – 2 ml of LA is injected where the nerve divides at the greater cornu of the hyoid.

(b) Cricothyroid injection. A 2-ml volume of 4% lignocaine is injected via the cricothyroid ligament after aspiration of air to confirm needle placement. This will elicit an explosive cough.

Anaesthesia for tracheostomy is achieved by simple infiltration. A cricothyroid injection as described above should reduce coughing when the trachea is incised.

3. *Ear.* Infiltration may be supplemented by:
(a) Auriculotemporal nerve block – 2 ml of lignocaine is injected anterior to the meatus.
(b) Greater auricular nerve block – 2 ml of lignocaine is injected 2 cm both anterior and posterior to the tip of the mastoid.

Further reading

Craft TM, Upton PM. *Key Topics in Anaesthesia*, 2nd edn. Oxford: BIOS Scientific Publishers, 1995.
Craig HJL. Anaesthesia for otolaryngology. In: Kerr AG (ed.) *Scott Brown's Otolaryngology*, Vol. 1, 5th edn. London: Butterworths, 1987; 585–611.

Related topic of interest

Anaesthesia – general (p. 20)

AUDIT

Audit is defined as the systematic appraisal of the implementation and outcome of any process in the context of prescribed targets and standards.

Clinical audit is the process by which medical staff collectively review, evaluate and improve their practice. This should include the assessment of patients' access to care, the process and outcome of care and financial and administrative efficiency. In the clinical setting the problem with this definition is what to define for each aspect of medicine as reasonable targets and standards, and this requires research. A working group of the World Health Organization defined audit as a seven-stage procedure, the most vital element being to ensure an improvement (indicating change) in care by reassessing results after the setting of criteria and standards.

The guidelines are:
(a) Problem identification.
(b) Setting priorities.
(c) Determining methodology.
(d) Setting criteria and standards.
(e) Comparing performance with standards.
(f) Designing and implementing remedial action.
(g) Re-evaluating the quality of care.

The reasons for performing audit are:
(a) To encourage modification and improvement in clinical practice.
(b) To allow peer review and support for clinicians.
(c) It is educational and raises the overall quality of care.

Research and audit

Research and audit are often confused, and it is important to clarify the difference. Clinical research tests hypotheses so that they may be accepted as scientific fact or refuted in order to establish what is the best clinical practice. It allows prescribed targets and standards to be defined and may allow a management policy for a specific condition to be drafted. Audit, on the other hand, seeks to determine whether good practice (the process) has been adopted or whether the prescribed targets and standards gained through research are being met (the outcome). In other words, audit tests either process or outcome after research has established that there is a link between them.

Important aspects of clinical audit are:
• Clinical audit meetings should be confidential and involve only clinicians specifically involved in patient care and anonymity of sensitive data must be secured. In this context it should be remembered that patients, relatives and their legal representative are allowed access

to medical but not audit records. Hospital managers are allowed access only to the conclusions of any meeting.

- Each meeting should attempt to provide a specific recommendation which when implemented improves clinical practice.
- Departments should set targets regarding appointments, investigations, admission and outpatient waiting times.
- The use of resources, for example beds, drugs, investigations and duty theatres, should be determined and, if appropriate, proposals made with the purpose of making them more efficient.
- Treatment policies should be reviewed to minimize morbidity and mortality and maximize quality of life.
- Clinical audit regularly undertaken may provide a basis for a successful medicolegal defence because it can be shown that treatment has been researched and reviewed.

National audit

This is necessary because each hospital, district and even region has a relatively small number of clinicians performing a proportionately small number of procedures compared with the national total. Type II errors in assessing clinical outcome might be averted.

The National Confidential Enquiry into Perioperative Deaths (NCEPOD)

Perioperative deaths are those which occur within 30 days of a surgical procedure, that is any procedure carried out by a surgeon or gynaecologist, with or without an anaesthetist, involving local, regional or general anaesthesia or sedation.

NCEPOD provides guidelines annually for specific clinical situations with the aim of improving surgical practice. The recommendations come from an independent body with representatives across the surgical specialty fields (the steering group) nominated by an elected body in that specialty (in otolaryngology it is a representative proposed by the British Association of Otolaryngologists). The guidelines are issued from information provided mainly by pathologists, who supply data regarding perioperative deaths in their hospitals. A sample of the reported deaths are reviewed in greater detail by the steering group by sending questionnaires regarding all aspects of the patient's care in each case of perioperative death to the consultant surgeon and anaesthetist in charge of the patient's care.

Further reading

Bull AR. Audit and research: complementary but distinct. *Annals of the Royal College of Surgeons of England*, 1993; **75**: 308–11.

Guidelines to Clinical Audit in Surgical Practice. London: The Royal College of Surgeons of England, 1989.

WHO Working Group. The organisation of quality assurance. *Quality Assurance in Health Care*, 1989; **1:** 111–23.

BENIGN NECK LUMPS

Classification

(a) Congenital (defined as present at birth): lymphangiomas, dermoids, thyroglossal cysts.
(b) Developmental: branchial cysts, laryngoceles, pharyngeal pouches.
(c) Tumours of the parapharyngeal space.
(d) Thyroid swellings.
(e) Salivary gland tumours.
(f) Reactive neck lymphadenopathy.
(g) Neck space infection.

The last four groups above are discussed as separate topics elsewhere in the book. This topic describes congenital, developmental and parapharyngeal space lumps.

Congenital

Lymphangiomas

These are simple and cavernous, arising principally in the lips, cheek and floor of the mouth. Cystic hygromas usually arise in the lower neck.

Dermoid cysts

These are midline swellings that do not move with swallowing or tongue protrusion. There are three types:
1. Epidermoid cysts, lined only with squamous epithelium.
2. True dermoids lined with squamous epithelium and all other normal skin appendages.
3. Teratoid cysts are lined by respiratory or squamous epithelium and contain ectodermal, endodermal and mesodermal elements, for example teeth, nails or thyroid tissue.

Thyroglossal cysts

These are cysts along the tract of the obliterated thyroglossal duct. They may contain elements of thyroid tissue and may even be the sole source of functioning thyroid tissue. Many experts therefore recommend a ^{99m}Tc or radioiodine (^{131}I) uptake scan prior to excision. Ninety per cent of thryoglossal cysts are midline and 9% left-sided, occurring between the body of the hyoid bone and the cricoid cartilage. Most occur in childhood (mean age 4 years). They move with swallowing and tongue protrusion as they are ultimately attached on their deep aspect to the larynx. Infection causes the rapid onset of diffuse swelling, pain and tenderness. Thyroglossal cysts should not be incised and drained as this may cause an ugly sinus which is difficult to excise *in toto* and in continuity with the deflated cyst. A long course of antibiotics and repeat aspiration of the cyst, if the child allows, are recommended. The tract may climb anterior or posterior to the body of the hyoid to the tongue base. The body of the hyoid and preferably a wedge of tongue base should therefore be included in the excision.

Developmental

Branchial cysts

Four theories regarding aetiology have been proposed.
1. They arise from elements of squamous epithelium within a lymph node. This is the current consensus view.
2. They arise from remnants of the first pharyngeal pouch.
3. They are remnants of the cervical sinus.
4. They are remnants of the duct connecting the thymus to the third pharyngeal pouch.

Branchial cysts are lined by stratified squamous epithelium and contain lymphoid tissue in their wall. They usually present in young adults, 60% on the left and 60% in males. Most arise along the line of the deep cervical lymph nodes deep to the anterior border of sternomastoid. They do not have a tract. A quarter become infected and should be managed similarly to an infected thyroglossal cyst. Excision should only be attempted when all inflammation has settled to minimize the risk of rupturing the cyst wall, which may lead to a recurrence or, if wall remnants are left, a fistula.

Laryngocele

Only about 30 occur each year in the UK, 80% in men with a mean age of 55. They arise from the laryngeal saccule, expanding internally to present in the vallecula or externally through the thyrohyoid membrane. In most subjects raising the intralaryngeal pressure causes no expansion of the saccule, but in those in whom the saccule expands, perhaps because of a wider than usual true cord to false cord distance (wide neck) or because the false cord is compressed against the saccule to create a one-way valve. Coughing, sneezing or trumpet playing may fully develop the laryngocele. They are occasionally associated with a ventricular carcinoma.

An intermittent neck swelling is the usual presentation, perhaps with a persistent cough or pain. It is usually impalpable but may become both visible and palpable on performing the Valsalva manoeuvre. Plain anteroposterior and lateral neck radiographs may show an air-filled sac. Laryngoceles may obstruct the larynx, so the safest treatment is excision, which includes the upper half of thyroid cartilage on the side of the laryngocele so that the neck can be ligated.

Tumours of the parapharyngeal space

This space is described in Neck space infection (p. 186). The common tumours are:

- Lipomas.
- Deep lobe of parotid tumours.
- Neurogenous tumours.
- Carotid aneurysm.

Parapharyngeal tumours expand either medially, when the tonsil will be displaced towards the midline, or laterally to present in the upper deep cervical region. It is therefore important to exclude a metastatic node as a cause of the swelling.

Neurogenous tumours develop from neural crest cells which have differentiated into Schwann cells or sympathicoblasts. Schwann cells give rise to neurofibromas and schwannomas, the sympathicoblasts to ganglioneuromas and chemodectomas (carotid body tumours, glomus vagale and glomus jugulare tumours).

(a) Neurofibromas arise from endoneural fibrous connective tissue and are composed of a mass of spindle cells which can entwine nerve fibres, sometimes causing weakness or paralysis of the involved nerve.

(b) Schwannomas are benign tumours of the neurolemma or sheath of Schwann and so tend to be encapsulated. Their expansion may compress the involved nerve, giving rise to reduced function, but paralysis is unusual. In the parapharyngeal space a painless neck mass is usually the only sign.

(c) Chemodectomas arise from paraganglionic tissue at three common sites in the neck. On the medial side of the carotid bulb are found highly vascular tumours arising from the carotid body cells; these *carotid body tumours* are rare except in high-altitude population centres such as Mexico City. Vagal paragangliomas arise from paraganglionic tissue within the perineurium of the vagus, the *glomus vagale* tumour, which, if it involves the ganglion nodosum just below the jugular foramen, is referred to as a *glomus jugulare*. The cells are not functionally active. Patients present with a slow-growing painless lump in the neck or a mass pushing the tonsil medially, although with the vagal nerve paragangliomas pulsating tinnitus, syncope and glossopharyngeal, vagal, accessory and hypoglossal nerve palsies may arise if the tumour expands at the skull base. Carotid body tumours may be pulsatile with an audible bruit. Malignant change rarely, if ever, occurs in chemodectomas of these three sites. Occasional reports of metastases in the literature may be confusing a chemodectoma with a large-cell neuroendocrine carcinoma. Chemodectomas may occur rarely at other sites, particularly the larynx.

A carotid aneurysm may be caused by atheroma, trauma or infection. If expanding or causing transient ischaemic attacks, it can be resected and replaced with a reversed saphenous vein graft.

Investigations   An MRI scan will assess the size and vascularity of the mass. If a carotid body tumour is suspected a digital subtraction angiogram will allow precise definition of the tumour circulation, its principal feeding vessels and the presence of a cross-circulation, all of which must be known prior to surgery. A fine-needle aspiration biopsy, if necessary under CT guidance, may allow a definite diagnosis to be made. Under no circumstance should either a Tru-cut biopsy or a biopsy from within the mouth be attempted because the vascularity of a carotid body tumour may cause a rapidly expanding parapharyngeal haematoma which might occlude the oropharyngeal airway.

Treatment

The mass will as a rule continue to expand so that symptoms may progress. A tissue diagnosis may not be possible. For these reasons, surgery is the treatment of choice for parapharyngeal masses, although in particular the vagus and the hypoglossal nerves are at high risk of injury. There is a small, but definite, risk of stroke from surgery. A significant proportion of young patients will refuse surgery if presented with all the facts. Recent publications have suggested that carotid body tumours may be radiosensitive and radiotherapy may be indicated either as adjuvant treatment or in those unfit or unwilling to have surgery.

Follow-up and aftercare

Review of all parapharyngeal mass patients postoperatively for 5 years, except those who had a lipoma, is indicated. Glossopharyngeal and vagal nerve injury may give rise to aspiration and a hoarse voice, although symptoms gradually settle, especially if an experienced speech therapist is involved in rehabilitation. A vocal cord palsy is treated as discussed elsewhere (see Related topics of interest).

Further reading

Ferlito A, Pesavento G, Recher G *et al*. Assessment and treatment of neurogenic and non-neurogenic tumours of the parapharyngeal space. *Head and Neck Surgery*, 1984; **7:** 32–43.
Jackson CG, Harris PF, Glasscock ME *et al*. Diagnosis and management of paragangliomas of the skull base. *American Journal of Surgery*, 1990; **159:** 389–93.

Related topics of interest

Neck space infection (p. 186)
Vocal cord palsy (p. 342)

CALORIC TESTS

Physiology

The semicircular canals are paired sensory structures responsible for the detection of angular acceleration. Each canal possesses a dilation at one end called the ampulla. Within the ampulla exists a saddle-shaped crista upon which sits a gelatinous cupula; the whole membranous canal is filled with endolymph. The inertia of the endolymphatic fluid means that there is a relative difference in the velocity of the canal and the fluid with head movements. This results in fluid being forced through the gap between crista and cupula and a deflection of the stereocilia which causes either an increase or decrease in the resting tonic discharge depending on the direction of deflection. The two labyrinths work in conjunction so that an increase in neural signals from one canal will be associated with a decreased discharge rate from the corresponding canal on the opposite side. As the three canals are mutually at right angles, complex three-dimensional information is provided.

Background

The caloric response can be used to test the integrity of this system and was first described by Robert Barany in 1906 and for which he was awarded a Nobel prize in 1914. He postulated that altering the temperature of the endolymph sets up thermally induced convection currents. This fluid movement leads to stimulation of the stereocilia and consequent nystagmus and vertigo. Caloric testing was further refined in 1942 by Fitzgerald and Hallpike when they described a standardized bithermal caloric test which remains an essential vestibular investigation to this day.

It has become apparent in recent years that thermal convection currents are not the only component in the caloric response. Positional alterations and the presence of a caloric response in microgravity have led to suggestions that a direct thermal effect on the sensory organs may account for as much as one-third of the response, although this in no way reduces the value of the test.

Procedure

The classic bithermal calorics utilize water at 30 and 44°C, kept at these temperatures in two heated tanks about 1 metre above the test couch. The patient reclines on the couch at 30° above the horizontal so as to bring the lateral semicircular canal into the vertical position. After checking that the external canals are clear of wax and debris and that the tympanic membranes are intact, cold water (30°C) is run into the left ear, via a siphon tube and 14G cannula, for 40 seconds. A stopwatch is used to time the period from the start of this manoeuvre to the point at which the nystagmus stops with the patient fixating on a point on the ceiling. This procedure is repeated for the right ear and then for both ears with the warm water (44°C).

A number of variations on this basic theme exist. Cold tap water can be used as a very basic single temperature screening test, and in patients with perforated eardrums air may be used to supply the thermal stimulus. Further refinements can be added by the use of Frenzel's glasses to remove optic fixation or measuring the nystagmus electrically (electronystagmography).

Interpretation

Bithermal calorics were developed to eliminate the effect of directional preponderance which may arise from any part of the peripheral or central vestibular system and represents a non-specific enhancement of nystagmus in one particular direction. By definition, the direction of the nystagmus is described by its fast phase. Cold stimulation leads to nystagmus with the fast phase to the opposite side, while warm stimulation leads to nystagmus with the fast phase to the same side. This is easily remembered by the mnemonic COWS (cold–opposite, warm-same). Various formulae exist, based on the recorded times for each part of the standard caloric test, to predict the degree of vestibular underactivity, so called canal paresis. By the nature of the test a canal paresis must be greater than 20–25% to be significant.

Clinical indications

Caloric testing forms the cornerstone of investigation for any vestibular pathology and is therefore useful in all patients with vertigo. It may still be of some value for the investigation of an acoustic neuroma, as the tumour usually arises from the superior vestibular nerve and leads to an ipsilateral canal paresis.

Further reading

Luxon LM. Methods of examination – audiological and vestibular. In: Ludman H (ed.) *Mawson's Diseases of the Ear*, 5th edn. London: Edward Arnold, 1988.
Stahle J. Controversies on the caloric response. *Acta Otolaryngologica*, 1990; **109**: 162–7.

Related topics of interest

CERVICAL LYMPHADENOPATHY

Cervical lymphadenopathy implies disease involving the cervical lymph nodes. In this topic a simple differential of these diseases is presented, but specific details are found elsewhere (see Benign neck lumps, p. 31). The remainder of the topic is confined to the problem of neck node metastases. A primary carcinoma arising in the upper aerodigestive tract may metastasize to the lymph nodes of the neck, so the control of regional metastatic disease constitutes a significant part of the management of head and neck cancer.

Differential diagnosis

Most cervical masses fall into one of four broad groups:

1. Congenital or developmental (thyroglossal, branchial and dermoid cysts).

2. Infectious (tonsillitis, infectious mononucleosis, tuberculosis, actinomycosis, HIV).

3. Inflammatory (sarcoidosis).

4. Neoplastic (primary arising from neck structures, metastatic secondaries, haematogenous).

The diagnosis is from the history, examination including endoscopy, radiology and laboratory tests. The specific investigations will be dictated by the differential diagnosis. Fine-needle aspiration (FNA) cytology is probably the single most useful diagnostic procedure if a neoplastic lymph node is suspected. False-negative and, very rarely, false-positive results can occur with FNA, so the information must always be used in conjunction with the clinical findings. An MRI scan is preferred to CT to delineate impalpable nodes. The scans can also reveal the integrity or involvement of the vasculature by a metastatic lymph node. A chest radiograph may show a primary carcinoma or evidence of secondary spread, as well as pulmonary tuberculosis or mediastinal gland enlargement.

Anatomy

The following definitions are recommended for the boundaries of cervical lymph node groups.

- Level I. Consists of the submental and submandibular lymph nodes within the triangle bounded by the anterior belly of the digastric, the hyoid bone, the posterior belly of digastric and the body of the mandible.

- Level II (upper deep cervical). Consists of lymph nodes located around the upper third of the internal jugular vein and adjacent spinal accessory nerve extending from the level of the carotid bifurcation to the skull base.
- Level III (mid deep cervical). Consists of lymph nodes around the middle third of the internal jugular vein extending from the carotid bifurcation superiorly to the cricothyroid notch inferiorly.
- Level IV (lower deep cervical). Consists of lymph nodes located around the lower third of the internal jugular vein extending from the cricothyroid notch to the clavicle inferiorly.
- Level V. Consists of the posterior triangle nodes which are located between the posterior border of the sternomastoid muscle and the anterior border of trapezius. The supraclavicular nodes are also included in this group.

TNM classification

The staging system in most common use in the UK is that proposed by the International Union against Cancer (UICC), which is based on data developed by the American Joint Committee (AJC) for Cancer Staging.

NX Regional lymph nodes cannot be assessed.
N0 Regional lymph nodes not palpable.
N1 Movable single homolateral node less than 3 cm in diameter.
N2 Movable homolateral or bilateral nodes.
    (a) Single ipsilateral node (between 3 and 6 cm in diameter).
    (b) Multiple ipsilateral nodes (up to 6 cm)
    (c) Bilateral or contralateral nodes (up to 6 cm).
N3 Nodes greater than 6 cm in diameter.

Although this system is useful, it has several inherent problems: clinicians will fail to agree on the presence of a palpable lymph node in as many as 30% of cases. In addition, it is generally acknowledged that the number of lymph nodes involved, the lymph node level and the presence of extracapsular spread are important prognostic parameters in metastatic disease of the neck and these are not included in the classification.

Treatment

The treatment of malignant neck nodes is by either some form of neck dissection or radiotherapy. Broadly speaking, lymph nodes of less than 2 cm diameter will be treated by radical radiotherapy and those greater than this size will be treated by a neck dissection with or without postoperative radiotherapy. The rupture of the lymph node capsule by tumour is a bad prognostic sign. Fifty per cent of nodes with a diameter greater than 3 cm exhibit this. Postoperative irradiation to the neck following radical neck dissection is mandatory in the presence of extra-capsular rupture.

1. N0. The performance of a radical neck dissection without palpable lymph nodes (prophylactic neck dissection) is considered by some to be of doubtful value. The argument supporting this concept is that some lymph nodes may be invaded by tumour (occult nodes) and still be impalpable. Prophylactic neck dissection may have some place in the patient who is unlikely to return for follow-up and has a primary tumour with a known high incidence of occult nodes (nasopharynx, tonsil, base of tongue, pyriform fossa, supraglottic larynx or oral cavity). Some form of treatment to the neck or at least first echelan nodes is essential in the treatment of tumours of these primary sites the treatment can be by selective neck dissection or by irradiation. For other sites the morbidity and mortality of the operation outweigh the potential benefit and many surgeons adopt a wait and watch policy.

2. N1. It is generally accepted that lymph nodes of less than 2 cm diameter can be sterilized by radiotherapy. This has the advantage that if a node reappears after a course of radiotherapy a neck dissection can be carried out, although the survival after such salvage surgery is poor. It must be confirmed that the node is metastatic as a high proportion of nodes in this category do not contain tumour and, even if they do, extranodal spread is uncommon, therefore a functional neck dissection can be used in these patients.

3. N2. Larger nodes (N2a) and multiple ipsilateral nodes (N2b) are best treated by a radical neck dissection because of the high incidence of extracapsular spread of the tumour and difficulty in sterilizing even small multiple nodes. Postoperative radiotherapy is indicated if there is extracapsular rupture or positive margins in the resection specimen. The incidence of further neck recurrence is probably reduced by postoperative radiotherapy, although overall survival is not affected. Patients with a supraglottic carcinoma and bilateral nodes do better than those with cancer of other primary sites at high risk of bilateral neck metastases (base of tongue and hypopharynx). The decision to treat should be taken very carefully as there is a considerable morbidity from a bilateral neck dissection which can be a simultaneous or a staged procedure. Most surgeons advocate either staged bilateral radical neck dissection or, if possible, a functional neck dissection on the least invaded side.

4. *N3.* These nodes used to be referred to as 'fixed', but size is now the criterion for staging. If the tumour invades the internal jugular vein, or the base of skull in the region of the mastoid process, or the brachial plexus, it is almost certainly incurable. Fixation to the skin can be treated by resection of the tumour with involved skin which is replaced with the use of flaps such as a pectoralis major myocutaneous flap. Invasion of the carotid artery can be treated with a bypass procedure performed with the resection, but there is a high operative mortality, and little chance of cure.

Palliation

Patients with inoperable neck nodes that have fungated through the skin can be treated with local dressings of kaltocarb and topical metronidazole. These will help prevent colonization by anaerobes and alleviate the odour from tissue necrosis. Death by carotid artery rupture will usually ensue. The patient should always be treated with appropriate doses of opiate analgesia and antiemetics. It is imperative that there is adequate social support and that the patient's family doctor is aware of the situation if the patient is to be cared for in the community.

Further reading

Jones AS, Roland NJ, Field JK, Phillips DE. The level of cervical node metastases: their prognostic relevance and relationship with head and neck squamous carcinoma primary sites. *Clinical Otolaryngology*, 1994; **19:** 63–9.
Snow GB, Annyas AA, Van Slooten EA, Bartelink H, Hart AAM. Prognostic factors of neck node metastasis. *Clinical Otolaryngology,* 1982; **7:** 185–92.
UICC, Hermanek P, Sabin LH (eds) *TNM Classification of Malignant Tumours,* 4th edn. Berlin: Springer Verlag, 1992.

Related topics of interest

CHOANAL ATRESIA

Congenital choanal atresia is due to the embryological failure of the primitive bucconasal membrane to rupture before birth. This results in the persistence of a bony plate (90%), membrane, or both, obstructing the posterior nares. The condition may be unilateral (most commonly) or bilateral. It occurs in about 1 in 7000 births, and there is a family tendency. About half of infants with congenital atresia display other abnormalities.

Embryology

The mouth, palate, nose and paranasal sinuses all develop from the cranial portion of the primitive foregut. The nose begins as two epithelial thickenings known as the nasal placodes, which appear above the stomatodeum about the fourth week *in utero*. The placodes deepen to form olfactory pits which lie between the medial and lateral nasal processes. The medial processes fuse to form the frontonasal process. This is compressed to form the nasal septum as the lateral nasal processes approach each other. The nasal septum will then grow posteriorly to divide the two nasal cavities. Each nasal cavity is closed posteriorly by the thinned out posterior wall of the nasal sac, called the bucconasal membrane. This usually breaks down around the sixth week *in utero*. Its persistence is thought to be the cause of choanal atresia.

Clinical features

A unilateral obstruction may be asymptomatic at birth but will later cause unilateral nasal discharge and obstruction. Examination of the nose will show a thick gelatinous secretion on the affected side, and no airway can be demonstrated by holding a cold plated spatula below the nares – only the clear side steaming the surface (mirror test). Older children may allow posterior rhinoscopy to view the occlusion.

Bilateral choanal atresia presents as an emergency at birth. The newborn is a near-obligate nasal breather and the nasal obstruction will therefore produce difficulty in breathing. The alae nasi dilate and the accessory muscles of respiration are used to no avail. There is pallor and cyanosis until the mouth is opened and after a few quick breaths are taken the infant cries. This sequence of events continues. The diagnosis should be suspected immediately and an oral airway inserted to assist respiration.

| Investigations | The diagnosis can be confirmed by the mirror test or by attempting to pass a catheter through the nose into the nasopharynx. This will not be possible if there is an obstruction. If there is still doubt the lesion can be demonstrated radiologically. A CT scan is the method of choice to delineate the nature and thickness of the obstruction. |

Management

In the case of the newborn the first priority is to insert and maintain an oral airway. The treatment of choanal atresia is surgical and two approaches are in common use.

1. Transnasal. This is the usual approach in infants. A membranous occlusion may require no more than perforation with a probe. This can also be accomplished with electrocautery or laser. In the more common bony occlusions it will be necessary to perform a trephine and remove the obstruction with a burr or KTP laser using the operating microscope. A stent should be inserted and a series of dilations of the choana will then be required to maintain an adequate lumen.

2. Transpalatal. This is preferred by some surgeons, particularly when the atresia is unilateral or if a previous transnasal opening has later closed. The palate is incised just in front of the posterior edge of the hard palate. The soft palate is retracted, and the occlusion removed together with part of the vomer and border of the hard palate.

Follow-up and aftercare

Maintenance of the opening following corrective surgery with regular bouginage is now mostly preferred to the use of indwelling tubes. Dilation will probably be necessary every 2 months initially, but this period can be extended as the child grows.

Related topic of interest

Paediatric airway problems (p. 234)

CHOLESTEATOMA

Definition

A cholesteatoma is a three-dimensional epidermal structure exhibiting independent growth, replacing middle-ear mucosa, resorbing underlying bone and tending to recur after removal. Put more simply, it is 'skin in the middle-ear cleft'.

Types

Cholesteatoma can be classified into congenital and acquired types. These are distinct pathological entities.

1. Congenital cholesteatoma. Congenital cholesteatoma has been shown by Michaels to be the result of the persistence of a small nidus of epidermoid ectoderm that occurs in the first trimester in the normal fetus and is normally resorbed. It usually manifests itself as an anterior attic pearl behind an intact drum in the first year or so of life. It may present later in childhood with extensive disease in an often cellular mastoid.

2. Acquired cholesteatoma. There is no definitive classification of acquired cholesteatoma, but it can be divided into three groups with reference to the tympanic membrane.
(a) Primary acquired cholesteatoma associated with a defect in the pars flaccida.
(b) Secondary acquired cholesteatoma associated with a defect in the pars tensa.
(c) Tertiary acquired cholesteatoma exists behind an apparently normal eardrum as a result of implantation or previous middle-ear infection.

Aetiology

There are a number of well-established, but unproven, theories regarding the aetiology of cholesteatoma.

1. Primary acquired cholesteatoma. This is the most common.
(a) The single most important fact about the skin of the eardrum is that in health it migrates from the centre of the drum outwards along the external ear canal, carrying keratin and wax debris with it. Therefore this skin is self-cleaning. Negative middle-ear pressure tends to pull the pars flaccida into the attic and may form a retraction pocket in which the epithelium, although initially self-cleaning, eventually loses its migratory capacity. The

pocket fills with epithelial debris, which in turn becomes infected and further expands under tension. As it expands the isthmus tends to narrow, compounding the problem and continuing the cycle.

(b) Direct invasion of migrating squamous epithelium through the pars flaccida may occur, either as papillae through a temporary defect or merely as a change in the direction of migration in the upper part of the tympanic membrane, with skin going in rather than continuing out along the ear canal.

2. *Secondary and tertiary acquired cholesteatoma.*

(a) Epithelium could migrate around the rim of a pars tensa perforation to cause a cholesteatoma.

(b) Acute otitis media may damage the fibrous layers of the pars tensa and a piece of squamous epithelium may be implanted should the tympanic membrane rupture. The drum may heal or there may be a permanent defect.

(c) Surgery involving trauma to the tympanic membrane (any middle-ear surgery or even grommet insertion) may occasionally allow squamous epithelium to be directly implanted.

(d) Metaplasia of middle-ear mucosa may occur secondary to episodes of chronic or recurrent acute otitis media.

Pathology

Macroscopically there is a rounded pearly white mass of variable size, often surrounded by friable granulations from infected bone or with polyp formation from infected mucosa. Microscopically, cholesteatoma is a benign keratinizing squamous cell cyst. In the centre are fully differentiated anucleate keratin squames, surrounded by an epithelium several cell layers thick, in turn surrounded by a matrix of inflamed subepithelial connective tissue. The epithelial matrix of acquired cholesteatoma has approximately 15 layers whereas that of congenital cholesteatoma has only about five layers. Electron microscopy shows normal epidermal cells plus Langerhan cells and Merkel cells.

A cholesteatoma invariably enlarges, but little is known as to how this growth is controlled. Infection with bacteria causes an increase in clinical progression. Initially the cyst of skin grows into the area of least resistance, usually into the mastoid antrum and then into the air cells. The epithelium, being naturally migratory, probably accounts for some of the growth, but other changes in the surrounding perimatrix, probably bought on by infection, lead to destruction of the bone locally. These changes include the activation of osteoclast and the production of lysozymes.

Clinical features

Symptoms depend on the activity of the disease and arise either from the disease itself or from the complications. The disease usually produces a discharge, which may be scanty or just a flaky waxy deposit, but is often foul and creamy. Deafness may occur, conductive secondary to ossicular erosion, or sensory, probably from toxins involved in chronic inflammation migrating through the round window. Dizziness may indicate a labyrinthine fistula.

The principal signs are an attic crust, a marginal perforation or a pocket of invading keratin debris. Marginal granulations and polyps protruding from the middle-ear cleft indicate osteitis and mucosal hyperplasia, respectively. Behind these may lie a cholesteatoma so that micro-otoscopic removal of an attic crust or aural polypectomy may allow the diagnosis to be made. A positive fistula sign is said to indicate erosion into the labyrinth (see Labyrinthitis, p. 144).

Complications may occur in acute exacerbation of the disease and are either within the temporal bone or intracranial. They are discussed under the topic Complications of CSOM.

Investigations

(a) Micro-otoscopy (with the removal of attic crusts and polyps for reasons stated above).
(b) Pure tone audiometry (with masking).
(c) Radiology. Plain radiographs may indicate the height of the middle fossa dura and site of the sigmoid sinus but usually give little information on disease extent. CT and MRI can both demonstrate the disease and give some idea of its extent. CT reveals a non-enhancing mass of eroding bone including ossicles with sharply defined smooth margins, isodense with CSF. MRI likewise shows a mass with a low intensity T1 weighted signal and a high T2 signal. In practice, it is often difficult on imaging to distinguish between cholesteatoma and pure mucosal disease.

Treatment

Suction clearance may control early disease, but the mainstay of treatment is surgical excision of the disease with reconstruction of the surgical defect and any conductive hearing loss. This usually takes the form of some type of mastoidectomy and tympanoplasty.

Further reading

Ferlito A. A review of the definition, terminology and pathology of aural cholesteatoma. *Journal of Laryngology and Otology*, 1993; **107:** 483-8.

McCabe BF, Sade J, Abramson M (eds). *Cholesteatoma.* Birmingham, AL: AESCULAPUS Publishing, 1977.

Palva, T. Cholesteatoma surgery today. *Clinics in Otolaryngology*, 1993; **18:** 245–55.

Related topics of interest

Chronic suppurative otitis media – complications (p. 55)
Mastoidectomy (p. 165)
Tympanoplasty (p. 328)

CHRONIC SINUSITIS

Chronic inflammation of the sinuses usually follows recurrent acute sinusitis, but in some cases the onset is more insidious. The incidence of this problem in the UK has been reduced by improvements in the general health of the population, diet, hygiene, and the introduction of antibiotics.

Predisposing factors

The commonest causes are nasal. Both the maxillary and frontal sinuses drain through narrow spaces and interstices into the middle meatus. The ethmoids also drain into this and the superior meatus. Any condition narrowing or blocking these may lead to secretion retention and poor ventilation, thus predisposing to consequent infection. Predisposing causes are similar to those for acute sinus infections and include:

1. Local.

- Recurrent acute sinus infections.
- Pre-existing rhinitis (allergic, intrinsic, rhinitis medicamentosa, etc.).
- Nasal polyps.
- Nasal foreign body.
- Recurrent upper respiratory tract infection (tonsillitis and adenoids).
- Nasal anatomical variations (septal deviation, abnormal uncinate process, middle turbinate or ethmoid bulla).
- Nasal tumour.
- Teeth (diseases of the upper premolars and molars).

2. General.

- Debilitation.
- Immunocompromised host
- Mucociliary disorders (e.g. Kartagener's syndrome).
- Atmospheric irritants (dust, fumes, tobacco smoke).

Pathology

There is an increase in vascularity and vascular permeability. This leads to oedema and hypertrophy of the mucosa which may become polypoidal. Goblet cell hyperplasia and a chronic cellular infiltrate will occur. Ulceration of the epithelium will result in the formation of granulation tissue. Multiple small abscesses occur in the thickened mucosa and fibrosis of the submucosal stroma supervenes. The changes in the mucosa over this time may be irreversible, and when the original cause of infection has been treated the lining will not revert to normal.

Clinical features

The cardinal symptoms are nasal congestion, nasal or postnasal discharge and pain. A headache over the forehead, the bridge of the nose and the face is usual. The patient may also suffer with anosmia, or even cacosmia (unpleasant smell), especially in infections of dental origin. Chronic irritation of the nasal airway and repeated rubbing may lead to a vestibulitis and epistaxis. Chronic pharyngitis and laryngitis with the patient complaining of a productive cough are often encountered. Clinical examination will usually show nasal inflammation or perhaps another obvious intranasal predisposing factor.

Differential diagnosis

It is not uncommon for general practitioners and those in other specialties to ascribe facial pain and headaches to sinus disease, sometimes when it is not. The ENT surgeon is confronted as a rule with three different groups of headache patients:

(a) Those with headaches clearly connected to a sinus problem, such as inflammatory disease, neoplasm, barotrauma or another readily identifiable cause.

(b) Those with headaches clearly traceable to non-sinus causes such as migraine, neuralgias, cervical spine disorders, temporomandibular joint diseases, glaucoma, hypertension, etc.

(c) Those whose problems are not clear and in whom there seems to be no overt indication of sinus disease. In this group of patients nasendoscopic examination with a high-definition coronal section CT scan may confirm that the symptoms are indeed sinus related.

Investigations

Sinus radiographs will show varying degrees of opacification of the involved sinuses with mucosal thickening. Mucosal thickening occurs in 30% of individuals and its detection is often meaningless. Opacification with a fluid level indicates an acute infection. Gross polypoidal changes may also show as an opacification. The radiographs should be carefully examined for any obvious predisposing factor such as dental disease. Some patients with sinogenic headaches may present with an atypical history and have negative findings on examination and plain sinus radiographs. This does not rule out a sinus cause for their problem. Many rhinologists now argue that only the combination of diagnostic endoscopy and high-definition coronal section CT scanning will provide the maximum information. One modality is said to enhance the accuracy of the other.

Management

The principal aims of treatment are to correct the predisposing cause, to ventilate the sinus and to restore normal mucosal lining in the sinus.

1. Medical. A course of broad-spectrum antibiotics in combination with a decongestant should be tried initially (though they should be avoided long-term). Any obvious predisposing factor, for example a rhinitis or nasal polyps, should be treated with medical therapy (e.g. antihistamines and/or a steroid nasal spray).

2. Surgery. Functional endoscopic sinus surgery (p. 119) is changing the way many surgeons approach this condition. The classical management is presented here.

If the maxillary sinus is affected, treatment of the maxillary sinus may allow the spontaneous resolution of the other sinuses. Antral lavage should therefore be the first step in surgical treatment. This clears away mucopurulent material from the sinus and may open the sinus ostium. However, the condition is liable to recur and several washouts may be necessary. Even better drainage and aeration of the sinus can be achieved by performing an inferior meatal intranasal antrostomy. Some of the thickened antral mucosa can be removed through the opening. The improved ventilation will often allow ciliary motion to be restored. Most of the mucociliary clearance will still be through the natural ostium.

If irreversible changes have occurred to the sinus mucosa then most surgeons would consider it necessary to remove it. A wide range of procedures are available, so the choice of operation should be tailored to the requirements of the individual patient. Each procedure has its own limitations and specific complications. Functional endoscopic sinus surgery is now an attractive alternative to the classical surgical approaches to chronic sinusitis. Those who advocate this procedure claim that more accurate surgery can now be undertaken and that injury to the eye, optic nerve or dura is less likely. Stepwise removal of the ethmoidal cells extending to the posterior ethmoid and sphenoid sinus can be undertaken. The natural ostium of the maxillary sinus in the middle meatus can be cleared, opened and enlarged, as can any disease of the frontonasal duct. However, the more radical procedures are still used and asked about in the examinations. They are listed below, but details of each procedure and its complications should be sought from an operative textbook.

- *Chronic maxillary sinusitis*: Caldwell–Luc procedure.
- *Chronic ethmoid sinusitis*: intranasal ethmoidectomy (considered a dangerous procedure).
  Functional endoscopic sinus surgery (FESS).
  Transorbital ethmoidectomy (Patterson's operation).
  Transantral (Horgan's operation).
- *Chronic frontal sinusitis*: external frontoethmoidectomy (Howarth's operation).
  Osteoplastic flap procedure (MacBeth's operation).
- *Chronic sphenoiditis*: via an intranasal ethmoidectomy.
  Transantral to the posterior ethmoids then to the sphenoid sinus.
  Via an external frontoethmoidectomy.

Further reading

Stammberger H. *Functional Endoscopic Sinus Surgery*. Philadelphia: B.C. Decker.
Stammberger H and Wolf G. Headaches and sinus disease: the endoscopic approach. *Annals of Otology, Rhinology and Laryngology*, 1988; Vol. 97 (Suppl. 134).

Related topics of interest

Acute sinusitis (p. 5)
Allergic rhinitis (p. 16)
Functional endoscopic sinus surgery (p. 119)
Intrinsic rhinitis (p. 141)
Sinusitis – complications (p. 285)

CHRONIC SUPPURATIVE OTITIS MEDIA

This can be subclassified into tubotympanic or safe disease and tympanomastoid (atticoantral) or unsafe disease. A classification gaining more prominence is chronic suppurative otitis media (CSOM) with or without cholesteatoma. CSOM without cholesteatoma is sometimes referred to as mucosal chronic otitis media and subdivided into active and inactive.

Tubotympanic CSOM

The essential features are a central tympanic membrane perforation and adequate atticoantral drainage. Disease is confined to the mucosa of the anteroinferior portion of the middle-ear cleft and the risk of serious complications is minimal. Most perforations arise when an acute perforation occurs during an episode of ASOM and, perhaps because of an inadequate dose, length or inappropriate choice of antibiotic, there is slow resolution. This allows sufficient time for squamous epithelium to migrate over the free edge of the tympanic layers to form a permanent perforation. The disease is described as quiescent during the first few weeks of a dry ear and inactive when the ear is dry long term and active when a mucoid or mucopurulent discharge within the middle ear is present. Pathogens gain entry to the middle ear either via the Eustachian tube, often triggered by an upper respiratory tract infection, or via the ear canal, when contaminated bath, swimming pool or sea water is the most common source.

Chronic mucoid discharge is associated with goblet cell hyperplasia, 'metaplasia' of middle ear mucosa to respiratory type and poor mucociliary function.

Clinical features

Deafness is proportional to the size of the perforation and not, as is often quoted, the site. An air–bone gap of more than 30 dB is unusual and suggests an ossicular discontinuity. The patient may notice that hearing improves when the ear discharges, indicating that there is an ossicular discontinuity which has been bridged by mucopus or a polyp. This finding is also common with atticoantral disease. Tinnitus, typically high pitched, and vertigo, typically momentary and initiated by sudden head movement, are usually associated with a high-tone sensorineural hearing loss. These may be secondary to toxins reaching the perilymph through the oval or round window.

Complications

On examination there is a wet or dry central tympanic membrane perforation. The term 'central' implies there is a rim of tympanic membrane around the perforation, and not that the perforation is centrally situated in the drum head. An infected polyp may protrude through the perforation and there may be signs of the complications of tubotympanic disease.

- Otitis externa.
- Ossicular erosion, especially the long process of the incus.
- High-tone sensorineural hearing loss.
- Vertigo. Typically mild and transient. Benign intermittent paroxysmal positional vertigo has been described.
- Tympanosclerosis.
- Middle-ear adhesions.

Intracranial and severe cochleovestibular symptoms are unusual, as is a lower motor neurone facial palsy.

Treatment

The principles of treatment are to obtain a dry ear, prevent reinfection and to minimize the disability of any hearing loss. The former is attained by frequent aural toilet, the application of appropriate topical antibiotic ear drops, eradicating any source of intercurrent or chronic upper aerodigestive tract infection, and prevention of water entering the external ear canal when swimming or bathing. The decision as to whether surgery or a hearing aid is more appropriate depends on the type and severity of the hearing loss, the hearing in the contralateral ear, the frequency of recurrent infection, the wish to swim, the patient's occupation, lifestyle and general condition (see Tympanoplasty, p. 328).

Atticoantral CSOM

This is also called unsafe as the ear is at risk of serious complications. It is caused by either cholesteatoma (see p. 43) or pure mucosal disease. It has been suggested that some subjects are predisposed to the latter because of a narrow epitympanic space, and indeed it has been shown by high-definition CT scanning of the petrous temporal bone that as a group these subjects have a gap between the scutum and medial middle-ear wall that is significantly narrower than in a matched group without CSOM. Inadequate atticoantral drainage causes the mucosa to become chronically inflamed and polypoidal, further compromising drainage. Osteomyelitis of bone lining the polypoidal mucosa is the inevitable result, sometimes causing florid granulation tissue formation. The incidence of intracranial complications is the same for ears with cholesteatoma or with pure mucosal disease.

Clinical features

Deafness may be conductive, sensorineural or mixed. The former occurs when an ossicular discontinuity occurs from ossicular erosion by cholesteatoma or chronically inflamed mucosa. Toxin penetration through the round window may be the mechanism of sensorineural loss. Scanty, smelly aural discharge, mild transient vertigo and high-pitched tinnitus are typical. Otoscopy may reveal no more than an attic crust, which must be removed if cholesteatoma, attic granulations or a perforation are to be revealed. A marginal or attic perforation surrounded by granulation tissue or a polyp is more usual. A sanguinous discharge, otalgia, lower motor neurone facial palsy, a unilateral headache, signs of meningitis or of raised intracranial pressure suggest a serious complication.

Pure tone audiometry varies from normal, if there is limited attic disease, to a severe mixed type of hearing loss in extensive disease.

Complications   See p. 55.

Management   The priority is to make the ear safe from intracranial complications. If cholesteatoma is not seen on examining the ear, perhaps because of florid granulations, an attempt must be made to dry the ear by means of regular aural toilet, antibiotic ear drops and systemic antibiotics. The antibiotics should cover anaerobes because they have been found in over 50% of cultures in children with CSOM. A high-definition CT scan of the petrous temporal bone will show the extent but not the cause of soft-tissue disease; in particular it does not distinguish between cholesteatoma, polypoidal disease or granulation tissue. An unsafe ear without cholesteatoma which continues to discharge in spite of intensive medical management requires surgery (see Mastoidectomy, p. 165). Exceptions to this rule may arise when the ear is the better or only hearing ear, in the very elderly or those medically unfit. Harker and Pignatari (1992) have shown that, in cases of lower motor neurone facial paralysis associated with CSOM, urgent surgery to eradicate all inflammatory disease is the priority. Facial nerve decompression is usually unnecessary. CSOM, unlike ASOM, rarely responds rapidly to intravenous antibiotics because the mucosal changes or cholesteatoma are long-standing and delay in surgical treatment may compromise facial nerve recovery. As with ASOM, the horizontal portion of the mastoid segment of the facial nerve is implicated as the site of involvement and the facial nerve palsy is a neuropraxia which recovers with eradication of the cause.

Further reading

Brook I, Burke P. The management of acute, serous and chronic otitis media: The role of anaerobic bacteria. *Journal of Hospital Infection*, 1992; **22** (Suppl. A): 75–87.

Harker LA, Pignatari SSN. Facial nerve paralysis secondary to chronic otitis media without cholesteatoma. *American Journal of Otolaryngology*, 1992; **13**: 372–4.

Related topics of interest

CHRONIC SUPPURATIVE OTITIS MEDIA – COMPLICATIONS

Complications of chronic suppurative otitis media (CSOM) are associated with a high morbidity and may be life-threatening. Cholesteatoma, atticoantral mucosal disease and acute suppurative otitis media (ASOM) (see p. 9) cause complications by spread of infection:

(a) Directly via the oval or round window to reach the labyrinth, through osteitic bone to reach the dura and lateral sinus or to affect a congenitally dehiscent facial nerve.

(b) By retrograde propagation of small foci of thrombophlebitis which may extend through the temporal bone and dura to the major venous sinuses to cause a lateral sinus thrombosis and by further extension a cerebellar or temporal lobe abscess.

(c) Along the periarteriolar spaces to cause a temporal or cerebellar lobe abscess.

Browning, in a retrospective study, has calculated that the risk of a patient with CSOM developing an intracerebral abscess is 1 in 3500.

The complications may be classified as:

1. Extracranial.

- Chronic *otitis externa* and meatal stenosis.
- *Ossicular discontinuity* from ossicular erosion.
- *Middle-ear adhesions.*
- *Tympanosclerosis,* which may spread from the tympanic membrane over the ossicular chain, causing ossicular chain fixation.
- *Squamous cell carcinoma* of the middle ear.
- Lower motor neurone *facial nerve palsy.*
- Serous or purulent *labyrinthitis.*
- *Petrositis* and *Gradenigo's syndrome.*

2. Intracranial complications.

- *Lateral (transverse and sigmoid) sinus thrombosis.* This may extend to involve the superior and inferior petrosal sinuses, the cavernous sinus, the sinus confluence, the superior sagittal sinus and the internal jugular vein.
- *Meningitis.*
- *Extradural, subdural, intracerebral* (cerebellar and temporal lobe) *abscess.*
- *Otitic hydrocephalus.*

Clinical features

Patients with acute intracranial complications usually present to the neurosurgeons and are most likely to be seen by an ENT surgeon after recovery from the acute episode. Patients with CSOM who present with unilateral or occipital headaches, visual disturbance, vomiting, clumsiness, forgetfulness or drowsiness should have a full neurological examination, looking in particular for signs of raised intracranial pressure, meningitis and localizing cerebellar and temporoparietal lobe signs. A deep throbbing otalgia and serosanguinous discharge may herald malignant change.

Investigations

A high-definition CT scan of the petrous temporal bone will show the extent of mastoid disease, although it may not distinguish cholesteatoma from mucosal disease. A gadolinium-enhanced magnetic resonance scan is now the investigation of choice for the diagnosis of an intracerebral venous thrombosis.

Treatment

Principles:
(a) High-dose intravenous antibiotics to commence after taking a culture swab of the aural discharge.
(b) Neurosurgeons to manage intracerebral abscess.
(c) Treatment of initiating otological disorder.

Subdural and extradural abscesses require a cortical mastoidectomy to provide adequate exposure before drainage. A lateral sinus thrombosis, if not responding to high-dose intravenous antibiotics, should have a cortical mastoidectomy and the lateral sinus exposed. The diagnosis should be confirmed by needling the sinus. After confirmation some authors propose tying the internal jugular vein high up in the neck to prevent infective embolization during evacuation of infected clot. The lateral sinus is opened, the clot evacuated and the sinus obliterated by packing with temporalis muscle reinforced by a BIPP mastoid pack.

A facial palsy secondary to ASOM is invariably a neuropraxia. The nerve does not require decompressing and should recover rapidly with aggressive treatment of the infection. The facial palsy in CSOM is usually secondary to compression from cholesteatoma or granulation tissue. Most otologists advocate an urgent mastoidectomy and decompression of the vertical segment of the facial nerve (this has recently been challenged by Harker and Pignatari; see Chronic suppurative otitis media, p. 51), although if there is an actively discharging ear others would observe for at least 48 hours on intravenous antibiotics, because in this instance the palsy may be due to neuropraxia of a dehiscent horizontal segment of the nerve, found in 6% of ears.

Further reading

Munz M, Farmer JP, Auger L, O'Gorman AM, Schloss MD. Otitis media and CNS complications. *Journal of Otolaryngology,* 1992; **21**: 224–6.

Related topics of interest

CLINICAL ASSESSMENT OF HEARING

Use of clinical tests

It is surprising how often a clinical assessment of hearing is omitted from the routine examination of the otology patient. Voice tests and tuning fork tests are the two main methods, but often only the Weber and Rinne tuning fork tests are performed. Clinical tests can be used to:

- Identify a hearing impairment.
- Determine the nature of a hearing loss (conductive or sensorineural).
- Grade the severity.
- Detect feigning or a non-organic hearing loss.

The main reason that clinical tests of auditory function are overlooked is that they have largely been superseded by more sensitive and reliable audiometric tests. However, audiometry on occasions may be inaccurate or unavailable. Furthermore, exaggerated thresholds may be missed if suspicion is not aroused by clinical testing. Proponents of clinical testing suggest that audiometry may be unnecessary if the hearing is normal or the results would not influence the management.

Masking

Masking is as important in clinical testing as it is in audiometric testing. The non-test ear should always be masked when clinically testing by air conduction, and in theory always when performing tuning fork tests, though this is not always practicable. There are two techniques in common use.

1. The tragal rub. Occlusion of the auditory canal by putting finger pressure on the tragus with a rubbing motion is the easiest method. Using this technique speech will be attenuated by approximately 50 dB. There is a risk of undermasking if the sound level of speech arriving at the test ear is greater than 70 dB A so a Bárány noise box should be used when testing an ear with a severe or profound impairment or when testing bone conduction with tuning forks.

2. Bárány noise box. This box produces a broad-band noise from a clockwork-driven source. The maximum sound output varies from approximately 90 dB A when a box is held at right angles to the ear and 100 dB A when held over the ear. These levels are sufficient to mask the non-test ear in all practical circumstances, but the main problem is cross-masking of the test ear. It should be used when a tragal rub does not provide adequate masking.

Voice tests

Difficulties in standardizing the technique and variability of the stimulus provided by the examiner have led to criticisms of this test. The easiest and best method of performing monaural free field voice testing is by using a whispered voice, conversational voice and then loud voice at 2 ft and then 6 inches. It is usual to start by testing the better hearing ear when there is one. The non-test ear is masked by a tragal rub unless a loud voice is required (use the Bárány noise box). The patient is asked to repeat as accurately as possible what the examiner says. Bisyllable words (e.g. bluebell, cowboy), numbers (e.g. 54, 37, 63) or combinations of numbers and letters (e.g. 4 B 7) can be used depending on the patient's age and understanding. The examiner starts using a whispered voice 2 ft away from the patient, which is the furthest away that is possible when masking the non-test ear. The sound level is increased in steps from a whispered voice at 2 ft, to a whispered voice at 6 inches, to a conversational voice at 2 ft, to a conversational voice at 6 inches, to a loud voice at 2 ft, and finally to a loud voice at 6 inches. The test finishes as soon as the patient repeats 50% of the words correctly at any one voice and distance level.

If a patient can hear a whispered voice 2 ft away from the ear, the pure tone thresholds are likely to be less than 30 dB (normal hearing). Patients who can hear a whisper at 6 inches or a conversational voice at 2 ft or 6 inches are likely to have thresholds in the range of 30–70 dB HL (mild/moderate impairment). Those patients who can only hear a loud voice are likely to have thresholds greater than 70 dB HL (severe/profound impairment).

Tuning forks

Tuning forks for audiological use are modified to include a finger grip on the stem and an expansion on the base of the stem to allow application to the skull. Ideally a 512- or 256-Hz tuning fork should be used. The duration of the stimulus decreases with increasing frequency, and it is difficult to activate forks with a frequency higher than 512 Hz sufficiently for them to be heard by those with a moderate or severe impairment. Forks with a frequency lower than 256 Hz can make it difficult for the patient to distinguish between hearing the sound and feeling it by vibration. A tuning fork should be set in vibration by a firm strike one-third of the way from the free end of the prong against a firm but elastic object (e.g. elbow or patella). This should produce a relatively pure tone with minimal overtones. It can then be presented by either air or bone conduction. For air conduction it should be held with its acoustic axis (a line joining two points near the tips of the two prongs) in line with and 2–3 cm from the external meatus. For bone conduction the base plate should be placed firmly on the skull, either mastoid process or vertex depending on the test. Although the tuning fork can theoretically be placed at any point on the skull for bone conduction, some points may give less reliable results.

A variety of tuning fork tests were developed to test absolute hearing thresholds (compared with the examiner), to differentiate real from feigned hearing loss, conductive from sensorineural, and cochlear from retrocochlear hearing loss. With the advent of newer and more sensitive forms of investigation, many of these tests are no longer in everyday use. However, a number of tests have stood the test of time and continue in current clinical practice.

The tests are based on two main principles:

1. The inner ear is normally twice as sensitive to sound conducted by air as to that conducted by bone.
2. In the presence of a purely conductive hearing loss, the affected ear is subject to less environmental noise, making it more sensitive to bone-conducted sound.

No single test is diagnostic but all can provide useful information when taken in context. Unfortunately, tuning fork tests are unreliable in children.

Weber test

This test is based on the principle that a conductive loss causes a relative improvement in the ability to hear a bone-conducted sound and the test is of most value in a unilateral hearing loss. The tuning fork is struck and placed on the vertex. The vertex is used as oppposed to the forehead as the reliability of the test is thus improved from 72% to 86%. (Further improvements can be achieved by using the upper incisors but these are not always available!) If a conductive loss of 10 dB or more exists, the sound should be heard in the affected ear. If a sensorineural hearing loss is present the sound will generally be heard in the normal ear. In the normal subject or some subjects with a long-standing sensorineural hearing loss, the sound will be heard in the midline.

Rinne test

This test examines each ear individually and is again based on the principle of improved bone conduction perception with a conductive loss. It can be performed in one of two ways. The subject can be asked to compare either the loudness of the tuning fork when presented by air conduction and bone conduction (placed on the ipsilateral mastoid process) or the duration of the sound when presented by both air and bone conduction. The normal response is to hear the sound as louder and longer with air conduction and is referred to as a Rinne positive. A positive response will also occur with a sensorineural hearing loss. A negative response (Rinne negative) will occur if there is a conductive loss of greater than 20 dB or if there is a severe sensorineural hearing loss. The former is referred to as a true-negative Rinne and the latter as a false negative. The two can be distinguished by using a Bárány sound box, in which case the false negative will become positive as the contralateral, minimally attenuated, bone conduction is masked.

Bing test

This test is similar to the Rinne and is based on the improvement in bone conduction perception in the normal subject when the external auditory meatus is occluded. The tuning fork is struck and placed on the subject's mastoid process. After the subject acknowledges hearing the sound, the ipsilateral meatus is occluded by the examiner's finger and the subject is asked if this makes the sound louder or quieter. Occluding the external auditory canal will block out ambient noise, and prevent some of the bone conduction sound which has emanated into the external auditory canal from escaping. If the sound becomes louder, the response is positive (and normal). If the sound does not change or becomes quieter, the response is negative, and usually indicates a conductive loss of 10 dB or more.

Stenger test

This test is used to differentiate a real from a feigned hearing loss and is based on the principle that, if two pure tones of equal intensity are presented to both ears at once, the sound will appear to originate in the midline. If the intensity of one side is increased, the sound will appear to originate from that side alone. In practice, the test is commenced by asking the subject to close his or her eyes to help concentrate on the sound. The tester works behind the subject. First a tuning fork is placed 15 cm from the good ear; the subject confirms hearing the sound. A tuning fork is then positioned 5 cm from the bad ear; the subject will deny hearing it. Finally, unknown to the subject, two tuning forks are used simultaneously: one 5 cm from the bad ear and one 15 cm from the good ear. If the hearing loss is real the subject will hear the sound in the good ear and report this. If the hearing loss is feigned, the subject will hear the sound loudest in the bad ear. Unaware that there is a previously audible sound present at the good ear, the subject will deny hearing anything and this suggests the diagnosis.

Further reading

Browning GG. *Clinical Otology and Audiology*. London: Butterworths, 1986; 23–37.
Committee for the Consideration of Hearing Tests. Report of the Committee for the Consideration of Hearing Tests. *Journal of Laryngology and Otology*, 1933; **48**: 22–48.
Golabek W, Stephens SDG. Some tuning fork tests revisited. *Clinical Otolaryngology*, 1979; **4**: 421–30.

Related topics of interest

Examination of the ear (p. 90)
Impedance audiometry (p. 137)
Non-organic hearing loss (p. 195)

Pure tone audiometry (p. 255)
Speech audiometry (p. 291)

COCHLEAR IMPLANTS

A cochlear implant is a device used to stimulate residual neural tissue in patients with a profound hearing loss. It is not a bionic ear, and the signal produced is a long way from normal sound. Their major benefits are as aids to lip-reading and in the recognition of some environmental sounds.

History

The use of electrical stimulation of the ears is not new, having been used, for various disorders, since the later part of the nineteenth century. However, it is only since the early 1960s that research into electrical stimulation of the inner ear and advances in electrical engineering and microsurgery have yielded practical benefits. In addition, cochlear implant development has been helped by advances in other biomechanical implants such as pacemakers and spinal stimulators.

Several groups around the world were initially active in developing cochlear implant programmes: North American groups, most notably the House group in Los Angeles and Michelson *et al.* in San Francisco, but also Clark *et al.* in Australia, Hochmair-Desoyer *et al.* in Austria and Chouard *et al.* in France. The success of these groups encouraged the emergence of many other interested researches in the late 1970s and early 1980s, including several in the UK.

Implant design

The implant consists of two parts: an implanted portion and an external portion. The external, body-worn, portion consists of a power source, microphone sound receiver and a microprocessor which filters, analyses and codes the sound and then passes it to an external transmitter. The implanted portion consists of a receiver with stimulating and ground electrodes. The external and internal portions can be connected directly by a percutaneous link or, more often, indirectly by a transcutaneous induction method. The transcutaneous method has the disadvantages of a less satisfactory electrical link and being heavier on the power source but has the advantages of being neater and presenting a lower risk of infection.

As the device is implanted it must be constructed from biocompatible materials. The electrode in particular must display a combination of suitable electrical characteristics, high tensile strength, resistance to corrosion, and low toxicity. At present platinum–iridium alloys seem to provide the best compromise. The stimulating electrode can be positioned in the round window, but is more often placed within the cochlea via the round window. Although both placings can operate a single-channel system, a multichannel system can only operate with an intracochlear electrode. A single-channel system means that only the frequency and intensity of stimulation of the single electrode can be altered to provide auditory information. A multichannel system has multiple active electrodes (up to 22) and can, in addition to the above variables, also stimulate at various sites within the cochlea. This system obviously allows the provision of far more auditory information. Unfortunately some patients have insufficient residual neural tissue to take advantage of these potential benefits.

Speech coding

Three basic schemes exist for speech processing:

1. *Analogue transformation (single channel only)*. In this method the received sound is filtered so only that between 200 and 4000 Hz is used. This sound is then transformed to modulate the amplitude of a high-frequency sinusoidal carrier wave. In effect, this system is trying to squeeze all the acoustic information available into a single channel.

2. *Multichannel filtering (multichannel only)*. In this method the processor separates the incoming sound into frequency bands. Each frequency band is represented by one of several active electrodes and the corresponding processed information is then sent to the appropriate electrode. This method tries to recreate normal auditory physiology.

3. *Speech pattern processing (single and multichannel)*. In this method the processor simplifies speech material by extracting only fundamental but important information such as intonation and voicing patterns. This technique assumes that the implant is to be used primarily as an aid to lip-reading and not as a replacement of hearing.

Preoperative assessment

This is the most crucial area of any implant programme. It is important for the success of the implant that only appropriate patients are selected. Factors involved in this selection are:

1. *Cause of deafness*. Patients with deafness due to a central cause are unsuitable for implantation. Different peripheral causes will leave varying numbers of residual neurones; function tends to be better with greater neuronal survival. (Bacterial labyrinthitis and vascular causes generally leave

few surviving neurones.) Patients deafened by meningitis tend to do less well, possibly as a result of some additional central damage.

2. *Timing of deafness.* Performance is better in postlingually deafened patients in whom there is some memory of speech and sound.

3. *Age.* There is no age limit as long as the patient is fit. There was initially controversy about implanting children, particularly regarding the assessment of hearing loss and the destruction of any residual hearing (not with a round window electrode), but now there are several paediatric cochlear implant programmes developing.

4. *General health.*

5. *Personality and psychological profile.* As normal hearing is not provided by an implant, it is important that the patient fully understands this and is motivated for the subsequent hard work of rehabilitation.

6. *Otological examination.* Middle-ear disease must be excluded and radiological assessment of the cochlea is important to demonstrate any barriers to electrode placement. A high resolution CT scan is mandatory.

7. *Audiometric assessment.* Pure tone audiogram, electrical response audiometry and tests of auditory discrimination (speech tests and recognition of environmental sounds) are essential. There is still controversy as to what level of hearing loss is appropriate for implantation. In general, the hearing loss should be at least 100 – 120 dB HL. Patients with a hearing threshold of less than 100 dB HL are best provided with a hearing aid rather than a cochlear implant. The potential benefits of an implant should obviously outweigh those of a suitable hearing aid before implantation is considered. For this reason many patients will require a preoperative trial of a hearing aid.

8. *Electrical stimulation of the cochlea.* Some centres still use this as a part of their preoperative work-up. A round window electrode placed through a small tympanotomy appears to provide more information than a transtympanic needle.

9. *Vestibular testing.* It is important not to destroy an only functioning labyrinth.

Not all of this information is required to make a decision on implantation but much of it is used in research and audit of the value of cochlear implant programmes.

Operative procedure

The implant is secured in the mastoid region and the electrode is then passed down to the round window by a posterior tympanotomy. A drill hole is made just above the round window into the basal turn of the cochlea and the sensor section of the implant fed through. Prophylactic antibiotics appear to be unnecessary.

Rehabilitation

Rehabilitation begins prior to surgery and involves a full explanation of the device and its limitations. Realistic postoperative expectations are fostered. After implantation an intensive programme of auditory and speech training is commenced, which takes several weeks to complete. This involves training the patient to recognize his or her own voice sounds, external speech and environmental sounds and to modulate and control speech, initially in quiet conditions and ultimately against a variety of background noise, both with and without familiar visual clues. It is often necessary for the patient to reside close to the implant centre during this period. It is also important to remember that the full benefit does not become apparent for up to 6 months. This is because of a combination of the healing process following surgery and a learning period to adjust to the novel stimuli.

Postoperative assessment

This takes place as part of the process of rehabilitation and involves many of the tests used as part of the preoperative assessment. These assessments have demonstrated a number of beneficial effects from cochlear implantation:

1. *Marked improvement in lip-reading ability.* This appears to be the main benefit of implantation with significant improvement in lip-reading skills reported by all groups.

2. *Identification of environmental sounds.*

3. *Relief of auditory isolation.* Most patients report a sense of relief and general improvement in psychological well-being in response to the new perception of sound.

4. *Improvement in speech perception.* Many patients are able to recognize some words without visual clues after

implantation. Some patients appear to hear almost normally in ideal conditions.

5. Improvement in patient's speech quality.

6. Tinnitus suppression.

Implant failure   Cochlear implants are by their nature delicate devices and failure can occur at many stages.

1. Preoperative. Damage sustained in transport, sterilization, preimplantation handling. The device should always be tested prior to insertion.

2. Operative. Rough handling during insertion, particularly bending or fracture of the electrode.

3. Postoperative. Migration of the device as a result of poor operative fixation; acquired infection.

Intrinsic component failure may strike at any time in the postoperative period, although it is most likely at the two extremes of the implant's lifetime; which may be upwards of 10 years.

Further reading

Gray RF. *Cochlear Implants*. London: Croom Helm, 1985.
The University College Hospital/Royal National Institute for the Deaf Cochlear Implant Programme. *Journal of Laryngology and Otology*, 1989 (Suppl. No. 18).

Related topic of interest

Evoked response audiometry (p. 85)
Hearing aids (p. 126)
Pure tone audiometry (p. 255)
Speech audiometry (p. 291)

CONGENITAL HEARING DISORDERS

We define the term congenital as existing at birth. Congenital deafness may be sensorineural, conductive or mixed and may occur in isolation or with other congenital abnormalities (the syndromes). Sensorineural deafness may be a hereditary degenerative deafness in which there is progressive loss of hearing, typically in late childhood, in subjects with a previously normal cochlea in both structure and function (*the abiotrophies*). There are a multitude of syndromes associated with congenital deafness. Below are those we consider to be the most important.

Autosomal recessive

1. Pendred's syndrome. Sensorineural hearing loss (SNHL) and a thyroid goitre.

2. Usher's syndrome. Retinitis pigmentosa and SNHL.

3. Jervell and Lange Nielson syndrome. Prolonged electrocardiographic Q–T interval and SNHL.

4. Refsum's disease. Retinitis pigmentosa, cerebellar ataxia, peripheral neuropathy and SNHL

Autosomal dominant

1. Waardenburg's syndrome. Telecanthus, pigment disorder (20% have a white forelock and 45% heterochromia iridis) with SNHL.

2. Treacher–Collins syndrome. Hypoplasia of the malar bones, maxilla and mandible. There may be microtia or multiple external and inner ear abnormalities.

3. Pierre–Robin syndrome. Hypoplastic mandible, cleft palate, glossoptosis. There may be external, middle or internal ear deformities.

4. Crouzon's disease. Hypoplastic mandible and maxilla, parrot beak nose, craniostenosis and exophthalmos associated with external and middle–ear abnormalities.

5. Apert's syndrome. Congenital fixation of the stapes footplate, acrocephaly, syndactyly, cleft palate, saddle nose, maxillary hypoplasia.

Dysplasias

The dysplasias describe four congenital abnormalities of the cochlea and often occur as a component of the hearing syndromes. They comprise:

1. *Michel's deformity*. The most severe 'dysplasia' (more correctly this is an aplasia) with agenesis of the labyrinth and total sensorineural deafness.

2. *Mondini's dysplasia*. Only the basal coil of the cochlea is present and the semicircular canals may be absent. There are islands of residual hearing, especially in the high tones.

3. *Bing–Siebenman dysplasia*. The bony labyrinth is normal but there is maldevelopment of the membranous labyrinth.

4. *Scheibe dysplasia*. The bony labyrinth is normal but the stria vascularis has alternating regions of aplasia and hypoplasia. There are few hair cells and the saccule is collapsed, hence its synonym cochleosaccular dysgenesis. Hearing loss is severe.

Congenital conductive hearing loss

The external ear canal develops from the first branchial cleft lying between the first and second branchial arches. These arches form the pinna (mesoderm and ectoderm), bony labyrinth (mesoderm), membranous labyrinth (ectoderm) and, from the dorsal end of cartilage within each arch, the ossicles (mesoderm). The ventral arch cartilage forms the mandible (first arch) and the hyoid bone (second arch). Anomalies of structures associated with these arches give rise to multiple deformities, for example Treacher–Collins and Pierre–Robin syndromes. The external and middle-ear anomalies are classified into three groups:

1. *Minor aplasia*. The external auditory meatus is narrow, the tympanic membrane functional, the pinna either normal or with a minor deformity and there may be ossicular fixation, usually of the stapes. Stapes surgery is difficult because of limited access and there is an increased risk of a perilymph gusher so that a small fenestra technique is recommended should stapedectomy be attempted.

2. *Major aplasia*. There is usually microtia with external ear canal atresia and fixation of an abnormal malleus and incus. The stapes is usually functionally normal.

3. *Major aplasia/atresia*. The external ear may be atretic, the tympanic cavity small, mastoid pneumatization absent and there is a significant risk of one of the cochlear dyplasias.

Classification of congenital sensorineural deafness	*1. Hereditary.*

Classification of congenital sensorineural deafness

1. Hereditary.

(a) Deafness present at birth. (i) Deafness alone. (ii) Syndromes associated with deafness.

(b) Deafness appearing in childhood. (i) Deafness alone. (ii) Syndromes associated with deafness.

2. Secondary to intrauterine disease.

(a) Infections: rubella, cytomegalovirus, toxoplasmosis, congenital syphilis.

(b) Ototoxic drugs (see Ototoxicity, p. 231).

(c) Metabolic disorders, e.g. maternal diabetes mellitus.

(d) Perinatal disorders, e.g. hypoxia, hyperbilirubinaemia, premature delivery, low birth weight.

Classification of congenital conductive hearing loss

1. Hereditary abnormal external or middle ear.

(a) Present at birth, e.g. Apert's syndrome, Crouzon's disease, Treacher–Collins syndrome, Pierre–Robin syndrome.

(b) Appearing in childhood, e.g. osteogenesis imperfecta, otosclerosis.

2. Congenital disorders predisposing to glue ear. Cystic fibrosis, cleft palate, Down's syndrome, Kartagener's syndrome.

3. Miscellaneous conditions. (i) Congenital cholesteatoma. (ii) Fibrous dysplasia. (iii) Goldenhar's syndrome.

Management

The congenital hearing loss may be suspected at birth because of the family history. These babies and those suspected of having one of the syndromes or dysplasias should be referred to a paediatric otologist or audiologist, who will be able to investigate the suspected hearing loss and institute, depending on the cause, appropriate surgery or/and rehabilitation.

Related topics of interest

Hearing aids (p. 126)
Ototoxicity (p. 231)
Paediatric hearing assessment (p. 241)

COSMETIC SURGERY

This chapter is confined to a description of rhinoplasty, pinnaplasty and facial reanimation.

Rhinoplasty

Indications

(a) Cosmetic: dorsal hump, dorsal saddle, too wide or too narrow dorsum, under- or overprojected tip, polly beak.
(b) Functional: nasal obstruction, snoring, sleep apnoea.

Much is written about the ideal nasal size and shape. This, however, depends on the dimensions of the upper, mid and lower thirds of the face, the thickness of the nasal skin and the race of the patient. There is no one perfect shape. It is not disputed, however, that a nose should be straight and have a uniform dorsal width from nasion to the tip. The nasolabial angle should be about 90° in males and 110° in females. It is important that patients state specifically what they dislike about their nasal shape and for surgeons to state exactly what deformities they are aiming to correct so that the patient will have a realistic expectation of the likely operative result. It is often the case that it is not possible to make an ugly nose pretty, but it is usually possible to correct specific defects so that the nose no longer brings attention to the face.

Technique

Most rhinoplasty surgery consists in a basic technique comprising nasal dehumping, medial and lateral osteotomies with in-fracture and excision of a cephalic rim of lower lateral cartilage. The latter technique is necessary if the tip requires cephalic rotation or narrowing. A dilemma in rhinoplasty surgery is what graft to use when augmentation is necessary. Again there is no ideal graft that fits all scenarios. Cartilaginous augmentation by manoeuvring quadrate cartilage into a new position or using conchal cartilage with perichondrium attached, bony dorsal augmentation using a rib graft (not a straight graft but it can be osteotomized), iliac crest (the bone here is cancellous). Silastic implants are easy to use but tend to extrude. In North America there is a current vogue for external rhinoplasty, which has the advantage of visualizing directly the osteocartilaginous vault during surgery.

Pinnaplasty

Most surgeons wait until the patient is at least 4 years old so that the ear is not too small to manipulate and for the full deformity (e.g. there may be an overlarge conchal bowl in addition to an absent antihelix) to become apparent. Ideally, surgery should be performed before infant school to prevent ridicule.

The two common techniques are:
(1) The anterior conchal scoring technique described by Stenstrom, allowing the concha to curl back to form an antihelix without suturing.
(2) The Mustarde technique in which the antihelix is folded and kept in position with mattress sutures.

Most surgeons will have their own modification of one of these techniques which works well for them (e.g. thinning the region of the antihelix fold in the Mustarde technique with a diamond drill to reduce cartilage tension and to allow a more natural curve). An important and often neglected portion of the procedure is the pressure dressing. Cotton wool should support the postauricular region and fill the conchal bowl, and a firm head dressing should be applied in such a way that it will not slip until it is removed 7–14 days later. The only indication to remove the dressing is increasing aural pain, which usually indicates that a subperichondrial haematoma has formed owing to inadequate pressure. It is unusual for the head dressing to be too tight, and then the main symptom will be a persistent headache, the operated ear being splinted and protected. Many surgeons state that it is better not to apply a head dressing than to apply one which is inadequate, as the trauma to the ear from repeated redressing will predispose to infection or haematoma.

Facial reanimation

Surgery to produce improved facial symmetry after a facial nerve palsy should not be undertaken until the surgeon is sure that there will be no spontaneous improvement. This may be immediate if trauma, either external or iatrogenic, has caused an immediate and total palsy suggesting nerve transection. It is recommended that 18 months post onset is taken as the minimum time to allow the nerve to recover maximum function after injury or following attempted reinnervation.

Facial nerve grafting The reinnervation procedure chosen will depend on the site of injury and the surgeon's personal preference. Direct apposition of the nerve ending using monofilament 9-0 nylon suture material should be attempted only if it is possible to avoid tension on the anastomosis. Otherwise, a cable graft using sural or great auricular nerve should be attempted. For more proximal injuries, such as those occurring after acoustic neuroma surgery, hypoglossal to facial and accessory to facial nerve anastomosis are the options. The latter uses the larger branch to the trapezius muscle with little loss of shoulder movement or strength. When only half the width of the hypoglossal nerve is anastomosed to the facial trunk, in order to preserve tongue movement, slightly less satisfactory facial tone occurs. Reliable results are obtained with this technique only if anastomosis is attempted within 1 year of the onset of a palsy, whereas the standard procedure is reliable when used up to 2 years after facial palsy.

Dynamic and static suspension

Dynamic suspension comprises transposition of the temporalis muscle to the submucosa or the orbicularis oris muscle in close proximity to the angle of the mouth. It improves the symmetry of the face at rest and on voluntary smiling in those with a permanent facial paralysis, but does not improve lagophthalmos. It can be complementary to facial nerve cable grafting or facial–hypoglossal anastomosis. The technique comprises placing the muscle sling lateral to the fascia overlying the muscles of facial expression to avoid the underlying facial nerve twigs. In some centres only the middle section of the muscle is transposed. Static suspension is achieved using a fascia lata sling from the zygomatic arch to the orbicularis muscle at the angle of the mouth. A second fascial sling can be positioned around the mouth. Sterile 1-mm-thick Gore-Tex Soft Tissue Patch can also be used for static suspension. The material is prestretched and so postoperative sagging is unusual, in contradistinction to fascia lata. The material is attached to the zygomatic arch and the orbicularis muscle to elevate the mid-facial and perioral region. Most series, however, report a high rate of extrusion and infection compared to fascia lata.

Eyelid procedures

A gold weight implant positioned over the tarsal plate and centred at the junction of the medial and middle third of the upper eyelid has been used for more than 30 years to rehabilitate the eyelid following facial nerve paralysis. Implants of different weights are taped to the upper lid preoperatively to determine the correct weight to just allow closure without ptosis. The main complications are infection and haematoma in the early postoperative period and extrusion, which can occur early or several years after implanting. To minimize extrusion rates it is recommended that a drill hole is fashioned through the implant and this used to attach it to the tarsal plate by a nylon or Prolene suture.

Further reading

Ebersold MJ, Quast LM. Long-term results of spinal accessory nerve–facial nerve anastomosis. *Journal of Neurosurgery,* 1992; **77:** 51–4.

Kunihiro T, Kanzaki J, O-Uchi T. Hypoglossal–facial nerve anastomosis. *Acta Otolaryngology,* 1991; **487:** 80–4.

May M, Drucker C. Temporalis muscle for facial reanimation: a 13 year experience with 224 procedures. *Archives of Otolaryngology Head and Neck Surgery,* 1993; **119:** 378–82.

Pickford MA, Scamp T, Harrison DH. Morbidity after gold weight insertion into the upper eyelid in facial palsy. *British Journal of Plastic Surgery,* 1992; **45:** 460–4.

Related topics of interest

DAY CASE ENT SURGERY

Definition

An ENT surgical day case patient is one admitted for operation on a planned non-resident basis but who requires facilities for recovery. Full admission procedures and records are required, which therefore excludes those operations and procedures undertaken in the outpatient or accident and emergency department.

The patient may be admitted into either a self-contained day surgery unit with its own admission suites, wards, theatres and recovery area, or less desirably a day case ward or unsatisfactorily a general ward. In a general ward booked admissions may be blocked by emergency admissions and this is an expensive option because the ward is not closed at night or at the weekend.

Patient selection

An adult must be available to supervise the patient during the evening and first night. A telephone must be accessible so that the hospital can be contacted in an emergency. The home should be within a 20-minute drive of the hospital if the patient is at risk of a primary haemorrhage, for example after adenoidectomy or submucosal diathermy. The patient must be taken home by an adult in a car or taxi on discharge. No mechanical device should be used or cooking undertaken, and legal documents should not be signed during the first 24-hour postoperative period, when alcohol is also forbidden. Driving is not advised within 48 hours of a general anaesthetic. Operations likely to take longer than 40 minutes are unsuitable because of the slow speed of recovery from general anaesthetic, and patients should normally be of ASA 1 or ASA 2 status, (The American Society of Anesthesiologists classification of physical status: class 1, the patient has no organic, physiological, biochemical or psychiatric disturbance and the pathological process for which surgery is to be performed is localized; or class 2, mild to moderate systemic disturbance caused either by the condition to be treated surgically or other pathophysiological processes, for example non-insulin-dependent diabetes mellitus or essential hypertension.) As a rule an upper age limit of 70 is recommended although older patients with a low biological age should be considered. The very obese are excluded.

Children's requirements

Special facilities for children are required. They should have their own designated area away from adult patients, with its own play area and parental waiting area. A preadmission visit allows familiarization. It is permissible to have a children-only operation day in a day surgery unit or day case ward if the required facilities are present. The children's area should be staffed by paediatric trained nurses.

Advantages

- Lower costs.
- Reduced in-patient theatre workload.
- Increased efficiency.
- Reduced disruption to life.
- Early mobilization.
- Less psychological preparation required.
- Anaesthetic administered allows rapid recovery.

Disadvantages

- Limited care available to the patient after discharge.
- In-patient admission, if needed, must be arranged at short notice.

Examples of appropriate operations

1. Ear. Excision of accessory auricles, skin tags, preauricular sinuses. Removal of impacted wax or foreign bodies. Wedge excision biopsy of pinna lesion, myringotomy with or without grommet insertion, aural polypectomy.

2. Nose. Reduction of nasal fractures, limited functional endoscopic sinus surgery, limited intranasal polypectomy, electrocautery of the nasal septum, submucosal diathermy of the inferior turbinate, septoplasty, submucosal resection of the nasal septum, bilateral antral puncture.

3. Head and neck. Adenoidectomy, tonsillectomy (controversial), Examination under anaesthetic (EUA) and biopsy of the laryngopharynx and oesophagus provided there is no risk to the airway. Selected patients requiring laser therapy, for example vocal cord polypectomy or nodule excision and laser excision of small tongue lesions. Other indications include the division of tongue tie and lymph node excision biopsy.

Further reading

Report of the Working Party on Guidelines for Daycase Surgery. Revised edition. London: The Royal College of Surgeons of England, 1992.

DISORDERS OF SMELL AND TASTE

There are three chemosensory portions to smell and taste:

- Olfaction.
- Gustation.
- Common chemical sensation.

Physiology

1. *Olfaction* (smell) is provided by a small area of olfactory epithelium in the vault of the nasal cavity. Odorant molecules are carried into the nasal cavity with (inspiratory and expiratory) airflow. They dissolve in the overlying mucus and may then combine with odorant-binding proteins. This complex then attaches to receptor proteins, resulting in the production of cyclic AMP as an intracellular secondary messenger, with subsequent cell depolarization and a neural action potential. Degradative enzyme systems appear to exist for stimulant breakdown after neural interaction. The olfactory neurones pass through the cribriform plate and sensory information passes to the olfactory bulb and then on to the thalamus, hypothalamus and cortex. Quite how this sensory information codes for smell is unknown. It is known, however, that different odorants have different rates and degrees of solubility in the overlying mucus. Not all olfactory receptors respond equally or at all to different odorants, neither are they equally distributed in the nasal cavity. It is likely that all these factors have a bearing on smell recognition.

2. *Gustation* (taste) is served by the taste buds, which are modified epithelial cells found throughout the oral cavity, although there are regional differences in their concentration and distribution. Bitter tastes are better perceived on the posterior tongue, sweet and salt on the anterior tongue and sour on the lateral border. Neural stimulation occurs after dissolving of the tastant in a similar fashion to olfaction although the neural pathways are more complex. Several different cranial nerves are involved, with their primary afferents synapsing in the tractus solitarius in the medulla, before sensation passes on to the thalamus and cortex.

3. *Common chemical sensation* (irritation) is served by free nerve endings of the lingual branch of the trigeminal nerve in the oral cavity and nose with a contribution from the

glossopharyngeal nerve in the oropharynx. These fibres are stimulated by any unpleasant mechanical, thermal or chemical stimuli. Information is ultimately passed to the cortex via the thalamus.

Pathology

It is uncommon for common chemical sensation or taste to be lost; there is much redundancy in the neural supply and the sensory distribution is relatively wide. It is more likely that olfaction may be lost or impaired. Most loss of taste that patients complain of are in fact loss of olfaction.

The main causes of disorders of smell and taste are as follows:

1. Sinonasal disease (20–30%). In most cases this is due to simple mechanical obstruction (polyps, mucosal swelling in rhinitis, etc.) preventing odorants from reaching the olfactory epithelium in the narrow nasal vault, although in some cases the local inflammatory response may alter the overlying mucus or the function of the receptor cells.

2. Following upper respiratory tract infection (15–20%). Probably due to damage of the peripheral olfactory receptors following infection with a neuropathic virus.

3. Head injury (20%). Serious head injury can result in shearing of the olfactory filaments as they pass through the cribriform plate or direct contusion of the olfactory bulb or cortex.

4. Diopathic (20%).

5. Others (15–20%). A multitude of other causes exist, including systemic disease, metabolic and connective tissue disorders, drug therapy, neurological conditions, toxin exposure, previous nasal surgery, radiotherapy and old age.

Clinical features

The patient may complain of loss (anosmia), diminution (hyposmia) or alteration, usually unpleasant (parosmia), in the sense of smell or taste. In this last case the patient is often confusing taste with flavour as taste is rarely lost. The majority of patients (60–75%) with sinonasal disease describe anosmia rather than hyposmia, as do those following head injury. Hyposmia is a more common symptom following an upper respiratory tract infection (URTI).

Investigations	A thorough history must be taken and any temporal relation to an upper respiratory infection or head injury noted. A full nasal examination including endoscopy will be required to establish any sinonasal disease. Radiological imaging (including CT scans) of the sinuses may be required. Further general investigations will be dictated by the clinical features. The sense of smell can be crudely tested using a variety of recognizable odours, e.g. peppermint, cloves, lemon or coffee. It is important that the test scents are not too pungent or irritant (e.g. bleach) as they may then be recognized by common chemical sensation. Some objective measure of olfaction is helpful. Commercial 'scratch and sniff' kits are available using a forced choice technique which greatly increase their sensitivity. For example they can be useful for assessing if a patient is suffering from anosmia or is malingering.
Management	Sinonasal disease should be managed as appropriate to the condition. It has the best prognosis in terms of response with treatment. Reassurance regarding the absence of serious pathology should be stressed to the post-URTI and head injury groups. A small proportion in both groups (10–20%) will improve with the passage of time. Management of any systemic causes is as for that condition and drug-induced problems may require a change of medication. Little is known about the idiopathic group and certainly no treatments are available, but some surgeons will see if the patient has any response after a trial of using a steroid nasal spray. Some authorities claim that a trial of zinc supplements should be administered.
Follow-up and aftercare	This should be as appropriate for the underlying cause.

Further reading

Mott AE, Leopold DA, Disorders in taste and smell. *Medical Clinics of North America*, 1991; **75**: 1321–48.

Related topics of interest

Allergic rhinitis (p. 16)
Halitosis (p. 124)
Intrinsic rhinitis (p. 141)
Nasal polyps (p. 172)

EPIGLOTTITIS

Acute epiglottitis is an uncommon but dangerous bacterial infection of the throat. There is an acute inflammation of the larynx which affects all the supraglottis, but predominantly the loose connective tissue of the epiglottis.

Aetiology

Haemophilus influenzae type B (HIB) is the usual causative organism, but this is not invariable. β-Haemolytic streptococci, pneumococci and staphylococci have also been isolated, especially in adult cases. Quite why the infection has a predilection for the epiglottis is not clear. Epiglottitis is usually seen in children between the ages of 2 and 6 years, with a peak incidence between the ages of 3 and 4. It may also occur in adults. In children under the age of 2 years *Haemophilus* tends to cause meningitis. It has been suggested that previous contact with *H. influenzae* in early childhood may later be followed by a type III Arthus hypersensitivity reaction which would account for the rapid onset of epiglottitis.

Prophylaxis

In recent years efforts have been focused on the prevention of HIB infections. There seems to have been a decline in new cases over the last 2 years, which may be attributed to the new conjugated HIB vaccine approved for administration to 2-month-old infants.

Clinical features

The disease may present at any time of the year but is more common in winter.

Initially the child usually complains of a sore throat and pain when swallowing. The inflammation and oedema will rapidly progress to cause muffling of the voice and respiratory obstruction. Inspiratory stridor then occurs. A critically ill, breathless child may then present to the casualty department having a toxic, flushed appearance and a high temperature (38–40°C). The child will usually sit up and lean forward dribbling saliva. The provisional diagnosis is made on the history and the examination of the child. Attempts to depress the tongue or indirect laryngoscopy should not be undertaken to confirm the diagnosis as this can precipitate laryngospasm. This can also occur if the child becomes distressed and starts to cry, so nothing that may be frightening should be allowed.

Investigations

Maintenance of the patient's airway is the primary consideration, and all investigations should be delayed until this is secure. In the early case a lateral soft-tissue neck radiograph may confirm a swollen epiglottis but is not essential and may be dangerous. The taking of a radiograph should never be done if epiglottitis is suspected and there are already signs of respiratory difficulty. Furthermore, no child should be sent for a radiograph without the continuous presence of someone skilled in paediatric intubation.

Treatment

The first requirement of treatment is to safeguard the airway. An experienced paediatric anaesthetist and otolaryngologist should be in attendance. The child is allowed to remain in an upright posture as sudden changes in position, especially lying down, may result in airway obstruction. Intravenous access is not attempted and the child should be moved to a quiet induction area with adjacent operating facilities. A gentle inhalation induction using halothane in oxygen is preferred. The oxygen saturation is closely monitored with pulse oximetry. A parent should be present and at all times the child is talked to and reassured. When the child is asleep, the parent is shown from the room. Direct laryngoscopy should be performed to establish the diagnosis and to pass an endotracheal tube. Oedematous aryepiglottic folds and a cherry red epiglottis are characteristic signs of the disease. An appropriately sized orotracheal tube is inserted to immediately restore the airway. This should then be replaced with a nasotracheal tube as they are more readily tolerated and more securely fixed. There may be difficulty establishing an endotracheal airway, and if intubation fails a rigid bronchoscope should be inserted immediately and subsequently replaced with an endotracheal tube. Rarely a tracheostomy may be necessary.

Once an airway has been established swabs are taken from the epiglottis and a blood culture is performed. An intravenous line is inserted for fluid replacement and antibiotic therapy. The current choice of antibiotic is chloramphenicol (100 mg per kg body weight per 24 hours) as up to 30% of *Haemophilus* strains are resistant to ampicillin. A nasogastric tube should be inserted for feeding. The sedated child is transferred to a paediatric intensive care unit for rehydration, antibiotics and humidified inspired gases.

Follow-up and aftercare

There is usually a prompt response to treatment with fluid replacement and antibiotics. As the epiglottic oedema settles an increasing leak around the endotracheal tube is expected. Once the child is afebrile and appears well, extubation can be considered. This is usually possible within 48 hours. Some surgeons advocate the use of corticosteriods before decannulation to help reduce oedema caused by the tube.

Further reading

Hugosson S *et al.* Acute epiglottitis — aetiology, epidemiology and outcome in a population before large scale *Haemophilus influenzae* type b vaccination. *Clinical Otolaryngology,* 1994; **19**: 441–5.

Kessler A, Westmore RF, Marsh R. Childhood epiglottitis in recent years. *International Journal of Otolaryngology*, 1993; **25**: 155–62.

Pascucci RC. Paediatric intensive care. In: Gregory GA (ed.) *Paediatric Anaesthesia*, 2nd edn. New York: Churchill Livingstone, 1989: 1327–37.

Related topics of interest

Paediatric airway problems (p. 234)
Paediatric endoscopy (p. 239)

EPISTAXIS

Aetiology

1. *Local causes.*

- Idiopathic (85%).
- Traumatic (fractures, foreign body, nose picking).
- Inflammatory (rhinitis, sinusitis).
- Neoplastic (tumours of the nose, sinuses and nasopharynx).
- Environmental (high altitude, air conditioning).
- Endocrine (menstruation, pregnancy).
- Iatrogenic (surgery, steroid nasal sprays).

2. *General causes.*

- Anticoagulants (warfarin, aspirin).
- Diseases of the blood (haemophilia, leukaemia).
- Familial haemorrhagic telangiectasia (Osler–Rendu–Weber).
- Hypertension.
- Raised venous pressure (whooping cough, pneumonia).

Blood vessels involved

The upper parts of the nose are supplied by branches from the internal carotid artery (anterior and posterior ethmoidal arteries) and the rest from branches of the external carotid artery (greater palatine, sphenopalatine, superior labial). Little's area (Kiesselbach's plexus) is the commonest site of bleeding, which may be more to do with its comparatively exposed position in the anterior part of the septum than the fact that this is where the vessels anastamose.

Clinical assessment

Always make sure that the patient is not in shock, especially when bleeding is brisk, but the instigation of immediate resuscitation is not usually necessary. It is important that nursing support is available in this situation to assist with management of the patient. Protect the patient's clothing and your own with an apron, and wear gloves. Take a full history and on examination try to localize the area from which bleeding is arising and any specific bleeding points. If the bleeding has been significant start an intravenous infusion. Investigations should include a full blood count (FBC) (check Hb, white cell count and platelets), clotting studies and blood for group and cross-match if necessary.

Management

The aims are to arrest the haemorrhage and to treat the underlying cause. The bleeding is usually stopped by one of the following methods:

- Pressure on the nostrils (can be supplemented with ice-cold packs and sucking ice cubes).
- Local cautery (chemical or electrocoagulation).
- Anterior nasal packing (paraffin gauze, bismuth iodoform paraffin paste (BIPP)).
- Packing of the postnasal space (gauze, Foley's catheter, Brighton balloon).

Calm reassurance coupled with sedation (i.v. diazepam) will relieve the patient's anxiety. If nasal packing is required, systemic antibiotics should be given to prevent otitis media from Eustachian tube blockage, and sinusitis. Examination under general anaesthetic may become necessary if the above measures fail, to allow better identification of the bleeding site and more effective cautery and packing. Further surgery is indicated only on the rare occasion when haemorrhage is not controlled by packing and cautery, or if a severe epistaxis recurs.

1. Submucosal resection.

2. Ligation or clipping of the maxillary artery in the pterygomaxillary fossa. A Caldwell Luc incision is made, the antrum entered and a window made in the posterior wall of the sinus. The artery is encountered in the pterygopalatine fossa and teased away from the fat pad. Each tortuous branch is clipped in turn.

3. Ethmoidal artery clipping is required for uncontrollable bleeding from the upper part of the nose, above the middle turbinate. The approach to the anterior ethmoidal artery is via a medial orbital incision with lateral displacement of the upper orbital contents. The artery is surrounded by periosteum about 2.5 cm deep to the orbital rim just above the level of the medial canthus and is readily controlled by clipping.

4. External carotid artery ligation in the neck may need to be performed if maxillary artery clipping is unsuccessful.

5. Embolization of vessels under radiographic control with gel sponge or beads is advocated in some centres, but because of the risks involved (e.g. cerebrovascular embolus) has not been fully accepted.

A specific problem in the management of epistaxis (and favourite examination topic) includes hereditary haemorrhagic telangiectasia or Rendu–Osler–Weber disease. Patients with this are easily recognized by red spots on the lips and the mucous membrane of the mouth, especially the tongue, as well as telangiectases on the face and nose. The condition may be complicated by the presence of lesions in the gut, which may bleed, or arteriovenous malformations in the lungs. In addition to repeated local treatment, other therapies include oestrogens, radiotherapy, sclerosants, lining mucosa with placenta or split skin grafts and laser therapy (argon or Nd–YAG).

Follow-up and aftercare   This depends on the cause and severity of the bleeding, but all patients who have required admission and treatment in hospital should be reviewed in the outpatient department. The patient is asked if there has been any further bleeding and a check haemoglobin performed before discharge.

Further reading

Shaheen OH. Epistaxis. In: Mackay I (ed.) *Scott-Brown's Otolaryngology*, Vol. 4, 5th edn. London: Butterworths, 1987; 272–82.

Related topic of interest

Examination of the nose (p. 93)

EVOKED RESPONSE AUDIOMETRY

In response to sound stimulation, electrical signals are produced by various parts of the auditory system from cochlea to cortex. Evoked response audiometry (also called electric response audiometry) is a technique designed to measure these signals. No conscious response is requires from the patient, so the tests are less open to the bias in results which arises in those tests requiring patient cooperation. However, the tests are not truly objective as a tester will have to interpret the complex tracings obtained from the procedure. In practical terms three main responses can be recorded:

- Electrocochleogram.
- Brainstem electrical response.
- Cortical electrical response.

Electrocochleography (ECochG)

Electrocochleography aims to measure the signal produced by the cochlea and cochlear nerve in response to acoustic stimulation.

Technique The patient lies comfortably in a soundproof room. A ground electrode is attached to the patient's forehead and a reference electrode to the ipsilateral mastoid. The active electrode is usually a trans-tympanic needle placed on the promontory (canal electrodes may be used but give a less satisfactory signal) after preparation with local anaesthetic (EMLA). The test signal can be produced using a loudspeaker or headphones (especially if acoustic conditions are less than ideal). As the amplitude of the evoked electrical response is small relative to the body's background electrical noise, a variety of filters and an averaging computer are used. Wideband clicks and high-frequency tone bursts are the usual stimulating test signals.

Physiology The signal recorded by ECochG is described as a compound action potential. It is diphasic at threshold and has a signal latency which decreases with increasing signal intensity and is made up of three parts:

(a) The cochlear microphonic. This signal is produced by the hair cells and resembles the pattern of the basilar membrane vibration. It has no threshold and increases in amplitude with the stimulus intensity. Its polarity follows that of the test signal.

(b) The summating potential. This complex potential is derived from a variety of sources but in essence is an alteration of the electrical potential baseline (usually negative) in response to a sound stimulus. It is also produced by cochlear hair cells and does not adapt in response to high stimulation rates.

(c) The action potential. This is the depolarization of the cochlear nerve and is similar in many respects to any neural depolarization. It has a threshold, is independent of signal polarity and exhibits adaptation.

Clinical indications

High-resolution computerized axial tomography and magnetic resonance imaging have superseded many older otological investigative techniques and consequently removed many of the indications for ECochG, particularly the search for an acoustic neuroma. In current practice ECochG may be used for:

1. Threshold testing. ECochG is the most accurate of the electrical response audiometric techniques for threshold testing and can predict to within 5–10 dB of the psychoacoustic threshold at 3–4 kHz. Unfortunately, it gives little low-frequency information (1 kHz) but has the advantage of being a non-aural test technique and is relatively resistant to minor muscular contractions which would preclude brainstem response audiometry and is unaffected by general anaesthetic. It is therefore particularly useful in very young children or those with neurological disorders.

2. Investigation of suspected Menière's disease. Typically there is an increase in the summating potential with a normal action potential in the affected ear.

3. Intraoperative monitoring during surgery around the inner ear and internal meatus.

Brainstem electrical response audiometry

Brainstem electrical response audiometry (BERA) records the signals produced in the brain stem detected by electrodes placed over the mastoid, forehead and vertex.

Technique

The patient reclines on a bed or couch. The electrodes are surface electrodes. The active electrode is attached to the vertex, the reference electrode to the ipsilateral (test ear) mastoid process and the ground electrode to the contralateral mastoid process. The hardware and test signals used (wideband clicks and high-frequency tone bursts) are identical to those used for ECochG, but the filter and time window settings are altered. The signals are usually presented using headphones to allow monaural testing. As the evoked responses are so small they are easily masked by other neuromuscular signals. It is therefore important that the patient stays as still as possible and, because of their size, several thousand responses are analysed as opposed to hundreds in ECochG. The results are analysed by looking at the absolute values for various wave latencies, the so-called I–V latency, and comparing results between the two ears. The accuracy of the I–V latency has been improved by combining ECochG with BERA to aid the detection of wave I.

Physiology

The signal recorded by BERA is made up of a five-wave complex, which is thought to represent successive synapses in the auditory pathway as follows (Jewett classification):

Wave site of generation latency (msec)
I   Cochlear nerve 2.0
II   Cochlear nucleus 3.0
III Superior olive 4.7
IV   Lateral lemniscus 5.3
V   Inferior colliculus 5.9

These potentials are very small and rarely reach more than 1 μV (potentials of 10 mV may be obtained in electrocochleography).

Clinical indications

1. Acoustic neuroma. One of the main indications for BERA is in excluding an acoustic neuroma (or other brainstem tumour) in patients with asymmetrical hearing loss. In this case the I–V interval in the affected ear should be prolonged by more than 0.4 msec when compared with the normal ear. However, useful results are virtually impossible if the affected ear has very poor thresholds (>70 dB), and gadolinium-enhanced MRI is a more sensitive and specific test for this condition.

2. Threshold testing. This is particularly useful in children as it is non-invasive and not influenced by anaesthetic, but it is not frequency specific.

3. Brainstem lesions. BERA can be used to define the site of a brainstem lesion depending on the presence or absence of successive waves. Unusual results may indicate multiple sclerosis.

4. Intraoperative testing. The technique may be used as a monitor during tumour surgery designed to preserve hearing.

Cortical electrical response audiometry

The cortical ERA (vertex or V potential) is a relatively late phenomenon and can be detected as a bi- or triphasic wave commencing after 50 msec and continuing beyond 200 msec. It is too late to be considered a primary cortical response and almost certainly represents a secondary, perceptual cortical phenomenon; as such its presence can be associated with clinical hearing. Unfortunately, it is strongly influenced by the patient's conscious level and attendance to the stimulus and so is only of value in the cooperative patient. If feasible it offers excellent frequency specificity.

Technique

The patient sits comfortably in a chair, staying both still and awake, as movement and consciousness level can easily influence the response. Surface electrodes are placed with active on the vertex, reference on either mastoid process and ground on the forehead. Tone bursts are the preferred test stimuli and are presented by headphones. Fewer than 100 responses need be sampled to achieve a useful result. Threshold is taken as the point at which the V-potential disappears.

Clinical indications

1. Threshold testing. In medicolegal cases this is restricted to 1, 2 and 3 kHz; any more would be too time-consuming.

2. Central deafness. In rare patients ECochG and BERA are normal but the V-potential is absent.

Further reading

Ballantyne D. *Handbook of Audiological Techniques*. London: Butterworth-Heinemann, 1990.
Beagley HA. Electrophysiological tests of hearing. In: Beagley HA (ed.) *Audiology and Audiological Medicine*, Vol. 2. Oxford: Oxford University Press, 1981.
Beagley HA. Fisch L. Bio-electrical potentials available for electric response audiometry: indications and contra-indications. In: Beagley HA (ed.) *Audiology and Audiological Medicine*, Vol. 2. Oxford: Oxford University Press, 1981.

Related topics of interest

EXAMINATION OF THE EAR

There is absolutely no doubt that you will be asked to assess an ear at some point during the course of any ENT examination. Time taken in practising your technique is therefore well spent. It is not just a question of spotting the particular clinical signs or disease process. The examiner will want to establish that you have an orderly and thorough technique, and that you are able to present your findings accurately and clearly. You will be asked how you would manage the patient, so be thinking about this as you present your examination findings.

Introduce yourself to the patient before starting the examination. Ask which is the better hearing ear. Always begin the examination with the better ear and never touch the patient before asking if there is any tenderness. Position the patient to one side of an electric lamp with the light source slightly above the level of the ear. The patient should be seated sideways to the surgeon, who sits opposite the ear to be examined and reflects light on to it.

The pinna

Examine the pinna in front and behind for signs of inflammation or skin lesions. The mastoid process should be carefully examined for scars, redness or tenderness. Be particularly careful not to miss a fading postauricular or endaural scar. Note any discharge from the external auditory meatus as well as any inflammation of the skin. Select a suitably sized speculum for insertion into the external canal. Common examination subjects include congenital lesions of the pinna, cauliflower ears, perichondritis and surgical scars.

The external auditory canal

To examine the external auditory canal, pull the pinna upwards, outwards and backwards. In infants, owing to non-development of the bony external meatus, the pinna has to be drawn downwards and backwards. Introduce the otoscope speculum just past the hairs of the outer canal, but avoid contact with the sensitive bony part of the canal. A good view of the tympanic membrane should then be possible. Common examination subjects include canal stenosis and exostoses.

The tympanic membrane

Look for the prominent lateral process and handle of the malleus. Examine all quadrants of the membrane. The long process of the incus is frequently observed behind and parallel to the handle of the malleus and it is sometimes possible to see it articulate with the head of the stapes.

If there is a perforation note its position, size and whether it is central or marginal. If you do discover a perforation then make sure you can describe what you see looking through it, for example the promontory, round window, incudostapedial joint, dehiscent Fallopian canal or some tympanosclerosis may be visible. A Siegle speculum or otoscope with a pneumatic attachment should be used to assess the mobility of the membrane. Immobility may be due to fluid in the middle ear, a perforation or tympanosclerosis. If the patient has had mastoid surgery determine the type of cavity, assess access (meatoplasty size and height of the facial ridge) and decide if the cavity is healthy or not. Perform a fistula test by applying pressure or with the pneumatic otoscope and look for nystagmus in the direction of the diseased side. Remember to tell the patient what you are doing beforehand.

Hearing tests

Perform free field speech tests by asking the patient to repeat words spoken with a whispered voice, conversation voice and shouted voice at 60 cm from the ear. The non-test ear is masked either by using a Bàràny noise box or by pressing the tragus backwards and rotating it with the index finger. The patient sits side on to the surgeon so that lip reading is not possible.

Use double figure numbers or bisyllable words as the words the patient is asked to repeat should not be easy to guess. The Rinne and Weber tuning fork tests, using a 512 kHz fork, should then be performed to help differentiate between a conductive and sensorineural hearing loss.

Other tests

The postnasal space should be examined to exclude a lesion and if possible to obtain a view of the Eustachian tube orifice. The cranial nerves should be formally examined if there is active ear disease. In a short case examiners will sometimes stipulate that they are only interested in facial nerve function, and this should always be routinely tested in examination of the ear.

Summary of examination of the ear

(a) Introduce yourself to the patient.
(b) Position the patient.
(c) Ascertain which is the better ear and start with this.
(d) Inspect the pinna, mastoid and external auditory meatus.
(e) Pneumatic otoscopic examination of the tympanic membrane.
(f) Fistula test.
(g) Free field voice tests.
(h) Tuning fork tests.
(i) Facial nerve.
(j) Postnasal space.

Further reading

Dale BA, Verr AI. Investigations of ear disease. In: Manan AGD (ed). *Logan Turner's Diseases of the Nose, Throat and Ear,* 10th edn. London: Wright, 1988; 237–45.

Related topics of interest

Clinical assessment of hearing (p. 58)
Examination of the nose (p. 93)
Examination of the throat (p. 96)

EXAMINATION OF THE NOSE

The diagnosis in nasal disease is often obvious after an accurate history has been taken. The essential symptoms are nasal obstruction, sneezing, rhinorrhoea, postnasal drip, headache and facial pains, abnormal sense of smell, epistaxis, snoring and cosmetic deformity. A previous medical history of trauma or allergy may also be relevant. Nasal disease is common, signs can be elicited quickly and management of the common diseases makes good discussion. Common findings are septal deviation, hypertrophied turbinates, septal perforation and nasal polyps. It is therefore essential that you are familiar with the aetiology, relevant investigations and treatments of these conditions. There may be a combination of signs (for example, a deviated septum and nasal polyps) so be thorough with your examination.

Position of the patient

Introduce yourself to the patient and sit opposite with an electric lamp at eye level over the patient's left shoulder. Sit with your knees together and to the right side of the patient's legs. This is more elegant than sitting with your legs astride the patient's.

Inspection of the external nose

Examine the nose in relation to the rest of the patient's face. Pay particular attention to its size and shape: the convexity or concavity of the dorsum, the width or projection of the tip, the deviation of the nose, the shape of the columella and nares. The thickness of the skin may be relevant if cosmetic surgery is contemplated. Look for swelling, bruising, erythema or for ulceration of the skin. An old examination favourite is a patient with the lupus pernio rash of sarcoid on their nose, with a septal perforation. Turn the patient's head to the left and then to the right to check the profile. Be especially vigilant to look for a fading lateral rhinotomy scar or hidden bicoronal incision wound behind the hairline. Lift the tip of the nose with the thumb to obtain a view of the nasal vestibules. The patency of the nasal airway is assessed by occluding each nostril in turn with the tip of the thumb and asking the patient to sniff or alternatively watching the shiny surface of a Lack tongue depressor held under the nose cloud over as the patient exhales.

The nasal cavity

Anterior rhinoscopy is carried out using a Thudichum speculum. Gently introduce this into the nose remembering that the nasal mucosa is very sensitive. If a lesion is immediately obvious, for example nasal polyps or a nasal tumour, note the position in relation to the turbinates and septum. Do not assume that they will be the only abnormality, be thorough in the rest of your examination.

Assess the mucosa; note its colour, vascularity and crusting. Examine the septum for its position in relation to the nasal airways; is it deviated to one side or is it dislocated off the maxillary crest? Examine the mucoperichondrium for its colour and vascularity. Note any lesions or perforation of the septum. Examine the lateral nasal wall and evaluate the size and colour of the inferior turbinate. If a better view is needed the nasal mucosa can be shrunk using 5 or 10% cocaine hydrochloride with 1:1000 adrenaline. In clinical practice a 0° nasendoscope can be used to inspect the lateral nasal wall and the anatomy and any pathology of the middle meatus.

Oral examination

Inspect and percuss the upper teeth. The floor of the maxillary sinus lies over the alveolar process of the maxilla and the roots of the second premolar and first molar teeth. Assess movement of the soft palate and if there is a bifid uvula be aware that this may signify a submucous cleft.

The nasopharynx

Explain to the patient what you are about to do. This is a difficult procedure and needs practice. Warm a small postnasal mirror and pass it through the mouth while gently holding the tongue down with a tongue depressor. Some patients have too strong a gag reflex to allow adequate examination. Report the problem to the examiner and suggest that in normal circumstances you would proceed to use a flexible fibreoptic nasendoscopy after applying topical cocaine to the nasal airway. Inspect the posterior end of the septum, the posterior choanae, through which the posterior ends of the inferior turbinates may be visible. In the lateral wall the tubal ridges of the pharyngeal ends of the Eustachian tubes can be seen. The fossae of Rosenmüller lie immediately above the tubal orifices and can be the site of a nasopharyngeal carcinoma.

The neck

Inspect and palpate the neck and look for the presence of lymphadenopathy. The lymphatic drainage from the anterior part of the nose is to the submandibular nodes and upper deep cervical nodes. Drainage from the posterior part is to the middle deep cervical nodes.

Summary of examination of the nose

(a) Introduce yourself.
(b) Position the patient.
(c) Inspect the external nose.
(d) Examine the nasal tip and vestibule and assess the nasal airways.
(e) Anterior rhinoscopy with a Thudichum speculum.

(f) Oral examination.
(g) Postnasal space examination.
(h) Neck.

Further reading

Murray JA. Investigation of nasal disease. In: Maran AGD (ed.) *Logan Turner's Diseases of the Nose, Throat, and Ear,* 10th edn. London: Wright, 1988; 13–20.

Related topics of interest

Examination of the ear (p. 90)
Examination of the throat (p. 96)
Nasal polyps (p. 172)
Nasopharyngeal tumours (p. 179)

EXAMINATION OF THE THROAT

The symptoms associated with throat disease include hoarseness, dysphagia, sore throat, lump in the throat, referred otalgia, cough, lump in the neck and weight loss. Throat is a vague term, unfortunately applied indifferently by some examiners to the pharynx and larynx. The technique outlined in this topic is ideal for a long case but may need to be modified for a short case. Listen carefully to the examiner and do what is asked. Unless clearly stipulated, do not assume that the examiner merely wants an indirect laryngoscopy performed. On the other hand, do not irritate the examiner by examining parts of the patient that have not been mentioned. However, if in doubt it is better to be thorough. There are a few scenarios.

Examine the patient's throat: systematically examine the patient's pharynx and larynx as you would any patient in clinic who complained of the aforementioned symptoms.

Examine the mouth: inspect and examine the oral cavity.

Examine this patient's neck: inspect and palpate the neck.

Common findings are patients with vocal cord paralysis, vocal cord oedema, vocal cord polyps, vocal cord nodules, laryngeal papillomas, occasionally patients with a neoplasm and laryngectomy patients.

Position the patient

The patient should sit opposite the surgeon with an electric lamp positioned at eye level over the left shoulder. The surgeon should sit with knees together and legs to the right side of the patient's. Ask edentulous patients to remove their dentures. Expose the whole of the neck up to and including the clavicles. Remove any neck scarf which may hide a wound or stoma.

The oral cavity

Inspect the lips for perioral lesions. Ask the patient if there is any tenderness in the mouth. Take two metal tongue depressors and insert them to retract the buccal mucosa on each side. Ask the patient to protrude the tongue and move it from side to side and then up to the palate and down. This should allow an inspection of the dorsal and ventral surfaces of the tongue, the tongue's lateral borders and the floor of the mouth; it also tests hypoglossal nerve function. The two tongue depressors are then used so that the buccal mucosa, teeth and alveolar ridges and the opening of the parotid ducts (opposite the upper second molar) can be examined. Then dispense with one of the tongue depressors and use the other to depress the tongue. Check over the palate, the tonsils and the posterior pharyngeal wall. Ask the patient to say 'aah' and check movement of the palate. Remove the tongue depressor and put a glove on. Bimanually palpate the floor of the mouth overlying the submandibular duct for calculi or masses. Palpate the base of tongue, as a tumour in this site may not be visible but easily palpable.

Postnasal space examination	Explain to the patient what you are about to do. Warm a postnasal mirror and pass it through the mouth while gently holding the tongue down with a tongue depressor. Ask the patient to breath gently through the nose. Look for any obvious lesion, but be particularly vigilant on inspection of the laterally placed Eustachian tube elevations, above which lie the fossae of Rosenmüller, the usual site of origin of nasopharyngeal carcinoma.
Indirect laryngoscopy	Explain to the patient what you are about to do. Warm a laryngeal mirror and check its temperature on the back of your hand. Ask the patient to protrude the tongue and gently grasp it with a swab held in the left hand. The patient should then be requested to breathe normally through the mouth as the mirror is introduced gently up to the soft palate. If the patient nose breathes and arches up the tongue, obstructing the view, it is possible to obtain some improvement by asking the patient to quietly make a 'hah' noise breathing in and out. Inspect the base of the tongue, the vallecula and the upper part of the epiglottis. Examine the posterior pharyngeal wall, and then both sides of the epiglottis, the aryepiglottic folds, the pyriform fossae, the arytenoids, the ventricular folds and the vocal cords. Note any inflammation, ulceration or exophytic lesion. The movements of the vocal cords are studied by asking the patient to say 'ee' followed by a deep breath and 'ee' again. Note any abnormal movement or fixation of the cords.

Some patients are unable to cope with an indirect laryngoscopy because of an overactive gag reflex. In these cases it may be possible after spraying the oropharynx with lignocaine. After a few minutes the soft palate and uvula will be anaesthetized. If the patient is still unable to tolerate the procedure spray the nose with 5–10% cocaine and use a nasendoscope. This is usually well tolerated and allows a more thorough inspection and assessment of vocal cord movement. Be sure to tell the patient to avoid food and drink for the next hour because the gag reflex is impaired. Nothing hot should be consumed for at least 2 hours, to avoid burning the throat and aspiration. Some patients still need to be assessed under a general anaesthetic. It is unlikely in an examination that the patient will have an overactive gag reflex as patients are specially selected.

Examination of the neck Check the neck for any obvious skin lesion or ulceration. Be careful not to overlook a fading wound. Check that the patient does not have a stoma. Ask the patient to swallow and watch the larynx move. A thyroid goitre may also be seen moving with the larynx. An enlarged neck mass may be visible: note its position and inform the examiner that you have seen it. Ask the patient to count to 10 and assess the voice. Get the patient to breathe deeply in and out through the mouth and note any stridor.

The neck should be palpated from behind and in an orderly sequence so that no areas are missed. Be gentle. Ask the patient if there is any tenderness. Start at the mastoid bone and palpate down the line of the trapezius muscle and in the posterior triangle down to the clavicle. Feel for supraclavicular and infraclavicular nodes. Then palpate down the line deep to the anterior border of the sternocleidomastoid muscle for deep cervical nodes. When your fingers reach the suprasternal notch, palpate up the anterior triangle, feeling the trachea, thyroid gland, laryngeal cartilages and hyoid bone. Loss of normal laryngeal crepitus (trotters sign) may indicate a postcricoid neoplasm. Feel for submental lymph nodes, submandibular nodes, the parotid gland, preauricular nodes and finally occipital nodes. If a lump is felt note its site, size, shape, consistency and fixation to adjacent tissues or skin. If you think a lump is pulsatile or attached to the carotid, auscultate and listen for a bruit. If a lump is palpated in the anterior triangle see whether it moves on swallowing. If you think a lump is cystic see if it transilluminates.

Summary of examination of the throat

(a) Introduce yourself to the patient.
(b) Position the patient and expose the neck down to the clavicles.
(c) Assess speech.
(d) Oral examination (oral cavity and oropharynx).
(e) Nasopharynx.
(f) Indirect laryngoscopy.
(g) Examination of the neck.

Further reading

Maran AGD. Investigation of laryngeal disease. In: Maran AGD (ed.) *Logan Turner's Diseases of the Nose, Throat and Ear,* 10th edn. London: Wright, 1988; 150–4.

Related topics of interest

EXTERNAL EAR CONDITIONS

Ear wax

Epithelial migration

In all other parts of the body, the superficial keratinized squamous epithelium is constantly shed, usually as a result of friction from clothing or washing. This is not possible in the external ear canal and so it has developed the property of epithelial migration. Squamous epithelium on the tympanic membrane moves radially until it reaches the canal walls, when it moves laterally. When it reaches the hair-bearing cartilaginous portion of the canal the superficial layer starts to separate. It then mixes with the secretion of the ceruminous and pilosebaceous glands and any collected debris to form what we recognize as ear wax. The glands are found in the skin of the outer third of the external acoustic meatus and secrete a liquid material at the base of the hairs. After secretion, evaporation occurs to leave a sticky, waxy substance that is able to trap dirt, squames and microbes with relative ease.

Wax

Wax can be secreted in one of two forms. Wet wax is produced by most Negroes and Caucasians and is familiar as moist, sticky and honey-coloured. The dry type is more common in mongoloid races and tends to be greyer in colour, less sticky, granular and brittle. The gene for wet wax is dominant. Regardless of type, ear wax tends to become drier with age as a result of reduced glandular numbers and activity. Wax is then normally loosened by transmission of movement from the temporomandibular joint from chewing or talking, allowing its passage out of the external auditory meatus. This natural process can be upset by a number of factors and cause wax impaction. Impaction is commoner in males owing to the presence of thicker, coarser hairs in the lateral part of the EAM. Narrow canals, zealous use of cotton buds and even a hearing aid mould may impede the normal flow of wax to the periphery. In some people no obvious cause is found to account for the impaction and it has been suggested that desquamation of the superficial layer of the meatal epidermis is impaired.

Clinical features

Impaction of wax can cause a sensation of obstruction, deafness, otalgia, vertigo and coughing (via the auricular branch of the vagus – Arnolds nerve), although wax impaction is a relatively rare cause of hearing loss. Most of these symptoms are improved by removing the wax, which can usually be accomplished easily by syringing.

Management

Syringing involves the use of a Higginson syringe to direct a jet of warm (body temperature) water along the roof or posterior canal wall so that it passes behind the wax and forces it outwards. Although relatively safe, complications may occur and include coughing, pain, local trauma, otitis externa and rarely tympanic membrane perforation and otitis media. Contraindications to syringing include frequent previous episodes of otitis externa, a known or suspected perforation and a difficult ear, often caused by a narrow and/or tortuous external meatus. In these cases removal under direct vision with an operating microscope using microsuction or wax-hooks is a more appropriate and safer alternative.

Keratosis obturans

This uncommon condition occurs when there is a failure of the normal process of migration. Keratinocytes and keratin debris collect in the deep part of the external auditory meatus. As with collections of keratin anywhere, this sets up a low-grade inflammatory response. Osteoclast-stimulating mediators are produced, resulting in a resorption of bone and usually a widening of the bony canal.

Clinical features

Patients usually present with an acute exacerbation of the inflammatory process. Otalgia is usually the dominant feature, although there is inevitably a conductive hearing loss from the occluded canal. The otoscopic appearances are similar to an acute otitis externa around impacted wax. The keratin takes this appearance because the part in contact with the air oxidizes and changes colour.

Management

Removal of the keratin plug is essential to control the inflammatory process. This is often difficult as the patient is usually in considerable pain and a general anaesthetic is not infrequently required. Topical antibiotic/steroid combinations are advised to prevent a secondary otitis externa. In the long term these patients require periodic monitoring and aural toilet.

Exostoses and osteomas

Osteomas are uncommon benign tumours of bone usually arising from the tympanosquamous or tympanomastoid suture line. Exostoses, on the other hand, are common. They are hyperostoses of the tympanic bone of the external canal. They appear to be caused by a periosteal reaction to exposure to cold, usually from swimming. In both conditions, although the lumen of the canal may be reduced, they rarely result in symptoms. If problems do occur they are usually related to impairment of the normal process of epithelial migration. In these cases surgical removal may be indicated. Osteomas can often be removed via the external canal, while exostoses will more often require a formal postaural or endaural approach.

Further reading

Hanger HC, Mulley GP. Cerumen: its fascination and clinical importance: a review. *Journal of the Royal Society of Medicine*, 1992; **85:** 346–9.
Sheehy JL. Diffuse exostoses and osteomata of the external auditory canal: a report of 100 operations. *Otolaryngology – Head and Neck Surgery*, 1982; **90:** 337–42.

Related topic of interest

Examination of the ear (p. 90)
Foreign bodies (p. 113)
Otitis externa (p. 210)

FACIAL NERVE PALSY

Although the detailed anatomy of the facial nerve will not be discussed, it is important to appreciate that there are supranuclear or upper motor neurone (motor cortex to pontine facial nuclei) and infranuclear or lower motor neurone causes of a facial nerve palsy. The infranuclear portion can be divided into cerebellopontine angle, meatal, labyrinthine, tympanic, mastoid and extracranial portions.

Communication with the vestibulocochlear nerve occurs within the internal auditory meatus, with the otic ganglion and sympathetic afferents from geniculate ganglion branches and with the auricular branch of the vagus nerve from a branch of the mastoid segment of the facial nerve. Extracranially there are communications with the glossopharyngeal, vagus, great auricular and the auriculotemporal nerves and multiple communications with branches of the trigeminal nerve. These interconnections explain the mastoid, ear, face and neck pain associated with herpes zoster and Bell's palsy, and the referred otalgia, face, occipital, throat and neck pain which may occur with malignant disease.

Injury may be classified into a neuropraxia, axonotmesis, neurotmesis, partial transection and complete transection. Evoked electromyography and maximal stimulation test response neurophysiological studies show that a neuropraxia injury gives normal results and an axonotmesis up to 10% of normal, but more severe injury gives no response. These studies can be used to provide a prognosis and to indicate if recovery is occurring.

Associated features

Altered facial nerve function occurs with a variety of conditions.

1. Synkinesis. The voluntary and reflex movement of groups of muscles that normally do not contract together, for example blinking, may be accompanied by movement of the corner of the mouth. This may occur after neurotmesis (or more severe injury) when the axons do not find their correct endoneurial sheath.

2. Hemifacial spasm. This is an intermittent spasm of the orbicularis oculi muscle which may spread to include other or all muscles of facial expression. It is thought to be usually caused by compression of the nerve by an artery in the posterior fossa, and if this is confirmed by an MRI scan and angiography the cause may be treated surgically. Cerebellopontine angle tumours may also cause this phenomenon.

3. Facial myokymia. In this condition there are multiple fine but asynchronous facial movements. It is associated with brain stem gliomas and multiple sclerosis.

4. Blepharospasm. This is unilateral or more commonly bilateral involuntary spasmodic eye closure. Injection of botulinum A toxin into the orbicularis oculi may provide temporary relief.

5. Crocodile tears. Lacrimation with eating can occur as a result of facial nerve injury in the region of the geniculate ganglion, where motor axons find the myelin sheath within the greater petrosal nerve.

Grading of palsy

The most commonly used system is that of House and Brackmann: grade 1, complete recovery without evidence of faulty regeneration; grade 2, mild weakness with minimal evidence of faulty regeneration; grade 3, obvious incomplete recovery with moderate faulty regeneration; grade 4, facial palsy and faulty regeneration both severe; grade 5, barely perceptible facial movement; grade 6, complete facial palsy.

Causes

1. Bell's palsy (55%). An acute lower motor neurone facial palsy of unknown aetiology and therefore a diagnosis of exclusion. It is probably a virally induced immune response that leads to inflammation, swelling and consequent impaired function of the facial nerve.

2. Ramsay Hunt syndrome (synonym: herpes zoster oticus) (7%). Caused by herpes zoster virus.

3. Trauma (19%). This may be external or iatrogenic.

4. Tumour (6%). These may arise from the nerve (facial nerve schwannoma), external compression of the nerve (vestibular nerve schwannoma), or invasion of the nerve (parotid adenoid cystic or mucoepidermoid carcinoma).

5. Infection (4%). A lower motor neurone facial palsy may occur with acute suppurative otitis media (in the 8% who have a dehiscent Fallopian canal), chronic suppurative otitis media either with or without cholesteatoma and malignant otitis externa.

6. Central causes, for example secondary to multiple sclerosis, gliomas or cerebrovascular accidents.

7. Other causes, for example sarcoid, drugs and Guillain–Barré syndrome.

Clinical features	In Bell's palsy the facial nerve palsy is usually of rapid onset and associated with otalgia, altered facial sensation and taste. It recurs in 12%, more commonly on the contralateral side. Severe otalgia with vesicles involving the external ear associated with crusting, external ear canal oedema, a sensorineural hearing loss, tinnitus and vertigo are all common in Ramsay Hunt syndrome. The communications of the facial nerve may allow the face, neck tongue, palate and buccal mucosa to become involved. It rarely recurs, but only 60% recover to House and Brackmann grade 1 or 2. When trauma has caused the palsy, it is important to know the severity of a palsy as soon as possible after nerve injury as this will influence the management. Facial nerve palsies caused by tumours and infection are discussed elsewhere (see Related topics of interest).

Clinical features

In Bell's palsy the facial nerve palsy is usually of rapid onset and associated with otalgia, altered facial sensation and taste. It recurs in 12%, more commonly on the contralateral side. Severe otalgia with vesicles involving the external ear associated with crusting, external ear canal oedema, a sensorineural hearing loss, tinnitus and vertigo are all common in Ramsay Hunt syndrome. The communications of the facial nerve may allow the face, neck tongue, palate and buccal mucosa to become involved. It rarely recurs, but only 60% recover to House and Brackmann grade 1 or 2. When trauma has caused the palsy, it is important to know the severity of a palsy as soon as possible after nerve injury as this will influence the management. Facial nerve palsies caused by tumours and infection are discussed elsewhere (see Related topics of interest).

Investigations

A high-resolution CT scan of the petrous temporal bone will exclude cerebellopontine angle tumours as a source of the palsy, necessary in suspected Bell's palsy as this is a diagnosis of exclusion. It may localize injury in cases due to trauma or chronic suppurative otitis media. An evoked electromyogram (EEMG), in which a stimulating electrode is placed adjacent to the stylomastoid foramen and recording electrodes are placed either on the skin over the facial muscles or through the skin into the muscles, is helpful. If the EEMG response remains above 10% of normal during the first 10 days after injury there is an excellent chance of grade 1 or 2 recovery (85%). The prognosis overall for those below this level is only a 20% chance of achieving grade 1 or 2 recovery, and many surgeons therefore now advocate surgical decompression of the nerve in these circumstances.

Management

1. *General.* Reassurance and explanation are essential for all patients. Eye care is mandatory in order to prevent corneal ulceration and comprises artificial tears, eye closure with tape on to which is applied a light pressure dressing of cotton wool, ointment at night and eye protection when outdoors on windy or hot dry days with an eye pad. In patients with marked symptoms a lateral tarsorrhaphy or the insertion of a gold weight into the upper eyelid may be necessary as a permanent or temporary manoeuvre to ensure adequate eye closure.

2. *Specific.*
(a) *Bell's palsy.* Although no placebo-controlled double-blind trial has been reported, many practitioners advocate

a short course of steroids provided there are no contraindications in the patient's medical history. Fisch advocates early decompression of the meatal portion of the facial nerve by a middle fossa approach, as this is the portion most often implicated as being affected in Bell's palsy.

(b) *Ramsay Hunt syndrome*. The commencement of acyclovir 800 mg five times daily for 7 days as early as possible during an attack may reduce the length of the infection and postherpetic neuralgia. Adequate analgesia is essential, and splinting the external ear canal with a pope wick expanded with antibiotic/steroid drops will reduce the otalgia.

(c) *Trauma*. If a complete lower motor neurone facial palsy is noted immediately after external trauma, this suggests that the nerve has been severed, and immediate exploration is indicated. It is preferable to anastomose the proximal to the distal stump after each has been prepared to present a clean surface. This must be performed without tension on the nerve, and should this not be possible after preparation of the stumps, perhaps because significant debridement was necessary or the injury involved a significant length of nerve, then a cable of sural or great auricular nerve is necessary. A partial palsy or a delayed onset of a palsy can be managed conservatively with sequential EEMG monitoring.

(d) *Tumour*. The facial nerve is usually sacrificed if it has been infiltrated by tumour which cannot therefore be teased off the nerve. A cable graft is indicated in these circumstances.

(e) *Infection*. The management in these circumstances is discussed elsewhere (see Related topics of interest). In summary, a palsy secondary to ASOM should be treated conservatively but that secondary to CSOM requires mastoid exploration to eradicate the underlying disease, although formal decompression of the nerve is probably unnecessary.

If no recovery of function has occurred within a year of injury in those with a severe or complete palsy (grade 5 or 6) a permanent facial reanimation procedure, e.g temporalis muscle sling or a gold weight for the upper eyelid, may be indicated.

Follow-up and aftercare

Adequate counselling regarding eye care is essential. Maximum recovery may take 12 months so that no decision regarding permanent facial reanimation procedures should be undertaken until then.

Further reading

Bradford CR. Facial reanimation. *Current Opinion in Otolaryngology and Head and Neck Surgery,* 1994; **4**: 369–74.

House JW, Brackman DE. Facial nerve grading system. *Otolaryngology and Head and Neck Surgery,* 1985; **93**: 146–7.

Related topics of interest

Acute suppurative otitis media (p. 9)
Chronic suppurative otitis media (p. 51)
Cosmetic surgery (p. 70)

FACIAL PAIN

The head and neck is an anatomically and neurologically complex region, and it is not surprising that pain arising there is often misunderstood, misdiagnosed and mistreated. In up to 50% of cases of facial pain no diagnosis is ever made, and the plethora of treatment options pays tribute to this statistic. For successful management it is essential to spend time with the patient. An accurate pain history is notoriously difficult to elicit. It is important to persuade the patient to use words that define the quality of the pain (e.g. burning, throbbing, stabbing) rather than its intensity (e.g. sore, agonizing, excruciating).

Classification

1. Primary neuralgias. Trigeminal, glossopharyngeal.

2. Secondary neuralgias. Resulting from intracranial, skull base or neck disease, including the cervical spine.

3. Vascular. Migraine and cluster headaches.

4. Musculoskeletal. Myofascial headache.

5. Referred pain. Otalgia from oral cavity, pharyngeal, laryngeal and skull base disease. Frontal and ethmoidal sinusitis may refer pain to the eye.

6. Local causes. From dental (e.g. root abscess, caries, fractures and neoplasms) paranasal sinus, temporomandibular joint, ear and eye (e.g. anterior uveitis, glaucoma) disease.

Primary neuralgias

The main sensory nerve to the head is the trigeminal nerve. Unsurprisingly, it is involved in most neurological head pain syndromes.

Trigeminal neuralgia (TGN) is an agonizingly painful condition, usually affecting people over 50. Before the 1950s, when effective remedies became available, it was associated with a high incidence of suicide. Diagnosis must contain three elements:

(a) Pain is within one or more divisions of the trigeminal nerve.

(b) Pain is described as a brief electric shock or knife-like sensation.

(c) Pain is elicited by normally innocuous stimulation of a trigger zone.

The maxillary division is most commonly affected, followed by mandibular and ophthalmic divisions. Acute stabs of pain usually last for a few minutes, subsiding to a dull ache before the next attack is triggered. Absence of a trigger zone generally excludes the diagnosis. Carbamazepine in the lowest effective dose is the first-line treatment (this pain is rarely sensitive to conventional analgesics, including morphine). If side-effects are troublesome, other antiepileptics such as sodium valproate or phenytoin may be tried. When drug therapy fails, destructive lesions to the Gasserian ganglion with alcohol injection or radiofrequency diathermy are usually effective, although the patient must be warned that symptom relief will be accompanied by sensory loss to the affected part of the face. Pain will probably return after 1–5 years and the treatment will need to be repeated. Magnetic resonance imaging is now of sufficiently high resolution to demonstrate in many cases an arterial loop compressing the trigeminal nerve root. It may also help to exclude other causes of these symptoms such as multiple sclerosis, base of skull tumours, acoustic neuroma and vascular anomalies such as aneurysms and vertebrobasilar atherosclerosis. Separation of this loop from the nerve with a small piece of foam usually results in symptomatic relief. However, posterior fossa surgery carries a significant morbidity, especially in the elderly, and less invasive treatments are the rule. Although much rarer, other cranial nerves may give rise to neuralgia whose manifestation is identical to TGN. The glossopharyngeal nerve is the most likely to be affected; pain is usually triggered by swallowing. This may be associated with a long styloid process, thought by some to be a source of irritation to the nerve. If drug therapy is ineffective, surgery should be considered, as malnutrition due to inability to swallow is a distinct possibility. Excision of the styloid process or a neurosurgical approach to divide the nerve as it emerges from the brain stem are the options.

Secondary neuralgias

That secondary to herpes zoster is the commonest.

1. Acute herpes zoster. Most people acquire varicella zoster virus during childhood. It is thought that the virus lies dormant in the dorsal root ganglia for many years and may opportunistically reactivate, causing an antidromic infection along a somatic nerve. Infection is commoner in the aged and the immunocompromised. It presents with pain, dysaesthesia or paraesthesia along the course of the affected nerve, followed a few days later by cutaneous vesicular eruptions. These form scabs within a week or so and heal within a month, though this may take longer in the immunocompromised. For reasons which are not understood the ophthalmic division of the trigeminal nerve and the fourth to the tenth thoracic nerves are more commonly affected than others. Treatment of acute zoster consists of pain relief and in speeding resolution of skin lesions. Analgesics and acyclovir should be given systemically. Pain in ophthalmic zoster is relieved by stellate ganglion block with local anaesthetic, although such relief is limited to its duration of action. To date there is little evidence that aggressive therapy reduces the incidence of postherpetic neuralgia, although early treatment with amitriptyline has been anecdotally claimed to reduce its severity. Constitutional upset frequently accompanies acute zoster and it may take weeks or even months for an elderly patient to recover fully.

2. Postherpetic neuralgia (PHN). Diagnosis of PHN is rarely difficult, but treatment often defies the efforts of the most determined physician. A recent history of herpes zoster infection is followed by the development of pain in the affected area. This pain is usually burning, but occasionally throbbing or stabbing. There is usually an accompanying sensory deficit and allodynia (pain caused by a normally innocuous stimulus) to light touch is often a feature. It is thought that this feature is caused by loss of the modulating effect of large-diameter sensory nerves (proprioception) at the dorsal root entry zone (i.e. the pain gate is held wide open) following viral damage during the acute infection. The ability of nerve fibres to repair themselves diminishes with age, which may account for the increased incidence of PHN with age. Treatment of burning pain and dysaesthesia is best achieved with tricyclic antidepressants such as amitriptyline in the lowest effective dose, since the incidence of dose-related side-effects is high in the elderly. The mechanism of action of these drugs is unknown, although they undoubtedly influence neurotransmitter systems high in the CNS. Antiepileptics such as carbamazepine and valproate may help lancinating pain, and techniques such as transcutaneous electrical nerve stimulation (TENS) and acupuncture may also be of value. Recently available is a topical preparation of capsaicin, a neurotoxin with some specificity for pain fibres which is extracted from chilli peppers. It is most effective in treating burning pain.

Vascular

1. Migraine. The prevalence of migraine headache in the general population is said to be 5–10%. Onset of symptoms is usually between puberty and the fifth decade. It is commoner in women and there is often a family history. Only about 10% of migraine headaches exhibit the classical signs of aura (most commonly a visual phenomenon, but may take the form of dysaesthesia in the ipsilateral limb or face and as a mood change) which precedes the headache by 10–60 minutes. The characteristic feature of migraine is its throbbing nature, which is usually unilateral in onset, but which may spread to involve the whole head and face and is accompanied by photo- and phonophobia and nausea. It lasts for 4–72 hours and the sufferer is free of pain between attacks. Precipitating factors include psychological stress, endocrine changes (such as menstruation) and dietary intake (especially tyramine-containing foods and irregular meals). The aetiology is not fully understood, although there is undoubtedly a vascular component. A rise in cerebral blood flow in the occipitoparietal cortex precedes the headache, and this is followed by a 25% reduction in flow spreading forwards from the occipital region. These changes seem to account for the symptoms of aura. The headache itself is probably due to the dilatation of cranial non-cerebral vessels. Treatment consists in symptomatic relief with analgesics and anti-emetics. An impending attack may be aborted with an ergotamine preparation taken orally or by inhaler. More recently available is sumatriptan, a cranioselective 5-HT$_1$ agonist, which is effective at any stage of an attack when given by subcutaneous injection. Prophylaxis consists largely in avoiding precipitating factors. Drugs such as β-blockers, pizotifen, diltiazem, methysergide and cyproheptadine have all been used in an attempt to stabilize the cranial circulation.

2. Cluster headache. This is a rare but important cause of unilateral facial pain. It takes its title from the grouping together of attacks into clusters, consisting of 1–8 headaches per day for 3–12 weeks. Symptom-free periods of 3–18 months separate the clusters. Age of onset is between 20 and 40 years and there is a male–female ratio of 7:1. The pain is deep and throbbing and is extremely severe. It may appear at the same time each day during a cluster and may wake the subject from sleep. There are always associated autonomic phenomena such as nasal congestion, injected conjunctivae and facial sweating. Each attack lasts for 15 minutes to 3 hours. Symptom relief during an attack may be achieved with oxygen, which causes transient cerebral vasoconstriction, ergotamine subcutaneously or by inhaler, or sphenopalatine ganglion block with intranasal local anaesthetic. For prophylaxis such drugs as prednisolone in a reducing dose, methysergide (long-term use may cause retroperitoneal fibrosis) and calcium channel blockers have all met with some success. Sumatriptan given by subcutaneous injection may relieve an attack.

Local

1. Temporomandibular joint (TMJ) dysfunction. When anatomical disturbance of the TMJ occurs, an associated myofascial syndrome commonly develops. TMJ problems manifest themselves as clicking or popping in the joint, pain on chewing or mouth opening and locking if the internal derangement is severe. Myofascial pain usually appears on the affected side, although it may in time become bilateral as a result of a general chronic tensing of head and neck muscles and assumption of a protective posture. A sensation of fullness or congestion in the ear may be mentioned. Diagnosis is confirmed by eliciting TMJ tenderness and clicking, and there will usually be trigger points in associated muscle groups, in particular the medial and lateral pterygoid muscles. Treatment consists of physical therapy to the painful muscles and a dental splint to reposition the mandible and prevent bruxism (teeth grinding), which is usually worn at night.

Musculoskeletal

Considering that muscle accounts for about 30% of body weight, it is overlooked surprisingly often as a source of chronic pain. Lack of a diagnosis rapidly results in frustration for the physician and loss of confidence in his or her abilities by the patient.

1. Myofascial headache (also called 'tension headache'). This is described as a deep, dull, aching, pressure-like pain which may be uni- or bilateral, and of gradual or sudden onset. There are no neurological abnormalities. Myofascial pain is always associated with trigger points in the muscle and its surrounding fascia, which refer either locally or to a distant site which is usually unrelated dermatomally or myotomally. Trigger points are palpable as tender bands within the muscle which, when pressed, will either reproduce the patient's pain or refer it to a characteristic reference zone. Trigger points are thought to arise following muscle trauma, either as a single event or a repeated microtrauma, such as poor posture or teeth grinding. Certain muscles appear to be particularly prone to developing trigger points, including sternomastoid, temporalis, ptergyoid, trapezius and neck strap muscles. Pain is often referred forward from the occipital region to the temple, forehead, orbit or ear. Treatment consists essentially in restoring normal function to the affected muscles by gentle stretching and mobilization. To permit this it is helpful to reduce discomfort in the muscle body with cooling spray, ice, local anaesthetic injection or acupuncture needling of trigger points. The assistance of physiotherapists may be useful. If the pain has remained undiagnosed for some time it is common for a degree of pain behaviour to have developed. In this situation psychological therapy may be required, coupled with such techniques as deep relaxation and counselling to improve the patient's insight into the condition. Chronic tension headache does not respond well to analgesics and the most effective medication may be amitriptylline. Tension headaches and migraine may be related and may co-exist.

Conclusion This is by no means a complete guide to diagnosis and treatment of facial pain. Careful consideration must be given to the history and symptomatology, and examination must always include full assessment of cranial nerve function.

Related topics of interest

FOREIGN BODIES

Foreign bodies in the nose

Nasal foreign bodies are most commonly found in 2- to 3-year-old children. They may be inorganic or organic. Inorganic foreign bodies include buttons, beads, metal, plastic from toys, stones, etc. They are often asymptomatic and may be discovered only accidentally during an examination for an unrelated complaint. Organic foreign bodies include sponge, rubber, paper, wood, peas, nuts, etc. These are irritant and the nasal mucosa usually becomes involved in an inflammatory reaction causing a nasal discharge. A unilateral nasal discharge is nearly always due to a foreign body. This is initially mucoid, but will eventually become mucopurulent and finally odiferous mucopus, which may be blood stained. Inflammation and infection of the paranasal sinuses may complicate the problem. Occasionally deposits of calcium and magnesium carbonates and phosphates takes place around a foreign body to form a rhinolith, which will require removal under general anaesthetic.

Management

Confirmation of the presence of the foreign body is from the history and examination of the child. Examination of the anterior nares is often possible with a head mirror, reflecting light on to the elevated tip of the nose with the child sat on either a parent's or nurse's knee. If nothing is visible then an auriscope may give a better view. It is possible in many children to remove the foreign body without the need for general anaesthesia. The child must be cooperative and the surgeon gently reassuring. Have good illumination and all the instruments possibly required to hand. The first effort will be the best and often the only attempt the child will allow. If this fails or if the foreign body is situated posteriorly in the nasal cavity then a general anaesthetic will be required.

Treatment

Removal is best accomplished with a wax hook or an old Eustachian tube catheter. It is passed point downwards above the foreign body, which is brought to the floor of the nose and raked anteriorly.

Cupped forceps are preferable for the removal of thin objects, such as buttons, or soft organic objects such as sponge.

In every case the nasal cavity must be examined afterwards as there may be a second foreign body more posteriorly. The child should be discharged with a supply of Naseptin nasal carrier cream and oral antibiotics if there is any obvious infection.

Foreign bodies in the ear

Foreign bodies are inserted into the ears more commonly by school children than by toddlers. The objects found can be organic (pieces of paper, rubber, pencil, seeds, peas and beans) or inorganic (beads, buttons, crayons and stones). Inorganic foreign bodies are often asymptomatic, but organic objects may give rise to otitis externa by local irritation of the epithelium of the meatal walls. One of the commonest causes of this is cotton wool, and it is not unusual to find this in adult patients who have been attempting to clean their ears.

Management

A foreign body in the external ear canal is usually easily seen on otoscopy. Removal may appear to be easy, but usually requires the skills and facilities of a specialist. Ill-directed attempts at their removal by the untrained may lead to complications. It is sometimes possible to remove the foreign body in the clinic, but a general anaesthetic may be required for children and sensitive adults.

Treatment

As a general rule, most foreign bodies can be removed by syringing. Objects of vegetable origin, such as peas, beans and nuts, are hygroscopic and should not be syringed. Large objects lying superficial to the external ear canal isthmus should not be syringed as there is a danger of wedging them in that area.

Suction or a fine hook may be used, with the object viewed with an operating microscope, to remove material of vegetable origin and large objects which lie superficial to the isthmus.

Forceps are useful for soft material such as paper, cotton wool or sponge. Forceps should never be used to remove smooth spherical objects such as beads, as they will tend to push them further down the ear canal.

Insects should be killed before syringing by instilling spirit drops into the ear canal. Maggots grip on the external ear canal skin, so must be killed or anaesthetized with chloroform water prior to syringing.

It is rarely necessary to extract a foreign body through the posterior canal wall after a postaural incision. This is useful if permeatal extraction is not possible because of swelling of the canal walls from irritation, or if a large object has lodged at the isthmus.

Once the object is out, the tympanic membrane should be examined to ensure it has not been damaged. If there is an otitis externa a swab should be taken, the ear should be cleaned, and antibiotic–steroid ear drops should be instilled.

Foreign bodies in the pharynx

Sharp and irregular foreign bodies may become impacted in the tonsils, base of tongue, vallecula or pyriform fossae. Small fish bones are the commonest and usually lodge in the tonsil.

Management

The patient, usually an adult, will be able to localize the side and site with reasonable accuracy. A thorough examination with light reflected from a head mirror, a tongue depressor and laryngeal mirror should reveal the offending bone. If the patient cannot tolerate indirect laryngoscopy and a foreign body is suspected in the vallecula or base of tongue, then examination with a nasendoscope is useful. In some patients there will be no abnormal findings and a lateral soft-tissue radiograph is indicated. If this too is normal they should be reassured and reviewed 2 days later. By this time the sensation will usually have passed, but if there are persistent symptoms the patient should be re-examined.

After the foreign body has been visualized, the pharynx should be anaesthetized with lignocaine spray. It is then often possible to grasp the foreign body with forceps and remove it swiftly and painlessly.

Some fibreoptic nasendoscopes have a side arm which facilitate forceps and can be used to remove foreign bodies.

In a patient anaesthetized with lignocaine spray and positioned on a flat bed with the neck and shoulders supported on a pillow it is sometimes possible to pass the blade of a McGill laryngoscope to depress the tongue. This has its own light source and may help locate a foreign body in the pharynx. The surgeon's free hand can then be used to remove the object with forceps.

General anaesthesia is required to remove a foreign body from the pharynx if the patient is young or unable to tolerate the above manoeuvres.

Patients who have been anaesthetized with lignocaine spray should be warned not to eat or drink for 2 hours as the pharynx will be relatively insensitive.

Foreign bodies in the oesophagus

Impaction of a foreign body depends chiefly on the size and shape of the object. The presence of an abnormality in the patient's aerodigestive tract, for example a stricture, will make impaction more likely. A large bolus of food swallowed hurriedly may become impacted even in a normal oesophagus. Mentally handicapped and some psychiatric patients are at particular risk. The commonest objects are coins in children and fish or meat bones in adults. Impaction is commonest at the level of the cricopharyngeus muscle, but may also occur at the level where the oesophagus is crossed by the left main bronchus or at the cardia.

Clinical features

Adults are usually aware of having swallowed something and can localize fairly accurately the level at which it is impacted. Children and psychiatric patients may not be so reliable. Discomfort or pain in the oesophagus and difficulty in swallowing are the cardinal symptoms. Dysphagia may be total. The foreign body may cause coughing and excessive salivation. Clinical examination may be normal, but pooling in the pyriform fossae on indirect laryngoscopy is sometimes evident. There may be localized tenderness in the neck and crepitus owing to surgical emphysema if there has been an oesophageal perforation.

Investigations

Lateral and anteroposterior soft-tissue radiographs of the neck and chest radiographs are mandatory. Some foreign bodies are easily identified because they are radio-opaque. The inexperienced may confuse calcification in the laryngeal cartilages with an opaque foreign body. Widening of the postcricoid space or a persistent air bubble in the oesophagus may occur. If the foreign body has caused a tear, surgical emphysema will be shown radiologically. Barium swallow as an investigation is condemned because it makes subsequent oesophagoscopy and identification of a foreign body more difficult, though Omnopaque 500 contrast medium can be used because it is clear.

Treatment

If the obstruction is due to an impacted food bolus, the safest treatment is to admit the patient and give a dose of intravenous hyoscine butylbromide and diazepam. This will usually allow the oesophagus to relax and permit the passage of the bolus. Some surgeons have suggested that the ingestion of cola fizzy drinks will encourage this process. The patient should have a barium swallow 2 weeks later to exclude an oesophageal neoplasm.

If there is sharp or bony object, the patient requires an oesophagoscopy as soon as possible. Using a rigid oesophagoscope the foreign body is identified and if possible drawn into the end of the scope using forceps. The scope and the foreign body should be withdrawn in unison under direct vision. The patient should remain in hospital for 24 hours postoperatively and receive nil by mouth for the first 4 hours and only water for the next 4 hours. If there is a mucosal injury the patient should have antibiotic cover. The neck should be examined to exclude surgical emphysema on the day of discharge. Perforation of the oesophagus should be treated with intravenous antibiotics and nasogastric feeding. Surgical repair should be considered depending on its site and extent.

Foreign bodies in the trachea and bronchi

Inhalation of a foreign object is most common in children under the age of 3 years. The event can easily escape a parent's notice. Any unexplained choking fit on the part of the child should be treated with suspicion, especially if any small object with which the child happened to be playing cannot be found. Adults usually give a clear history of foreign body inhalation. Most inhaled foreign bodies enter the right main bronchus, which is larger and more vertical than the left.

Clinical features

After the initial inhalation, which causes choking and coughing, and sometimes cyanosis, the foreign body may pass symptomless into the trachea. For this reason, if there is a good history suggestive of inhalation of an object, the child should have a bronchoscopy. There may, however, be a cough with inspiratory and expiratory stridor, or a wheeze. A foreign body which is causing a complete obstruction of a bronchus will produce a collapse of that lung segment, followed by consolidation. A foreign body may partly occlude the bronchus and act like a valve so that the partly obstructed lung becomes overinflated. Vegetable foreign bodies are particularly dangerous (nuts, pips, vegetables, fruits) as they will cause an intense inflammatory reaction of the bronchial mucosa leading to a pneumonitis.

Investigations

Lateral and anteroposterior chest radiographs are mandatory. Opaque objects are easily identified. Radiolucent objects are suspected when there is unexplained atelectasis, obstructive emphysema, mediastinal shift or consolidation of the lung.

Treatment

Bronchoscopy should be performed as soon as possible. A senior ENT surgeon and anaesthetist are required. A variety of bronchoscopes, suction tubes and forceps appropriate to the nature of the foreign body and size of the patient need to be readily available. Storz or similar instruments with Hopkins rod telescopes should be available with young children.

Removal via a thoracotomy is sometimes necessary if the foreign body cannot be retrieved by endoscopic methods.

Antibiotics and physiotherapy may be necessary if there is any sign of pneumonitis. A tracheostomy may be needed if there is oedema or obstruction of the larynx, either prior to or after bronchoscopy.

Related topics of interest

Paediatric airway problems (p. 234)
Paediatric endoscopy (p. 239)

FUNCTIONAL ENDOSCOPIC SINUS SURGERY

Most infections of the sinuses are rhinogenic, i.e. disease spreads from the nose to the paranasal sinuses. In most cases of frontal and maxillary sinus disease the underlying causes are not found in the affected sinuses themselves, but in the lateral nasal wall. There, narrow clefts of the anterior ethmoid hold a key position for normal sinus function and pathophysiology. They are regarded as prechambers of the dependent frontal and maxillary sinuses, providing them with ventilation and drainage. Functional endoscopic sinus surgery (FESS) is based on the premise that treatment of disease in the ethmoidal prechambers is more logical and beneficial to the patient than treating the secondarily involved larger sinuses. The underlying principle is that the sinus mucosa is preserved and will return to its normal functioning state once obstruction is relieved and ventilation and drainage are re-established.

Pathophysiology

Mucus produced in the maxillary sinus is transported by the ciliary beat from the floor of the sinus, along the sinus walls to the natural ostium. The frontal and maxillary sinuses communicate with the nose through a complex system of narrow clefts which provide their drainage and their ventilation. These prechambers – the frontal recess in the case of the frontal sinus and the ethmoidal infundibulum in the case of the maxillary sinus – are parts of the anterior ethmoid system. These clefts are only a few millimetres wide and contain mucosal areas with ciliated respiratory epithelium that face each other. If extensive contact of opposing mucosal surfaces occurs, whatever the cause, the ciliary activity may be impeded so that the spaces are completely blocked. Locations for the contact areas in the nose include the frontal recess and the ethmoidal infundibulum, the cleft between the uncinate process and the middle turbinate, between the ethmoid bulla and the middle turbinate (in the so-called turbinate sinus) or in the lateral sinus above and behind the ethmoid bulla. Anatomical variants of the uncinate process, ethmoidal bulla and the middle turbinate further narrow the clefts. These can act as a focus for infections which may spread to the dependent larger sinuses. Thus, even relatively limited disease in the ethmoidal infundibulum or the frontal recess may severely affect the sinus.

Indications for FESS

Enthusiasts for the technique propose the following indications. Most probably these will be refined as results in each condition are accurately audited and published:

- Polypoid sinusitis.
- Recurrent acute and chronic sinusitis.
- Nasal obstruction.
- Headaches.
- Postnasal drip.
- Anosmia.
- Mucoceles.
- Retention cysts.
- Sinus mycoses.
- Adjuvant surgery to allergy treatment.
- Orbital disease.
- Antrochoanal polyps.

Certain relative contraindications also exist concerning the use of endoscopic techniques in the treatment of chronic sinusitis. These are the absence of specific ostiomeatal abnormalities, osteomyelitis, inaccessible lateral frontal sinus disease, frontal sinus disease accompanied by a stenosed internal os and threatened intracranial or intraorbital complications.

Investigations

The definitive radiological investigation is the coronal CT scan. A normal standard radiograph of the sinuses does not rule out a sinogenic origin to the patient's problems. When evaluating the CT scan it is important to look for mucosal thickening, soft-tissue masses or for opacification inside the sinus air cells and spaces. It is equally important to recognize and identify contact areas or other stenoses in key positions even if they are not diseased at the time the scan was performed. Axial CT will allow the orientation of the internal carotid artery and optic nerve in the lateral wall of the sphenoid sinus.

Surgical technique

The procedure may be performed under local anaesthetic with topical vasoconstriction and intravenous sedation, but a general anaesthetic is more usual in the UK. The anterior ethmoid is entered by resection of the uncinate process, which opens the ethmoid infundibulum – so-called infundibulotomy. The general aim of surgery is to clear diseased ethmoid clefts and compartments under guidance of the rigid endoscope and to re-establish ventilation and drainage of the diseased larger sinuses through their physiological routes. Stepwise removal of the ethmoidal cells extending to the posterior ethmoid and sphenoid sinus can be undertaken. The natural ostium of the maxillary sinus can be cleared, opened and enlarged, as can disease of the frontonasal duct.

Complications	1. *Peroperative.*

- Anaesthetic reaction.
- Bleeding (ethmoidal artery injury).
- Penetration of the ethmoid roof or the lamina papyracea.
- Nasolacrimal duct damage.
- Optic nerve injury.

2. *Immediate postoperative.*

- Intraorbital bleeding (orbital haematoma).
- Blindness.
- Diplopia.
- Epistaxis.

3. *Early postoperative.*

- CSF leak (sometimes from an unrecognized cribriform plate or ethmoid roof penetration).
- Intercranial injection (menigitis, brain abscess).

4. *Late complications.*

- Synechiae between the middle turbinate and lateral nasal wall or the nasal septum.
- Recurrent disease.

Follow-up and aftercare

Depending on the pathology present, the ethmoid cavity usually heals within 2–3 weeks after surgery; the dependent larger sinuses, especially in cases of diffuse polyposis, may need up to 6 weeks to heal. Meticulous care of the nose and the cavities is proposed by some authorities, removing crusts and excess wound secretions using the endoscope in the outpatient department. Topical steroid treatment may be appropriate in some cases. Some place patients on systemic steroids and antibiotics. Care must be taken to prevent adhesion and scar formation between the middle turbinate and the lateral nasal wall.

Further reading

Sillers MJ *et al.* Surgery of the nose and paranasal sinuses. *Current Opinion in Otolaryngology and Head and Neck Surgery*, 1994; **2**: 42–7.

Stammberger H, Posawetz W. Functional endoscopic sinus surgery: concept, indications and results of the Messerklinger technique. *European Archives of Otorhinolaryngology*, 1990; **247**: 63–7.

Related topics of interest

Acute sinusitis (p. 5)
Chronic sinusitis (p. 47)
Sinusitis – complications (p. 285)

GLOBUS PHARYNGEUS

Globus pharyngeus (globus syndrome, globus hystericus) is the sensation of a lump, discomfort or foreign body in the throat for which there is no obvious cause.

Pathophysiology

A number of organic aetiological theories have been proposed; the two most strongly supported are the suggestion that it represents a manifestation of reflux oesophagitis or is a disorder of pharyngeal and oesophageal motility. Disorders of motor function have certainly been demonstrated in globus patients, including elevation of cricopharyngeal sphincter pressure, mid-oesophageal dysmotility and poor lower oesophageal sphincter relaxation, but there is still debate as to whether these are primary or secondary phenomena. Pharyngeal pH measurements tend to be normal in such patients. What is undisputed is that globus patients have much higher levels of psychological distress in the form of anxiety, somatic concern, neuroticism and even depression. Many people suffer from globus sensation for whatever underlying reason at some time in their life. It is the patient's psychological profile that dictates whether it becomes a problem. In this group of patients a vicious cycle is created where somatic concern and anxiety only serve to further aggravate the symptom, thus further increasing anxiety and concern.

Clinical features

Patients are more often women, usually in their fifth decade. The complaint is typically of a lump in the throat, usually at the region of the sternal notch, although it may be felt higher and to be unilateral. Although patients may complain of some subjective difficulty in swallowing, true difficulties are never a feature. The sensation is often intermittent and variable in severity. Many patients seem anxious and introspective. Physical examination is normal, although one must be alert for any physical cause for the symptom such as a postcricoid carcinoma, a foreign body or an inflammatory cause. In particular, a neoplastic lesion should be excluded, which is what many of these patients are most concerned about.

Investigations

Most clinicians would perform a chest radiograph and a barium swallow in spite of a typical history and a normal clinical examination. The radiologist should be encouraged to pay particular attention to the hypopharynx during the examination. In those patients with persistent or suspicious symptoms, rigid endoscopy is indicated. Ambulatory pH measurement and manometry are research tools and are unlikely to offer much in the clinical situation.

Management

There is no specific treatment for globus pharyngeus. Strong and appropriate reassurance at all stages is invaluable. Reflux oesophagitis should be treated with medication to speed gastric motility (e.g. cisapride), antacids, H_2 antagonists (e.g. ranitidine) or a proton pump inhibitor (e.g. omeprazole). Relaxation therapy can be suggested for those who are tense and over-anxious. Antidepressants may be required for those patients who are clinically depressed. Smoking should be discouraged.

Follow-up and aftercare

Most patients are happy once reassured that they do not have cancer or other serious pathology, and follow-up is not usually required.

Further reading

Wilson JA. Globus sensation. *Clinical Otolaryngology*, 1992; **17**: 105–6.

Related topics of interest

Hypopharyngeal carcinoma (p. 133)
Pharyngeal pouch (p. 246)

HALITOSIS

Aetiology and pathophysiology

Halitosis is a problem that not uncommonly presents to the ENT surgeon and may be subjective or objective. The causes can be divided into three broad categories: local, general and drugs. Local and general causes overlap when general or systemic conditions give rise to a dry mouth.

1. Local causes. Saliva plays a crucial role in the oral cavity and is involved in taste, lubrication, water balance and oral hygiene. Saliva acts as a mechanical cleansing agent, its contained buffers combat acid/alkali excesses and the secreted immunoglobulins have an important anti-infective function. Any significant reduction in salivary flow allows an increase in the local bacterial flora. These micro-organisms break down proteins with the production of odiferous volatile gases and consequent halitosis as well as leading to an increase in dental caries and periodontal disease, in themselves a cause of halitosis. A decrease in saliva production can occur temporarily, as during sleep and with anxiety, or more permanently as a result of previous radiotherapy, cardiac and renal failure and some autoimmune conditions (Sjögren's syndrome). Any local inflammatory lesion is likely to become secondarily infected and lead to halitosis. Examples include any oral ulcerative lesion (from aphthous to neoplastic), tonsillitis, pharyngitis and nasal and sinus infections.

2. General causes. Certain foods, alcohol and cigarettes all give rise to a characteristic unpleasant smell on the breath. A reduction in food intake during any systemic illness will lead to ketosis and typical ketotic breath. Diabetes can lead to a sweet acetone smell, uraemia a smell of ammonia, liver failure a smell of decaying blood and chest infections a peculiarly foul anaerobic smell. The latter is particularly common in brochiectasis.

Reflux of partially digested stomach contents into the oesophagus as a result of hiatus hernia is another cause. There are some patients who complain bitterly of halitosis for which there is no objective support. This may represent a monosymptomatic hypochondriacal condition, and these patients may be severely depressed.

3. Drugs. Drugs can cause halitosis by several mechanisms: they may cause a dry mouth (anticholinergics), they may alter the normal oral flora (antibiotics) or their metabolites may be excreted by the lungs (chloral hydrate, iodine-based medications).

Clinical features

Halitosis is usually due to local causes. It is commonest in those with poor dental hygiene and peridontal disease. There is a natural decline in salivary flow and increase in dental disease with age. A full history should be taken to establish any possible systemic or drug causes. Clinical examination should establish objective evidence of halitosis. A useful manoeuvre is to ask the patient to breathe through the mouth and the nose separately; if the smell is still present when breathing through the nose, an extraoral cause should be suspected.

Investigations

Investigations should be directed at the suspected cause and might include a chest radiograph and blood tests to exclude systemic disease.

Management

Management should obviously be directed at the underlying cause and will often fall outside the remit of the ENT surgeon. Those with systemic causes and severe chest disease will require referral to an appropriate physician. Patients with a psychological problem may require referral to a psychiatrist. Periodontal disease will require the services of a dental practitioner. Most oral inflammatory conditions will resolve spontaneously, but any that persist demand biopsy and subsequent definitive treatment. Pharyngitis, tonsillitis and sinonasal disease can all be treated appropriately by the ENT surgeon.

Follow-up and aftercare

These will be dictated by the underlying cause.

Further reading

Symposium on dry mouth and halitosis. *The Practitioner*, 1990; **234**: 603–19.

Related topics of interest

HEARING AIDS

A hearing aid is any device that amplifies sound or assists the hearing-impaired individual, but in the present context will be taken to mean an electroacoustic device used to amplify sounds. Cochlear implants can be included in this definition, but they are described in a separate topic.

Design

It is important to be familiar with the basic design of the hearing aid as many patients attending the ENT department are prescribed them. There is a good chance you will be handed one and asked to describe it in an examination. The basic components of any hearing aid are a receiver (microphone and/or induction coil), an amplifier (a variety of which can be used to amplify sound in various ways in terms of frequency response and intensity), a sound transmitter (earphone, bone conductor) and a power source (primary cell). The external controls are usually a selector switch and a volume control. The selector switch has three markings; O is for off, T is for a television or telephone induction coil and M is for the microphone. Internal controls on the amplifier are often available to alter the frequency response and spread of volume control available to the user. Most current aids amplify sounds in the frequency range of 250 – 4000 Hz.

In order to avoid the problem of excessive amplification of loud sounds which may cause discomfort to the user, amplifiers can use one of two methods of reducing sudden peaks of sound.

(a) Peak clipping. In essence this system basically chops the tops off the peaks of sound. It has the advantage of being simple and instant but does result in some distortion.

(b) Automatic gain control. This system involves some complicated circuitry that picks up the signal and compresses it so that the maximum sound peak is never above a set maximum value. The system is relatively new and a little more complicated but produces less distortion.

Types

1. Postaural aids. In most common usage are the standard behind-the-ear (BE) aids, available on the NHS. The body of the aid sits behind the wearer's ear and is normally connected by a hollow plastic tube to an ear mould, which allows sound passage to the ear. There are three main groups of BE aids, the 10, 30 and 50 series, with the power of the aids increasing correspondingly. Within each series are a number of models with differing patterns of frequency response. All contain an induction coil which can be used with telephones, televisions and in theatres and cinemas, fitted with induction loops, to bypass much of the unwanted background noise.

2. In-the-ear aids. These commonly available commercial aids sit in the concha or canal. Their external shell is usually of acrylic and conforms to the shape of the wearer's ear. They are less obtrusive than the standard BE aids but are expensive and occasionally prone to feedback problems.

3. Body-worn (BW) aids. These rather cumbersome, ugly aids are usually worn with a strap around the neck and the body of the aid on the patient's chest. By virtue of their size they can be made very powerful, and the distance between microphone and earphone means that, even with high amplification, feedback is rarely a problem. They are, however, prone to picking up the sounds of rustling clothes. There are two series available on the NHS: BW 60 and BW 80.

4. Bone conduction aids. These are very similar to the standard body-worn aid but feed their output to a bone conductor rather than an earphone. They are indicated because of meatal discharge or stenosis, or subjective preference for bone conduction reception.

5. Osseointegrated hearing aids. Conventional bone conduction aids have drawbacks, such as bulkiness and discomfort. In addition, the skull cannot be vibrated directly, but only through the energy-absorbing skin and soft tissues. Bone-anchored hearing aids largely overcome these problems.

There are two devices in clinical use, both relying on the transmission of mechanical vibrations to the bone of the skull.

(a) In the bone-anchored hearing aid (BAHA) a percutaneous titanium abutment is fixed to a titanium screw implanted in the mastoid. A vibrator is then mounted directly on to the abutment, which is fed either from a microphone and circuit in a small box with the vibrator or from a body-worn hearing aid (for higher output power).

(b) The Xomed audiant bone conductor consists of an encased rare earth magnet implanted completely under the skin and fixed into bone with a titanium screw. Externally, another magnet serves to hold its surrounding induction coil in place over the implanted magnet. By passing electric currents (derived from what is essentially a hearing aid) through the induction coil, an electromagnetic field is set up that causes the implanted magnet, and hence the skull, to vibrate.

6. *Spectacle aids.* These involve modification of standard spectacle frames to incorporate a hearing aid. They can then be used in a number of ways: as a standard hearing aid, as a bone conductor or for contralateral routing of signal (CROS). In this last variation, sound is picked up from one side of the head and fed to the contralateral side, which is often the good side.

Choice of hearing aid

Many factors will influence the choice of hearing aid. The actual degree and nature of the hearing loss will dictate the amplification characteristics. The cause of the deafness will influence the type of aid chosen, as will vanity and available finance. It is important to establish the patient's requirements and to remember that an aid will not cure the underlying disease.

1. *Type.* A spectacle-type aid is useful for those people who regularly wear glasses as they are relatively inconspicuous. They are often chosen when there is one very deaf ear and a requirement for contralateral signal routing. A bone conduction aid is ideal in those cases where a hearing loss exists in association with active outer ear or middle-ear inflammatory pathology. A body-worn aid is useful for anyone with a profound hearing loss. For most NHS patients an ear-level aid will be found to be suitable.

2. *Amplification characteristics.* The pattern of frequency response chosen depends very much on the shape of the audiogram. As for amplification, a hearing aid must function in a relatively narrow dynamic range, providing adequate amplification to overcome the hearing loss, but not overamplifying sound and causing recruitment and consequent discomfort and intolerance. In an effort to overcome this problem, a number of formulae have been developed to calculate the appropriate amplification for the

patient's hearing loss (half-gain rule, Berger's procedure, POGO 2, NAL-R, etc.). All formulae give differing importance to differing frequencies, with maximum importance for hearing loss at the main speech frequencies of 1000 and 2000 Hz. Many patients with deafness have a high frequency loss with comparative sparing of the lower frequencies. Most hearing aids can be adjusted to alter their frequency response, for instance high tone boost and base tone cut. A vented mould or modified horn (feeding the sound to the ear) will also effectively reduce the lower frequency amplification.

3. Ear moulds. A number of modifications can be made to the ear mould. These may be made for both auditory and medical reasons. Venting the mould will reduce the low-frequency response. In patients prone to otitis externa, it is useful to ventilate or even skeletonize the mould to provide aeration. Unfortunately, feedback becomes more likely with a high-power aid if the mould is vented.

4. General. Although it is preferable to provide binaural aids in cases of bilateral hearing loss, this is rarely possible in the NHS on the grounds of cost. Which ear to fit the aid in will then depend on a number of factors, including patient preference, available dynamic range and discrimination scores in each ear and the presence of any active inflammatory process in either ear, as well as other medical factors such as manual dexterity relating to arthritis, strokes, amputations, etc.

Follow-up and aftercare   After the initial fitting, a period of support and rehabilitation is essential to allow the patient to gain confidence, iron out early teething troubles and achieve useful function with the hearing aid.

Further reading

Ballantyne D. *Handbook of Audiological Techniques*. London: Butterworth-Heinemann, 1990.
Rosen S. Implantable electroacoustic prostheses. *Current Opinion in Otolaryngology and Head and Neck Surgery*, 1994; **2**: 209–16.

Related topics of interest

HIV INFECTION

Aetiology

Acquired immunodeficiency syndrome (AIDS) is caused by two of five human retroviruses: human immunodeficiency viruses (HIV) 1 and 2. (The other three are T-cell leukaemia viruses and are associated with lymphomas and leukaemias.)

Pathology

HIV-1 is prevalent worldwide, while HIV-2 is found mainly in West Africa. HIV infects cells bearing the CD4 antigen, which acts as a virus receptor. These cells are the monocyte, macrophage and T-helper cells. The HIV-1 glycoprotein, gp120, binds to CD4 and allows virus to enter the cell. Viral replication may occur in cells in which HIV-1 DNA has been integrated (productive infection), although in some cells containing integrated HIV-1 DNA the virus does not replicate except when the cell is activated by antigenic stimulation (latent infection), for example by Epstein–Barr virus or cytomegalovirus infection. Ultimately, a functional impairment and depletion of T-helper cells occurs, but to a degree that is disproportionate to the number of cells infected. The mechanism of this has yet to be elucidated, but the ultimate consequence is a compromise of the host immune system. Immunosuppression places the victim at risk of developing opportunistic infections and unusual malignancies, particularly B-cell lymphoma and Kaposi's sarcoma. Although the time to development of AIDS is variable, it is possible that everyone infected with HIV will ultimately develop the condition. It is invariably fatal, with nearly two-thirds of reported sufferers in the USA already dead. There are various methods of transmission, but all demand close contact with infected body fluids, particularly blood. High-risk groups include intravenous drug users, homosexual males, heterosexual contact with an infected partner and children of infected mothers. Although transfusion of blood products, particularly in haemophiliacs, resulted in a significant number of cases, the screening of all blood products for HIV-1 and HIV-2 antibody has greatly reduced but not irradicated the risk because it may take up to 4 months for seroconversion (the interval between infection and the appearance of antibody).

Clinical features

AIDS is defined as the development of a complication of immunosuppression such as malignancy or opportunistic infection in an HIV-positive individual. The T-cell CD4 count is less than 200/mm^3. AIDS-related complex (ARC) comprises persistent fever lasting longer than 3 months, weight loss, leucopenia, anaemia and diarrhoea. The T-cell CD4 count is less than 400/mm^3. Typical patients are in one of the high-risk groups and, excluding children, are usually between the ages of 20 and 40. Between 40 and 70% of patients will have head and neck manifestations. Certain conditions characterize the AIDS patient.

1. Otological. Otitis media and externa (particularly fungal) are more common. Kaposi's sarcoma of the pinna or external auditory meatus may occur.

2. Rhinological. Chronic rhinosinusitis may occur because of the debilitated state of the patient. Acute sinus infections may occur and unusual organisms such as yeasts and fungi are not uncommon. Kaposi's sarcoma and lymphomas may be found in the nasopharynx.

3. Oropharyngeal. The oral cavity is one of the most commonly affected sites. Kaposi's sarcoma is not uncommon. Severe candidiasis is frequent and may spread to involve the pharynx and larynx. Herpes simplex ulceration is also common and tends to be widespread and severe. Xerostomia is a frequent complaint and epiglottitis is reported to occur more often.

4. Neck. Neck abscess may occur and tends to be deep. They often culture unusual organisms, e.g. atypical mycobacteria.

Generalized cervical lymphadenopathy is a frequent finding in all AIDS patients.

Investigations

The diagnosis of HIV infection depends on detecting the virus or the host response to it in the blood. Usually this is done by identifying a specific antibody, using first an enzyme-linked immunosorbent assay (ELISA) as a screen, followed by Western blot confirmation. Once HIV infection is confirmed, the most useful investigation is monitoring of the CD4 T-cell count as a measure of immune function. Opportunistic infections are diagnosed by appropriate sampling and microbiological culturing. Neoplastic lesions are confirmed histologically on biopsy. Other investigations (e.g. radiology) are dictated by the clinical conditions.

Management

The management of HIV infection as it presents to the ENT surgeon and the management of the patient so as to avoid the risks of infection pose separate problems.

The occurrence of unusual organisms requires a high index of suspicion to make the diagnosis followed by appropriate therapy. Radiotherapy and chemotherapy may be used for Kaposi's sarcoma and lymphomas.

Risk of infection

The risk of infection to a health care worker from an HIV-positive patient is extremely low and invariably relates to blood exposure. To reduce this risk, two sets of commonsense recommendations have developed.

- Universal precautions should be adopted for all patients and involve the use of gowns and gloves to avoid blood contamination. All non-intact skin surfaces should be covered and sharps should be handled with appropriate caution.
- Theatre precautions apply to any invasive procedure on a proven or suspected HIV-positive patient. A high level of discipline is required in these cases. The most senior or experienced surgeon/clinician should operate and theatre/ancillary staff should be kept to a minimum. All staff should be fully gowned and double gloved and boots and eye protection should be worn. Drapes should be disposable and double bagged at the end of the procedure. The patient need not be last on the list, but the theatre should be thoroughly cleaned with hypochlorite solution prior to the next case. There is no evidence of infection risk from the anaesthetic system, but sensible hygienic measures should be employed.

Should inoculation occur, zidovudine, the only drug considered to offer any degree of HIV prophylaxis, may be taken for 28 days. Appropriate serological monitoring is then required over a period of several months.

The General Medical Council recommends that an HIV-positive clinician should not perform invasive procedures.

Follow-up and aftercare

In general terms these patients are best cared for in a centre with a team with a particular interest in AIDS.

Further reading

Gold JWM. HIV-1 infection: diagnosis and management. *Medical Clinics of North America*, 1992; **76**: 1–18.

Joint Working Party of the Hospital Infection Society and Surgical Infection Study Group. Risk to surgeons and patients from HIV and hepatitis: guidelines on precautions and management of exposure to blood or body fluids. *British Medical Journal*, 1992; **305**: 1337–43.

Lucente FE. Otolaryngologic aspects of the acquired immunodeficiency syndrome. *Medical Clinics of North America*, 1991; **75**: 1389–99.

HYPOPHARYNGEAL CARCINOMA

The hypopharynx extends from the lower limit of the oropharynx at the level of the hyoid bone down to the lower level of the cricoid cartilage at the opening of the oesophagus. For the purposes of tumour classification the UICC recognises three anatomical sites:

1. *Pyriform fossa.* This extends from the pharyngoepiglottic fold to the opening of the oesophagus. It is bounded medially by the aryepiglottic folds and laterally by the inner surface of the thyroid ala.
2. *Postcricoid.* Extends from the level of the arytenoid cartilages and connecting folds to the inferior margin of the cricoid cartilage.
3. *Posterior pharyngeal wall.* Extends from the level of the floor of the vallecula to the level of the crico-arytenoid joints.

Pathology

More than 90% of tumours of the hypopharynx are squamous cell carcinoma. Other epithelial and mesodermal tumours of benign and malignant behaviour do occur, but they are rare.

Carcinoma of the hypopharynx in itself is an uncommon disease with a prevalence of less than 1 per 100 000 population. It is a disease of the elderly and the incidence is higher in men than in women. In the postcricoid site the reverse is true. Although tobacco smoking and alcohol have been implicated as aetiological agents, the association is not as clear as with other upper aerodigestive tract tumours. Approximately 2% of patients with the Paterson–Kelly syndrome (iron deficiency anaemia, glossitis, angular stomatitis, pharyngeal web, koilonychia and splenomegaly) will develop postcricoid carcinoma. A few patients who had irradiation for thyrotoxicosis many years ago are now presenting with a pharyngeal carcinoma after a latent period of 25–30 years.

Hypopharyngeal tumours are sometimes so advanced when first seen that it is difficult to determine the site of origin, but the pyriform fossa (60%) is the most common site, with postcricoid carcinoma (30%) and posterior pharyngeal wall tumours (10%) occurring less often. Tumours of the posterior pharyngeal wall and the upper pyriform fossa tend to be exophytic, whereas an ulcerated lesion is typical of the other parts of the hypopharynx. Tumours of the lateral wall of the pyriform fossa may invade the thyrohyoid membrane and present as a palpable neck mass which may represent direct extension of the tumour rather than an enlarged lymph node. Medial wall tumours invade the aryepiglottic fold and into the paraglottic space, causing fixation of the vocal cord and consequent hoarseness. Dissemination of hypopharyngeal tumours in the submucosal lymphatics leads to a high incidence of 'skip lesions'. More than 10% of patients have a second tumour in the oesophagus. Hypopharyngeal tumours also have a propensity to metastasize to cervical lymph nodes. The pyriform fossa has the richest lymphatic drainage, and more than two-thirds of these patients will have lymph node metastases at presentation, with half of these being bilateral. Postcricoid tumours have a tendency to spread to paratracheal nodes.

Clinical features

Early symptoms include the sensation of a lump or discomfort in the throat. Later the patient will usually present with dysphagia, at first for solids then for fluids. Hoarseness may occur as a result of invasion of the larynx or vocal cord paralysis. The patient with advanced disease may have anorexia and weight loss. There may be a history of food sticking and repeated aspirations which will cause pneumonia. Indirect laryngoscopy may reveal an obvious tumour or oedema of the arytenoids with pooling of saliva in the pyriform fossa. There may be vocal cord fixation. The neck must be examined for lymph node metastases. Laryngeal crepitus is lost in postcricoid tumours and occasionally a direct extension of the tumour through the thyrohyoid membrane is palpable.

Investigations

1. Laboratory tests. A full blood count to exclude anaemia and biochemical tests are required as electrolyte disturbances are not infrequent.

2. Radiography. A soft-tissue neck radiograph is of limited value, but it may show a shadow posterior to the trachea. This can be regarded as abnormal if it is wider than the thickness of a vertebral body. Every patient who presents with swallowing difficulty or the sensation of a lump in the throat should have a barium swallow, which will usually demonstrate the presence and extent of any hypopharyngeal tumour or oesophageal lesion. MRI is preferable to CT scanning in delineating the extent and spread of tumour. A chest radiograph is mandatory to exclude metastases and to demonstrate any consolidation due to aspiration.

3. Endoscopy. Direct laryngoscopy and oesophagoscopy should be performed in every patient who has an abnormal barium swallow or persistent symptoms despite a normal barium swallow. This allows staging of the tumour and a representative biopsy to be taken. Bronchoscopy should be performed to look for any spread to the trachea. The extent of the lesion, particularly its upper and lower limits, need to be assessed. Digital examination of the tumour is appropriate if there is superior spread, and all patients should have their necks palpated again while they are under the general anaesthetic. Management of the patient will depend on, among other factors, the site and extent of the disease.

Management

Hypopharyngeal carcinoma generally has a poor prognosis even with extensive surgery, and 60% of patients are dead within a year of diagnosis. Because of the low survival and high recurrence rate the choice of treatment is particularly important. The optimal treatment modality should provide the best chance of cure, the lowest mortality and morbidity, the shortest hospital stay and the highest chance of good upper aerodigestive tract function (speech and swallowing).

Treatment may consist of radiotherapy, surgical resection, combined therapy or palliative therapy.

1. Radiotherapy. Early hypopharyngeal cancer may be treated with radiotherapy, with the option of salvage surgery if recurrence supervenes. Radiotherapy may be reserved for the patient without enlarged lymph nodes, but it has been proposed that in selected cases radiotherapy can be given to the primary tumour and a radical neck dissection carried out for nodal metastases.

2. Surgery. Surgical resection is preferred for large tumours or in the presence of bulky cervical metastases. A lateral pharyngotomy can be performed for posterior wall tumours and the defect repaired with a radial forearm free flap. Extensive and circumferential lesions will require total pharyngolaryngectomy and then reconstruction of the residual defect. A variety of techniques to reconstruct have been used including skin grafts, cervical and deltopectoral skin flaps, myocutaneous pectoralis major and latissimus dorsi flaps and visceral interposition of stomach, jejunum or colon. The main complications are failure of the graft or flap, postoperative fistulae and stenosis, which are all more likely if there has been previous radiotherapy. There is also a significant mortality rate of 1% for skin flaps and revascularized loops and 10% for gastric transposition. Many surgeons would agree that for smaller lesions a free jejunal loop is the best treatment, with gastric transposition reserved for larger tumours.

3. Combined therapy. Postoperative radiotherapy is carried out within 6 weeks of surgical resection as a combined treatment, with the aims of destroying metastases and maximizing the recurrence-free life interval. It is indicated if surgical resection margins are close to or involved in tumour and in most large tumours requiring surgery.

4. Palliation. This therapy is for those patients with advanced end-stage disease, severe intercurrent illness, poor general condition, distant metastases, or those who refuse treatment.

Follow-up and aftercare   On the 10th postoperative day, if there is no evidence of graft failure or leak, the patient can be tested with a methylene blue or gastrograffin swallow. If there is no evidence of extravasation, the patient can be commenced on fluids and then soft diet. Most patients will require thyroid, calcium and calciferol replacement for life. Speech rehabilitation is difficult in these patients, but there are some encouraging reports with low-pressure speech valves (e.g. provox). Patients should be regularly reviewed in the clinic and their nutritional status and swallowing ability should be monitored along with a careful examination for primary and secondary recurrence.

Further reading

Jones AS. The management of early hypopharyngeal cancer: primary radiotherapy and salvage surgery. *Clinical Otolaryngology*, 1992; **17**: 545–9.
Stell PM, Swift AC. Tumours of the hypopharynx. In: Stell PM (ed.) *Scott-Brown's Otolaryngology,* Vol. 5, 5th edn. London: Butterworths, 1987; 250–63.
UICC, Hermanek P, Sabin LH (eds) *TNM Classification of Malignant Tumours,* 4th edn. Berlin: Springer Verlag, 1992.

Related topics of interest

IMPEDANCE AUDIOMETRY

Sound perception

The ear responds equally, not to equal increments, but to equal multiples of sound intensity. In other words, intensity is exponentially related to loudness perception and therefore a logarithmic scale in measuring loudness is necessary. The bel is the log to the base 10 of the ratio of the sound intensity being measured to a reference intensity which is constant, and is measured in W/m^2. The decibel is 10 times this ratio. Therefore:

$$\text{Sound intensity in dB} = 10 \log_{10} \text{intensity}$$

Since sound intensity is proportional to the square of the sound pressure then:

$$\text{Sound pressure in dB} = 10 \log_{10} \text{pressure}^2 \text{ or}$$
$$= 20 \log_{10} \text{pressure}$$

$\log_{10}2$ is about 0.3, so doubling sound intensity corresponds to a 3 dB increase. Each 10 dB increase represents a 10-fold increase in the intensity of sound ($\log_{10} 10 = 1$), a 3.3-fold increase in sound pressure, but the perception of only doubling the loudness.

Impedance

The middle-ear and mastoid air cells communicate with the nasopharynx via the Eustachian tube. As a closed system, air is being continually absorbed by the lining mucosa but is periodically replaced when the Eustachian tube opens, during the act of swallowing. Sound transmission from the external to the inner ear is optimal when the compliance of the middle-ear system is maximal, i.e. when the pressure in the middle ear is equal to the pressure in the external auditory meatus. Compliance (or admittance) is the measure of this system to allow the passage of sound energy through it, and is inversely related to impedance, which is the resistance to the passage of sound energy. The mass, stiffness and frictional resistance of the medium through which the sound wave travels contribute to the impedance, which at low frequency is stiffness dominated. Strictly speaking, compliance is the reciprocal of stiffness so that impedance measurements at low frequency are usually referred to as the compliance.

Basic principles	Impedance audiometry consists of three tests: tympanometry, acoustic reflex testing and static compliance. All three tests work on the same basic principle. The test probe consists of a sound producer, a sound receiver and a device for altering the air pressure within the external auditory meatus (EAM). The probe has a soft plastic or rubber tip to allow an airtight seal in the EAM. A test tone is made (220 Hz, 65 dB) into the EAM, of which some will be absorbed (admitted) by the middle-ear system ('drum and ossicles) and some reflected. The reflected sound energy is measured by the probe microphone. The compliance, that is the amount of sound absorbed by the middle-ear system, can be determined either by measuring the reflected sound level in the ear canal or more commonly by measuring the amount of energy required to keep the sound level constant at varying ear canal pressures. The compliance will be maximal when the ear canal pressure is equal to middle-ear pressure, that is when there is no pressure differential across the tympanic membrane. A tracing of the compliance as ear canal pressure alters allows this and other parameters to be determined.

Clinical uses

1. Tympanometry. This test is the most commonly used aspect of impedance audiometry and is particularly useful in evaluating children with otitis media with effusion. Here compliance is measured continuously while the pressure in the EAM is automatically varied from +200 to −400 mmH_2O. This gives a graphical result which can be classified into one of three groups.

Type A. Maximal compliance occurs when the pressure in the EAM is between +50 and −100 mmH_2O. A normal maximal compliance value is between 2 and 4 ml. A low value for maximal compliance indicates stiffness of the middle-ear system as in tympanosclerosis or otosclerosis. A high or unrecordable peak of compliance indicates excess mobility of the middle-ear system as in ossicular discontinuity or atelectasis.

Type B. A low-value flat or horizontal compliance trace occurs, implying persistently low compliance. This is usually taken to indicate fluid in the middle-ear cavity, and in young children (< 7 years) with glue ear can be correlated with audiometric hearing loss. A type B tympanogram will also occur in the presence of a perforation in the tympanic membrane but the ear canal volume will be large (> 6 ml) because it is measuring that of the middle-ear cleft too. It can occasionally be useful in confirming this diagnosis or to test the patency of a ventilation tube.

Type C. This group give a peak compliance when the pressure in the EAM is <-100 mmH$_2$O. This indicates a significant low pressure in the middle-ear system and is a sign of Eustachian tube dysfunction. The C curve can be subdivided into C1, when the peak is between -100 and -199 mmH$_2$O, and C2, when the peak occurs at less than 200 mmH$_2$O.

2. Acoustic reflex measurement. Acoustic reflexes are measured at the ear canal pressure producing maximum compliance, which corresponds to middle-ear pressure. Ipsilateral reflexes are recorded using the tympanometry probe; contralateral reflexes use a monaural headset to deliver sound to the non-probe ear. It is usual to test at 0.5 kHz and then at either 1 or 2 kHz. A sound intensity of 70–90 dB above the pure tone threshold at that frequency is required to elicit a reflex in a normal-hearing subject, although in one who has a recruiting sensorineural hearing loss a reflex may be present only 10 dB above threshold. The compliance, which is constant for the ear canal pressure selected, is recorded as a horizontal line and shows a dip on contraction of stapedius muscle, representing a reduction in compliance. The stapedial reflex is a complex crossed reflex and demands an intact afferent arm, brain stem and VIIth cranial nerve. As such, the acoustic reflex can provide diagnostic information with regard to the site of a neurological lesion based on the pattern of response to ipsi- and contralateral testing.

It is important to remember that a conductive hearing loss of only 5 dB may result in an absent ipsilateral and contralateral (for reasons that have not been satisfactorily explained) reflex, although it is not until there is a 15 dB air–bone gap that the reflex is absent in 50% of cases.

Adaption (stapedial reflex decay) is determined by producing a persistent tone in the test ear and measuring the reflex in the contralateral ear. Normal adaption occurs only after 10 seconds, decay being no more than 50%.

Summary of the value of measuring the acoustic reflex:
(a) Assesses the integrity of the facial nerve up to the branch to stapedius tendon.
(b) Assesses recruitment and stapedial reflex decay, the latter in particular being an accurate pointer in distinguishing a

cochlear (recruiting) from a retrocochlear (abnormal decay) lesion.

(c) Assess the presence of a conductive hearing loss.

(d) Assess brainstem function.

3. Static compliance. The least used of the three tests. The compliance is measured with an air pressure of +200 mmH$_2$O in the EAM, and this figure is subtracted from the maximal compliance, regardless of the pressure in the EAM at which this occurs. The normal range for this is from 0.3 to 1.6 ml. A figure greater than 2.0 ml implies the presence of a tympanic membrane perforation.

Conclusion

Impedance audiometry is rapid and easy to use. It provides an objective measure of middle-ear function, can help to distinguish cochlear from retrocochlear hearing loss, as well as localizing brainstem and facial nerve lesions. It is, however, essential that the results are interpreted in the context of other clinical findings.

Further reading

Ballantyne D. *Handbook of Audiological Techniques*. London: Butterworth-Heinemann, 1990.

Jerger J, Hayes D. Clinical use of acoustic impedance testing in audiological diagnosis. In: Beagley HA (ed.) *Audiology and Audiological Medicine*, Oxford: Oxford University Press, 1981.

Related topics of interest

Acoustic neuroma (p. 1)
Clinical assessment of hearing (p. 58)
Facial nerve palsy (p. 102)
Otitis media with effusion (p. 214)
Pure tone audiometry (p. 255)
Speech audiometry (p. 291)

INTRINSIC RHINITIS

Intrinsic rhinitis (IR) is an inflammatory condition of the nasal mucosa which is probably better described by the title non-infective, non-allergic rhinitis. There is a combination of nasal obstruction and watery rhinorrhoea of unknown aetiology.

Pathology

IR can be divided into two types, eosinophilic and non-eosinophilic, on the basis of the numbers of eosinophils found in the nasal secretions, and to some extent the clinical features.

1. Non-eosinophilic rhinitis is twice as common as the eosinophilic type and is felt to be due to an imbalance in the autonomic nerve supply. Underactivity of the sympathetic system leads to nasal obstruction, while overactivity of the parasympathetic leads to rhinorrhoea.

2. Eosinophilic IR is probably an intrinsic mucosal disorder of prostaglandin metabolism. In this type there is an association with aspirin hypersensitivity, asthma and nasal polyposis.

There is glandular hyperplasia and submucosal vascular dilation in both types. The nasal mucosa becomes hyperaemic and hypertrophic. Eosinophil-laden polyps are more common in IR than in allergic rhinitis. Hypertrophy of the inferior turbinates is common.

Predisposing factors

- Familial tendency.
- Preceding infection (nasal mucosal hyper-reactivity following viral or bacterial rhinitis).
- Psychological and emotional factors.
- Endocrine (puberty, menstruation and pregnancy).
- Drugs (hypotensive agents, e.g. beta blockers and methyl dopa, aspirin, oral contraceptives).
- Pollution (atmospheric pollution, fumes, dust, industrial detergents and cigarette smoke).
- Atmospheric conditions (changes in humidity and temperature).
- Alcohol.
- Smoking.

Clinical features

IR accounts for 40–70% of all cases of perennial rhinitis and becomes more common with increasing age. All patients exhibit nasal obstruction and rhinorrhoea or postnasal space discharge, but itching and sneezing are less common than in allergic rhinitis. Characteristically, eosinophilic IR produces more nasal obstruction and less discharge than the non-eosinophilic variant. Conversely non-eosinophilic IR is characterized by watery nasal secretions. There may be associated nasal polyps in the eosinophilic form and anosmia is more likely. Examination generally reveals wet, and particularly in eosinophilic IR, hypertrophic inferior turbinates, which are usually red, with a consequent reduction in the airway.

Investigations

IR is a diagnosis of exclusion, and the aim of investigations is to identify other causes of rhinitis. IgE estimation by PRIST and RAST and skin testing can be used to indicate an allergy. Radiographical examination of the sinuses may help diagnose sinus infection. Nasal cytology brushings can be performed to assess the proportion of eosinophils, and a neutrophilia suggests infection.

Management

1. Medical.
(a) Intranasal steroids. The eosinophilic variant responds well to topical intranasal steroid preparations (e.g. beclomethasone dipropionate, fluticasone, betamethasone). In contrast, the non-eosinophilic variant responds little if at all.
(b) Antihistamines are useful in some cases. Older preparations such as chlorpheniramine have anticholinergic effects and are to be preferred.
(c) Topical ipratropium bromide is useful, especially in reducing rhinorrhoea.
(d) Systemic sympathomimetics can be helpful (e.g. pseudoephedrine), though they may produce unpleasant side-effects such as dry mouth, constipation and excitability. They should not be used long term or in children.
(e) Local nasal decongestants. Self-medication with topical vasoconstrictors (e.g. xylometazoline, ephedrine) is common and initially successful in bringing relief to the patient with enlarged inferior turbinates by reducing blood flow in them. Unfortunately, when the effects wear off, there is a reflex vasodilatation causing increased blood flow and turbinate engorgement (rebound phenomenon). Prolonged use leads to an aggravation of symptoms, which eventually become unresponsive to the decongestant, and rhinitis medicamentosa may supervene. The treatment is to stop the decongestant and prescribe topical nasal steroids.

2. *Surgical.* Surgical treatment is useful for the control of symptoms, particularly nasal obstruction, when medical treatment becomes ineffective.

(a) Treatment of concomitant problems. Associated nasal polyps are treated with excision or topical intra-nasal steroids as appropriate. Correction of septal deflections and spurs should be considered to relieve an obstructed airway.

(b) Turbinate surgery. Most procedures are aimed at reducing the bulk of the inferior turbinate to improve the airway. Submucosal diathermy, linear diathermy, laser cautery, cryosurgery and multiple out-fractures are all successful in the short term, but obstruction recurs after 1–2 years. Inferior turbinectomy is associated with slightly higher morbidity from postoperative haemorrhage but is more successful for long-term symptom control. The theoretical risk of atrophic rhinitis has not materialized.

(c) Vidian neurectomy. This operation divides the parasympathetic nerve supply to the nose as the nerve of the pterygoid canal (Vidian nerve) enters the pterygopalatine fossa. Initial enthusiasm for Vidian neurectomy for the relief of rhinorrhoea without nasal obstruction waned when it became apparent that over 50% of patients relapsed within 1 year.

Further reading

Jones AS, Lancer JM. Vasomotor rhinitis (editorial). *British Medical Journal*, 1987; **294**: 1505–6.

Related topics of interest

Allergic rhinitis (p. 16)
Examination of the nose (p. 93)
Nasal polyps (p. 172)

LABYRINTHITIS

Labyrinthitis is an inflammation of the labyrinth and may be classified into serous labyrinthitis, suppurative labyrinthitis, perilabyrinthitis and paralabyrinthitis. Three important definitions are provided to aid their understanding.

Labyrinthine fistula

A labyrinthine fistula is a bony erosion of the labyrinthine capsule to expose but not breach the endosteum of the labyrinth. A breach will usually result in a dead ear. A fistula most commonly occurs in the dome of the lateral semicircular canal.

Tullio phenomenon

The Tullio phenomenon is defined as vertigo in the presence of loud sounds. The phenomenon occurs when sound energy is transmitted from a mobile stapes footplate to the labyrinth, which is distensible only when there is a fistula. Historically the phenomenon occurred in patients with syphilis or if a fenestration procedure was performed in the presence of a mobile footplate, this scenario arising in the 1950s in patients with severe adhesive otitis. The phenomenon may also arise in those with endolymphatic hydrops, when it is thought to be secondary to sound energy transmission from the footplate to the distended saccule, which may be touching the undersurface of the footplate in advanced cases.

The positive fistula sign

In the presence of a labyrinthine fistula, raising the ear canal pressure of the affected side may cause conjugate deviation of the eyes away from the affected ear. The mechanism is pressure transmission to the labyrinth, causing endolymph movement and stimulation of the labyrinthine sense organs. This occurs either directly if there is labyrinth endosteum exposed to the ear canal after mastoid surgery or indirectly if endosteum is covered by disease that can transmit the pressure wave, such as cholesteatoma. On occasion it may occur by a similar mechanism to the Tullio phenomenon. Releasing the pressure allows the deviated eyes to return to the midline.

Perilabyrinthitis

Perilabyrinthitis is a *syndrome* caused by a labyrinthine fistula after mastoid surgery in the presence of retained labyrinthine function. The fistula may have been present but silent before surgery, for example when secondary to cholesteatoma, the mass of the cholesteatoma sac preventing distension of the labyrinthine endosteum. Alternatively, the fistula may be iatrogenic. The hallmarks of perilabyrinthitis are the *Tullio phenomenon* and a *positive fistula sign*. Vertigo may also arise in perilabyrinthitis on windy days when the relatively cooler wind produces a thermal gradient across the labyrinth and a difference in the density of endolymph at each end of the semicircular canal to cause circulation of the endolymph within the canal.

Treatment consists in occluding the meatus with cotton wool when outdoors or grafting the fistula with temporalis fascia, sealing the graft with fibrin glue and a temporalis muscle flap.

Paralabyrinthitis

This is vertigo occurring in the presence of CSOM when inflammation close to the endosteum of the labyrinth causes an irritative nystagmus, that is a nystagmus towards the affected ear.

Serous and suppurative labyrinthitis

Serous labyrinthitis is a retrospective diagnosis and depends on there being some recovery of cochlear and vestibular function after an attack of postulated bacterial labyrinthitis. The symptoms and signs are identical to suppurative labyrinthitis, except that in the latter the loss of inner ear function is irreversible.

Clinical features

The labyrinthitis is usually secondary to CSOM but may also be a complication of ASOM via the round window, meningitis or rarely be blood borne. In the presence of the clinical features of the precipitating cause there is an acute onset of violent, overwhelming vertigo that is so severe it inhibits the perception of tinnitus and hearing loss. There may be a short period of irritative jerk nystagmus towards the affected ear, but soon a paralytic jerk nystagmus to the healthy ear ensues. Tiny movements of the head exacerbate the vertigo so that the patient prefers to lie completely still on one side, and in the presence of a paralytic nystagmus the affected ear will be uppermost. In this position the patient will tend to look voluntarily in the direction of the affected side (especially in the presence of visitors), reducing the drive from the unaffected ear so that the corrective nystagmus and therefore the vertigo will be less severe. This can be understood when we explain that the normal labyrinth causes conjugate deviation of the eyes to the opposite side so that if one labyrinth is paralysed the opposite labyrinth will become dominant and deviate the eyes to the side of the affected ear, the nystagmus occurring as a corrective measure. Initially there is third-degree nystagmus, that is nystagmus in any direction of lateral gaze. As compensation occurs, second-degree nystagmus develops (nystagmus when gazing straight ahead or looking in the direction of the nystagmus) and then first-degree nystagmus (nystagmus only when looking in the direction of the nystagmus). Finally there is absence of nystagmus on optic fixation.

Investigations of labyrinthitis

The diagnosis is made from the clinical features occurring in the presence of a precipitating factor. If possible, the ears should be examined under the microscope, and after removal of all debris a labyrinthine fistula may be visible. If there are no features to suggest a meningitis, the important diagnosis not to miss is a cerebellar abscess, of which the symptoms and signs are different but may be difficult to recognize in a patient continuously vomiting. An enhanced MRI CT scan will be necessary in these circumstances. Sequential pure tone audiometry and ENG will allow the monitoring of recovery, although hearing loss and vestibular failure are permanent with purulent labyrinthitis.

Management of labyrinthitis

Treatment of both the precipitating factor and the labyrinthitis is necessary.

- An ear culture swab and appropriate antibiotics, broad spectrum until results of the swab are available.
- Bed rest, avoiding head movements.
- Vestibular sedatives.
- Intravenous fluids if vomiting.
- If the precipitating factor was CSOM, exploration of the mastoid after recovery from the acute symptoms should be considered. A labyrinthine fistula may have arisen from chronic osteitis or cholesteatoma. The chronic disease should be eradicated, and if a fistula is identified the treatment is as described above.

Follow up and aftercare

After recovery from the acute infection, Cooksey–Cawthorne exercises may accelerate central compensation. A walking stick may be useful. Counselling is a necessary but often overlooked part of the management. Even with complete central compensation, patients with unilateral labyrinthine failure will still be unsteady in the dark, if they develop a severe illness (allows inhibition of central compensation) or if they should develop a neuropathy affecting the peripheral proprioceptors.

Further reading

Shepard NT, Telian SA, Smith-Wheelock M, Raj A. Vestibular and balance rehabilitation therapy. *Annals of Otology Rhinology and Laryngology*, 1993; **102:** 198–205.

Related topics of interest

Chronic suppurative otitis media – complications (p. 55)
Vertigo (p. 334)
Vestibular function tests (p. 338)

LARYNGEAL CARCINOMA

Pathology

Squamous cell carcinoma of the larynx is the commonest head and neck cancer in the Western world and represents approximately 1% of all malignancies in men. In some areas of India and Malaysia it is the most common cancer and is probably related to variations in smoking habit. It is about five times commoner in males than in females. The incidence increases with age, but the peak age of presentation is in the seventh decade. The cause of cancer of the larynx is not known, but persons who smoke tobacco and drink alcohol are predisposed to the disease. It is very rare in non-smokers. Alcohol on its own is probably not a cause of laryngeal cancer but it is highly synergistic with smoking. Verrucous carcinoma is a distinct variant of well-differentiated squamous cell carcinoma. Adenocarcinoma, adenoid cystic carcinoma, fibrosarcoma, chondrosarcoma and lymphomas are all rare.

For classification purposes, the larynx is divided into three regions which each include a number of sites:

1. Supraglottis. This comprises the larynx superior to the apex of the ventricle. It includes the ventricle, vestibular folds, arytenoids, aryepiglottic folds and the laryngeal surface of the epiglottis. The lingual surface of the epiglottis and the vallecula are in the oropharynx.

2. Glottis. This comprises the vocal cords and the anterior and posterior commissures. It extends from the apex of the laryngeal ventricle to 1 cm below. Some authorities hold that the superior and inferior borders of the glottis correspond to the superior and inferior arcuate lines, respectively.

3. Subglottis. This extends from the inferior border of the glottis to the lower border of the cricoid cartilage.

Laryngeal tumours are diverse in their behaviour and prognosis and thus there have been many endeavours to classify them. Clinical staging attempts to group together features which may share a level of prognosis or a certain treatment. In cancer of the larynx, clinical staging is the only generally reliable criterion of any prognostic significance, and even with this standard there is considerable variability. The TNM system is based on the number of sites affected and the mobility of the vocal cords. It is slightly different for each site but, in summary, a tumour can be described as either:

T1(a) Limited to one site.

T1(b) In two sites but within one region.

T2 Affecting two or more regions, but vocal cords mobile.

T3 Confined to the larynx with a fixed vocal cord.

T4 Spread outside the larynx.

The presence of palpable lymph nodes is the most important factor in determining prognosis, but assessment of lymphadenopathy is subjective. About one-third of patients with no palpable lymph nodes have histologically invaded nodes, and a similar number of palpable nodes are not invaded by tumour. The supraglottis has a rich lymphatic drainage, and a high proportion of these tumours spread to cervical lymph nodes. The subglottis drains to paratracheal and mediastinal nodes in addition to the cervical lymph node. The glottis has virtually no lymphatic drainage, so metastases usually only occur when the tumour has spread to involve the supraglottis and subglottis in the so-called transglottic tumour. Some authorities maintain that transglottic tumours arise from the laryngeal ventricle.

Clinical features

The clinical features of malignant disease are dictated by the primary tumour, secondary deposits and the general effects of cancer. The symptoms and signs of a laryngeal tumour depend on the way in which it is related to the upper aerodigestive tract. Hoarseness is the commonest and often the only presenting symptom. Dyspnoea and stridor are late symptoms and almost invariably indicate an advanced tumour. Pain is an uncommon symptom but is most typical in supraglottic tumours. Patients with a cancer in this site may complain of a unilateral sore throat. There may be referred otalgia. Dysphagia indicates invasion of the pharynx. Swelling of the neck may be due to direct penetration of the tumour outside the larynx or to lymph node metastases. Cough and irritation of the throat are occasional symptoms. The general symptoms of anorexia, cachexia and fetor imply advanced disease.

There should be a general examination to identify distant metastases and an assessment of the overall physical status of the patient. Indirect laryngoscopy should allow an inspection of the primary tumour site and size. Vocal cord mobility should also be assessed. There are three areas which are difficult to examine by this technique: the subglottis, the laryngeal surface of the epiglottis and the laryngeal ventricle. All patients should, therefore, also undergo fibreoptic laryngoscopy. The neck should be carefully palpated for the presence of enlarged lymph nodes. Examination must include an assessment of the number, mobility and level of the nodes. Laryngeal tumours usually metastasize to the upper deep cervical lymph nodes, but supraglottic tumours may cause bilateral nodes, and some subglottic tumours may spread to the upper mediastinal nodes.

Investigations

A chest radiograph, full blood count and serum analysis are baseline investigations prior to a general anaesthetic. The serum analysis should be inspected to uncover deranged liver function raising suspicion of liver metastases, or hypoproteinaemia, which may indicate malnourishment and a possibility of poor wound healing. The chest radiograph should be carefully examined to exclude metastases or to assess intercurrent lung disease. MRI or CT scans of the larynx and neck provide further information about the primary tumour. Imaging may also uncover the presence of impalpable or occult nodes. A CT scan of the chest may be indicated if suspected lung metastases need further delineation. An ultrasound scan of the liver is required if hepatic metastases are suspected and in some units this is routine prior to major surgery. An isotope bone scan is indicated only if symptoms suggest bony metastases or there is a raised serum calcium or alkaline phosphatase. Distant metastases are unusual in laryngeal carcinoma at presentation (1%).

Direct laryngoscopy under general anaesthesia is mandatory. In addition, the patient should have a full parendoscopy including bronchoscopy. The incidence of a synchronous second primary tumour in the head, neck or lung is in the region of 1%. All the larynx sites should be inspected systematically. The tumour's position and extension should be recorded by means of a diagram in the case notes. Biopsy material should include an adequate amount of representative tissue to obtain a definitive diagnosis of malignancy, identification of the tumour type and tumour differentiation. Cord mobility should be assessed if not done already. While the patient's neck muscles are relaxed under general anaesthetic the neck should be palpated for nodes which may not have been noted previously.

The information from the investigations of the patient allow the surgeon to 'stage' the tumour according to the TNM classification and manage it accordingly.

Management

Each patient will fall into one of the following treatment categories depending on their age, general condition, and stage of the tumour: curative treatment or palliative treatment.

1. Curative treatment may involve radiotherapy, surgery or a combination of these two modalities. As a general rule, small tumours are treated by radical radiotherapy in the first instance, with surgery reserved for recurrence. Large tumours are treated with primary surgery, usually with postoperative radiotherapy.

(a) Glottic tumours: in the UK, radiotherapy is the conventional treatment of choice for T1 and T2 glottic tumours, giving cure rates in excess of 90%. Alternatively, small tumours confined to one vocal cord can be treated by cordectomy. Many T3 glottic tumours are treated in the first instance by radiotherapy, but larger tumours causing stridor will need a total laryngectomy, sometimes as an emergency procedure. T4 tumours will be treated by total laryngectomy and a radical neck dissection if there are any nodal metastases.

(b) Supraglottic tumours: T1 and T2 tumours are usually treated by radiotherapy, but larger tumours will require treatment by either a supraglottic laryngectomy or total laryngectomy.

(c) Subglottic tumours: pure subglottic cancer is very unusual. The subglottis becomes involved in extensive glottic and transglottic carcinoma. Small tumours may be treated by radiotherapy, but these tumours often present late and the patient needs a total laryngectomy. It is important that the upper mediastinum is included in the radical treatment regimen.

2. Palliative treatment includes pain relief, tracheostomy, palliative radiotherapy, chemotherapy and occasionally surgery.

Follow-up and aftercare   Patients who have had potentially curative treatment should be carefully examined for signs of primary recurrence, neck node spread and distant metastases, and have their weight recorded in the outpatient clinic on a regular basis. This should be monthly for the first 12 months, then every 2 months for 6 months, every 3 months for 6 months, then 6 monthly for the next 3 years. Some units continue to monitor patients as the incidence of second primary tumours is in the region of 10–20%. Patients who have had a laryngectomy will require speech therapy. They will also require monitoring of their thyroid function and calcium levels if there has been a thyroid gland excision.

Further reading

DeSanto LW. Cancer of the larynx. *Current Opinion in Otolaryngology and Head and Neck Surgery*, 1993; **1**: 133–6.

Stell PM. Review. Prognostic factors in laryngeal carcinoma. *Clinical Otolaryngology*, 1988: **13**: 399–409.

UICC, Hermanek P and Sabin CH (eds) *TNM Classification of Malignant Tumours,* 4th edn. Berlin: Springer Verlag, 1992.

Related topics of interest

LARYNGEAL PAPILLOMA

Squamous cell papilloma is by far the commonest benign tumour of the larynx. Adenomas, chondromas, fibromas, haemangiomas and other neurogenic and mesodermal benign tumours are all rare and will not be considered further.

Aetiology

The aetiology of laryngeal papillomas is now known to be infection of the epithelial cells with human papillomavirus (HPV), particularly HPV types 6 and 11. It is thought that in some patients the disease is transmitted at the time of delivery from a mother infected with genital warts. Electron microscopy and immunofluorescent techniques have shown that human papillomavirus DNA is incorporated into the host's cellular DNA. Polymerase chain reaction is now the most sensitive technique available to show evidence of HPV infection. Apparently normal mucosa cells adjacent to the papillomas also contain viral DNA, which may become activated to form a recurrent lesion. This partly explains the difficulty in curing the disease.

Pathology

Squamous papillomas usually occur at any age from birth to 5 years. They may grow anywhere in the respiratory tract from the lips to the lungs, but the vocal cords, anterior commissure and vestibular folds are the commonest sites of involvement. The lesions have a predilection for points of airway constriction, where there is increased airflow, drying, crusting and irritation. Laryngeal mucus is thought to behave as a protective blanket in some sites, for example the interarytenoid area. The growths may present as scattered single lesions or clusters or as a huge exuberant mass. They can be sessile or pedunculated and are characteristically non-keratinizing with a connective tissue core.

Clinical features

Hoarseness of voice or an abnormal cry is the usual presenting symptom. Respiratory obstruction and increasing stridor are late manifestations of the disease process.

Investigations

Endoscopy is required to establish the diagnosis, obtain tissue for confirmatory histology and to assess the extent of the disease and potential risk to the patient's airway. Treatment can also then be initiated.

Treatment

The aim of treatment is to remove the papillomas as they appear, to maintain a safe patent airway and laryngeal function, without damaging the larynx in the process, and to wait for resolution of the condition. Remission can take place at any age and does not seem to be related to treatment. It is most likely to occur if the disease presents between the ages of 6 and 10 years and if the disease is confined to the larynx.

1. Surgery is the most satisfactory treatment of this condition. The treatment of choice is the removal of all the lesions using a laser, and repetition of this procedure at intervals. This increases the remission rate to approximately 50% in patients below 16 years of age. If disease is found to involve the anterior commissure, two operations 4 weeks apart are required to avoid web formation, treating first one cord then the other. Tracheostomy should be avoided if possible as the papillomas can become implanted into the trachea and bronchi.

2. Non-surgical treatments. Alpha interferon has been shown to significantly reduce the growth rate of papillomas in one-third of patients. Isotretinoin (13-*cis*-retinoic acid) produces a significant response in about two-thirds of patients. Because of treatment side-effects and uncertain response these treatments should be reserved for cases requiring frequent (i.e. more than 1–2 monthly) laser treatment, or if the trachea and bronchi become involved. It has been claimed that the antiviral drug ribavirin is a useful adjuvant to surgery, but further trials are required to substantiate this. Radiotherapy was used in the past, but should be avoided as it predisposes to malignant change. Squamous cell carcinoma and verrucous carcinoma are also more likely to occur in adults if the patient smokes.

Single papilloma

Single papillomas are usually seen in adults, arising from the free edge of a vocal cord. It is liable to recurrence and malignant degeneration. The papilloma should be removed at direct laryngoscopy. The patients should be followed up for 5 years because of the risk of recurrence and malignant change.

Follow-up and aftercare

Laser laryngoscopy is repeated as often as necessary to preserve the airway and the voice in those cases which do recur.

Further reading

Eicher SA, Taylor-Cooley LD, Donovan DT. Isotretinoin therapy for recurrent respiratory papillomatosis. *Archives of Otolaryngology and Head and Neck Surgery,* 1994; **120:** 405–9.

Leuenthal BG, Kashima HK, Mounts P *et al.* Longterm response of recurrent respiratory papillomatosis to treatment with lymphoblastoid interferon alpha-n1. *New England Journal of Medicine,* 1991; **325:** 613–7.

McGlennen RC *et al.* Pilot trial of ribavirin for the treatment of laryngeal papillomatosis. *Head and Neck,* 1993; **15:** 504–13.

Terry RM *et al.* Demonstration of human papillomavirus types 6 and 11 in juvenile laryngeal papillometosis by *in situ* hybridisation. *Journal of Pathology,* 1987; **153:** 245–8.

Related topics of interest

Lasers in ENT (p. 161)
Paediatric airway problems (p. 234)
Paediatric endoscopy (p. 239)
Stridor and stertor (p. 301)

LARYNGECTOMY

The choice between surgery and radiotherapy as treatment for carcinoma of the larynx should be made according to the likely effective control of the cancer, the general health of the patient and the relative consequences of the treatment. With both a laryngectomy and radiotherapy there is invariably some or total loss of normal voice and compromise of airway protection and function. Radiotherapy has the advantage of vastly reduced morbidity compared with surgery. In general in the UK, radiotherapy is reserved for smaller tumours (T1 and T2), whereas surgery is considered more effective for larger tumours (T3 and T4) and where there are secondary deposits of carcinoma in the lymph nodes of the neck. It has been shown that T3 laryngeal tumours can be treated initially by radiation with salvage surgery for any subsequent recurrence without a reduction in the overall cure. The other less common malignant neoplasms of the larynx (adenocarcinoma, verrucous carcinoma, fibrosarcoma, chondrosarcoma, etc.) are invariably treated by laryngectomy.

Types of laryngectomy

1. Vertical partial resection.
(a) Cordectomy.
(b) Hemilaryngectomy.

2. Horizontal partial resection.
(a) Epiglottectomy.
(b) Supraglottic laryngectomy.

3. Total laryngectomy.

Investigations

A panendoscopy should always be performed by the surgeon prior to operation. This will allow a representative biopsy to be obtained, the tumour to be staged and the appropriate operation planned.

The patient should be investigated to allow surgery to proceed and to exclude distant metastases. A CT or MRI scan of the larynx should be obtained. A chest radiograph and liver ultrasound scan are essential (in addition many authoriites would advocate a chest CT scan). Serum urea and electrolytes, liver function tests and a full blood count will be required. The patient should be cross-matched for 2 units if a total laryngectomy is proposed. Written confirmation of the histological diagnosis must be in the case notes or the surgeon should have personally spoken to a senior pathologist to confirm the diagnosis of cancer when a frozen section result is presented.

Patient preparation

The patient should have a clear explanation of the diagnosis and what it means. The operation should be described and the patient should have knowledge of the wounds, drains, nasogastric tube and sutures, etc. It should be remembered that this situation will be distressing for the patient, who should have a relative or close friend present. The patient should be warned before any treatment that there is no guarantee of cure. Specifically for a laryngectomy the patient must be warned that the voice box will be lost and a new technique to speak will need to be learned, a permanent end tracheostome will be necessary, and thyroid and parathyroid supplements may be needed for life following the operation. The explanation and warnings should be logged in the case notes. The speech therapist should see the patient preoperatively.

Cordectomy

This is indicated for a T1a cancer of the glottis which does not reach the anterior commissure or the arytenoid cartilage. Excision can be performed using the KTP or CO_2 laser. It is now performed much less frequently in the UK owing to the equally effective results achieved by radiation. It remains a suitable operation for the removal of benign laryngeal tumours.

Hemilaryngectomy

This technique can be used to remove tumours confined to the vocal cord, with an adequate margin of healthy tissue. It involves removal of half of the thyroid cartilage, with the false and true vocal cords, part of the supraglottis and the upper half of the cricoid cartilage. The resulting gap is closed by the strap muscles, fashioned so as to form a new fixed vocal cord. This procedure therefore has the advantage of allowing some protection for the airway and a reasonable voice for the patient. However, if on histological examination there has been incomplete resection of the lesion, either postoperative radiotherapy or total laryngectomy should be performed. Consent for total laryngectomy should always be obtained before embarking on any partial resection.

Supraglottic laryngectomy

This is indicated for cancer of the supraglottis (epiglottis and laryngeal vestibule). The technique involves removing the entire supraglottis from the vallecula to the ventricle, and joining the lower half of the larynx to the base of the tongue. Cricopharyngeal myotomy is considered an essential manoeuvre to make swallowing easier. The operation is not suitable if the tumour extends to the base of tongue or vocal cords, if the patient is over the age of 65 years or if there is intercurrent lung disease. It should be preceded by direct laryngoscopy to assess the extent of disease and likelihood of successful resection. If the operation is to be carried out for post-radiotherapy recurrence, it is important that the extent of the original lesion is known.

Total laryngectomy

Total laryngectomy is indicated for the curative treatment of laryngeal carcinoma when the tumour is considered to be unsuitable for either radiotherapy or a partial resection. It is also indicated as salvage surgery in failed radiotherapy, as a palliative measure in some advanced cases of carcinoma and as a last resort in those who have no voice and chronic aspiration due to palsy of the IXth, Xth and XIth cranial nerves. The technique involves removing the hyoid bone, thyroid and cricoid cartilages and several rings of the proximal trachea and an ipsilateral thyroid lobectomy or total thyroidectomy. The main disadvantages of this procedure are that the patient's normal voice is lost and a permanent end tracheostome is required. All patients having a total laryngectomy should have a speech valve inserted at the time of the operation.

Emergency laryngectomy

An emergency laryngectomy is a laryngectomy performed on a patient with airway compromise due to carcinoma, within 24 h of presentation, without a prior tracheostomy.

The rationale for this procedure is based on the dismal prognosis for any patient who develops a tumour recurrence in their tracheostome: so-called stomal recurrence. Performing a tracheostomy for the relief of airway obstruction due to carcinoma prior to any definitive treatment is associated with a high rate of stomal recurrence. This could be due to tumour seeding at the time of tracheostomy, to inadequate resection or to a second primary. A number of solutions have been offered to this problem. Some groups have argued that if definitive treatment is undertaken within 48 hours of the tracheostomy the rate of stomal recurrence is not increased. This has never been properly substantiated. More recently, the laser has been used to debulk the tumour and improve the airway, after laryngoscopy and biopsy. This has the advantage of avoiding any surgical disturbance of the regional anatomy, yet secures the airway while the biopsy results are awaited, the patient counselled and further treatment planned.

Emergency laryngectomy was developed to provide definitive treatment for both the airway obstruction and the laryngeal carcinoma at the same sitting. However, the patient and surgeon have little time to prepare for major surgery in which the normal voice will be lost, and the diagnosis is based on frozen section biopsy. Despite this the stomal recurrence rate (<5%), overall morbidity and mortality are no different to those of elective laryngectomy. For these reasons emergency laryngectomies will continue to be performed.

The presumptive diagnosis and the management plan must be explained to the patient, and any accompanying family, as early as possible. The principle of attending hospital and within 24 hours losing your larynx is daunting. Despite this, because of the long prior history of hoarse voice and sometimes dysphagia, and the intercurrent airway compromise, most patients are more than willing to undergo the surgery.

After the investigations have been performed an anaesthetic assessment is required and a senior, experienced pathologist should be contacted to examine the frozen section biopsies.

During the waiting time prior to theatre, as much psychological and rehabilitative preparation as possible should be performed. This should include time for the patient to talk to family, the medical and nursing staff, and the speech therapists who will be attending the patient in the postoperative period.

Once in theatre, a laryngoscopic assessment of the tumour size and extent should be made; biopsies are then taken and submitted to frozen section analysis. If squamous carcinoma is confirmed a standard laryngectomy is performed. The difficulties occur if, despite repeated frozen section biopsies, a carcinoma cannot be found. In these cases it is essential to wait for the paraffin sections. The real dilemma is what to do for the patient's airway. It is safer to debulk the tumour, using a laser if available, to temporarily improve the airway until definitive treatment can be undertaken. If a definitive diagnosis can be made and treatment instituted within 48 hours, it may be justifiable to perform a tracheostomy.

Follow-up and aftercare
Voice rehabilitation and periodic surveillance for recurrence or second tumour are the main features of follow-up. Thyroid function and calcium levels should be checked appropriately.

Further reading

Jones AS, Cook JA, Phillips D, Soler Lluch E. Treatment of T_3 carcinoma of the larynx by surgery or radiotherapy. *Clinical Otolaryngology,* 1992; **17:** 433–6.

McCombe AW, Stell PM. Emergency laryngectomy. *Journal of Laryngology and Otology,* 1991; **105:** 463–5.

Robin PE, Olofsson J. Tumours of the larynx. In: Stell PM (ed.) *Scott-Brown's Otolaryngology,* Vol. 5, 5th edn. London: Butterworths, 1987; 186–234.

Stell PM, Maran AG. *Head and Neck Surgery,* 3rd edn. London: Heinemann, 1994.

Related topics of interest

LASERS IN ENT

Laser is an acronym for light amplification by the stimulated emission of radiation.

Historical

The theoretical foundations for lasers were postulated by Einstein in 1917. In essence, he proposed that electromagnetic radiation (including light) could be produced by an electron of an atom jumping from a high-energy atomic shell to a lower energy shell, thereby releasing a photon of energy. The wavelength of the photon would depend on the energy difference between the two energy shells and so would be identical for all atoms of a specific element or molecule. Should this photon strike an atom or molecule identical to that which released the photon and which is in a high-energy state, another photon will be released, travelling in the same direction as that which stimulated the emission, the electron which released the photon dropping to a lower energy level. The electron must first be stimulated into the higher energy shell by an external energy source, usually electrical. In 1955 microwaves were produced in this fashion and in 1960 the first laser was built by Dr T. Maiman using synthetic ruby crystals.

Technical background

All currently available medical laser devices work in a similar fashion. An optical resonating chamber has a fully reflective mirror at one end and a partially reflective, partially transmitting mirror at the other. Through this chamber is pumped the laser medium, which is stimulated by an electrical current. This results in emitted photons, which bounce around the inside of the chamber; only those parallel to the long axis of the resonating chamber are able to escape through the partially transmitting mirror as laser light. This light is monochromatic (same colour), collimated (parallel and unidirectional) and coherent (intense and in phase) and therefore represents an extremely powerful, high-energy beam. It may then be passed through a lens system for focusing. As this whole process results in the production of heat, the optical chamber is surrounded by a water jacket cooling system.

Types

The carbon dioxide laser produces light in the far-infrared range (wavelength 10 600 nm). Consequently it is invisible to the human eye and the system is usually provided with a low-power helium–neon laser carried coaxially to act as a sighting beam. The Nd-YAG laser has a crystal of neodymium doped-yttrium aluminium garnet stimulated by a krypton arc lamp, produces light of wavelength 1064, in the near-infrared range, and so is also invisible. The argon laser produces visible blue/green light with light at a number of wavelengths but mostly 488–514 nm.. A modification of the Nd-YAG laser is the KTP, in which a crystal of potassium titanyl phosphate is stimulated by a krypton arc lamp to produce a beam of 532 nm visible green light. The wavelength of light produced, and so its tissue effects, depend on the laser medium used.

Tissue effects

All the effects of lasers are due to the local absorption of energy and the subsequent production of heat in the tissues. This laser burn is extremely accurate, and will cause tissue damage which varies with its penetration. The energy of the CO_2 laser is strongly absorbed by any water-containing tissues, regardless of pigmentation, and its effects are extremely localized (0.3 mm penetration). It kills cells by boiling the water content of cells (80% water), which causes a sudden increase in volume and vaporization. The advantage of this is that it can accurately destroy small volumes of tissue with minimal surrounding tissue injury, but its disadvantage is that its poor penetration will certainly not coagulate blood vessels more than 0.5 mm in diameter. When excising lesions in tissue with larger vessels, such as the tongue, a bloodless field will only be gained with a more penetrative laser, the KTP being ideal. Energy from the argon laser is particularly well absorbed by pigmented tissues, notably haemoglobin, which is advantageous in areas where small haemorrhages will prove disastrous, such as the retina of the eye. Tissue penetration is about 1 mm and so it will accurately and reliably coagulate vessels of this diameter. The Nd-YAG laser is prone to light scattering and so tissue effects may be evident 2–4 mm from the target site. It is therefore less precise than the other lasers but will coagulate vessels 1.5–2 mm in diameter. It is mostly used in fibreoptic bronchoscopy and oesophagoscopy, although the KTP laser, by being more precise, may gradually take over this work.

Total energy delivery to the tissues is dependent on the power density of the beam and the duration of exposure. It can be controlled by three methods. The total power of the beam (watts) is set at the laser control panel. The area of the spot is altered by adjusting the focus of the beam. Exposure time (seconds) can also be set at the control panel in pulsed mode or left as continuous mode.

Safety

Medical lasers are class 4 and their use requires extreme caution. A number of protective measures are required and include:

1. Environment. The operating theatre should be designated a laser area and appropriate warning signs displayed. It should be equipped with remote door-locks to prevent non-essential personnel straying into theatre during laser use.

2. Personnel. Access should be limited to essential personnel only and there should be nominated laser users who are fully conversant with the operation and risks of the laser. All theatre personnel are required to wear eye protection.

3. Anaesthetic. There is a potential explosion risk with volatile anaesthetic agents and oxygen. To protect the endotracheal tube, metal tubes, coated tubes and even jet venturi are used.

4. Patient. All exposed parts of the patient adjacent to the operating area are covered with damp swabs to prevent any burns.

Clinical uses

- *Ear.* The argon laser can be used in stapedectomy to divide the crura and fashion a stapedotomy. It has also been used to spot weld tympanoplasty grafts in place.
- *Nose.* The CO_2 laser has been used to perform linear cautery to the inferior turbinates and turbinectomy, in the symptomatic treatment of rhinitis, as well as removing a variety of localized benign intranasal mucosal lesions. However, the KTP laser will be less likely to cause troublesome bleeding in these instances and will vaporize tissue more efficiently but is very expensive. This laser has been used with some success to perform endoscopic dacrocystorhinostomy.
- *Throat.* The CO_2 laser has found most application in ENT in the treatment of laryngeal conditions. Treatment with this laser results in minimal injury to surrounding tissue and minimal postoperative oedema so there is less chance of postoperative airway compromise. Scar tissue formation is also minimized and so the CO_2 laser is the method of choice in the excision of benign lesions from

the vocal cord. These include papillomata, which may be vaporized at a high power setting, polyps, nodules and the division of webs. It can be used to perform an arytenoidectomy and cordectomy in airway compromise due to vocal cord palsy. Recent studies have shown that cordectomy for T1 vocal cord squamous cell carcinoma provides a similar prognosis to radiotherapy regarding tumour recurrence. It provides at least as good voice preservation after healing. Carefully controlled trials are needed to confirm these preliminary findings. Obstructing laryngeal and tracheobronchial tumours may be debulked with this or the KTP laser, and on occasion small tumours have been completely excised. Although the CO_2 laser may be used for excising lesions of the tongue and oral cavity, the KTP laser is the method of choice as bleeding is minimal because of its better penetration.

Photodynamic therapy

This technique has found its greatest use in the treatment of skin cancers. A photosensitive haematoporphyrin derivative which shows preferential uptake by the tumour is administered to the patient. A gold vapour laser emitting a red light is used to activate the photosensitizer, which is stimulated to release singlet oxygen atoms. These are extremely cytotoxic and result in tumour necrosis. This technique has not found a significant application in ENT although its potential for treating laryngeal cancers is currently being investigated.

Related topics of interest

Laryngeal papilloma (p. 153)
Laryngectomy (p. 156)
Otosclerosis (p. 226)
Vocal cord palsy (p. 342)

MASTOIDECTOMY

Mastoidectomy is an operation undertaken on the mastoid air cells to remove disease within the middle-ear cleft. The disease is usually infective but may occasionally be neoplastic. It may also be performed as part of a procedure for access to deeper structures, for example endolymphatic sac surgery.

Incisions
Either an endaural or postaural incision is used. Both are equally popular in the UK. A properly performed endaural incision will allow good access to the attic, tegmen and sigmoid sinus even in well-aerated mastoids. It will not allow sufficient posterior access for a subtotal petrosectomy; this degree of bone removal is routinely performed by some if there is mastoid disease to allow the postauricular soft tissues to fall into the smooth defect, obviating the need for an obliteration procedure. Neither will the endaural incision allow an adequate angle of approach to the middle ear in those who perform a posterior tympanotomy (required for combined approach tympanoplasty and to access the round window in cochlear implants).

Cortical mastoidectomy

This is also know as the Schwartze operation and is used for the treatment of the acute non-cholesteatomatouas mastoiditis when medical treatment has failed or complications have set in. If cholesteatoma is found, the posterior canal wall may be removed and the procedure converted to a modified radical mastoidectomy. A cortical mastoidectomy can also be used as treatment for chronic suppurative otitis media when there is no cholesteatoma, to clear granulation tissue from the mastoid air cells and the antrum. A myringoplasty is performed at the same time, if indicated. Occasionally a cortical mastoidectomy is performed for severe glue ear.

Procedure
A postaural incision is made at least 1 cm behind the skin fold down to the periosteum, which is elevated to expose the whole of the mastoid, including the tip. A high-speed drill is used to remove the outer cortex of the mastoid bone and then all air cells, leaving cortical bone over the sigmoid sinus and middle fossa dura. The posterior canal wall is left intact and the middle-ear contents are not disturbed.

Modified radical mastoidectomy

The routine procedure for cholesteatoma is a modified radical mastoidectomy. This is an operation to remove all middle-ear and mastoid disease, exteriorizing both into a common cavity. Disease-free remnants of the tympanic membrane and ossicular chain are preserved. If all the tympanic membrane, the malleus and incus are removed, the procedure is termed a *'radical mastoidectomy'*.

Procedure

In a modified radical mastoidectomy the disease is either approached from behind or followed back from the middle ear. When approached from behind, a cortical mastoidectomy is performed and the bridge of the posterior canal wall drilled away to continue removal of the disease from the antrum, attic and middle ear (atticoantrostomy). When followed backwards, the attic is removed first, the middle ear explored and then the antrum opened and the bone removed only as far back as the disease. This has the advantage that the cavity is only as big as the extent of disease. Some cases require an atticotomy only. There are a large number of modifications in the way this operation is performed, for instance some surgeons try to remove the canal wall in one piece and then replace it at the end of the procedure.

There are even more variations in the way the reconstruction is done to minimize the chances of chronic or repeated discharge and maximize the hearing. The basic reconstruction involves including the Eustachian tube opening in a reconstructed middle ear using a fascial graft. The graft, usually temporal fascia, is placed under the drum remnant and often over the whole of the mastoid cavity. This appears to encourage squamous epithelium to cover the cavity and it may allow air from the Eustachian tube to fill deep to it and effectively reform a soft posterior canal wall and a near-normal ear canal. The cavity can also be obliterated with bone dust, muscle flaps, artificial substances, e.g. hydroxyapatite, or free muscle. The bony work on the cavity itself is of greater importance than the obliteration substance. All air cells should be removed, the cavity edges must be well saucerized, the mastoid tip removed as far medially as the digastric ridge, the facial ridge lowered to the level of the inferior canal wall and a decent meatoplasty fashioned. These procedures will improve the chance of a dry ear and are especially useful in revision surgery. When all the cells of the mastoid are removed, in particular those in Trautman's triangle, the perifacial, the retrosigmoid, the zygomatic root, and all perilabyrinthine cells, the operation is called a subtotal petrosectomy. This may be combined with Eustachian tube obliteration, closure of the external auditory meatus and filling the cavity with free abdominal fat graft in particularly difficult ears.

Hearing reconstruction   The reconstruction of hearing is dealt with elsewhere, but has to be considered at the same time as the primary surgery even if the tympanoplasty is done as a second stage. Most British surgeons prefer to accept a type III tympanoplasty with the new eardrum in direct contact with the head of the stapes if it is present. This gives a 5–25 dB conductive loss but profers long-term stability. This type III can be encouraged if the posterior annulus is medialized when lowering the facial ridge so that the head of the stapes is relatively more prominent. It is also useful if an edge of bone is formed for the new tympanic membrane to take off from. If the stapes superstructure is not present, the hearing reconstruction is best left to a second stage. Many patients opt for no further surgery or a hearing aid if given the choice. If a second stage is done, a deep middle ear is helpful and this should be encouraged at the first stage by leaving a lateral annulus. At the second stage a piece of bone or an artificial total ossicular chain prosthesis is placed between drum and footplate.

Combined approach tympanoplasty

This operation removes disease from the mastoid and middle ear. A cortical mastoidectomy is extended to remove bone posteriorly over the lateral sinus to allow an adequate angle to visualize the middle-ear contents via a posterior tympanotomy in which the posterior part of the middle ear is entered lateral to the mastoid segment of the facial nerve in the angle between it and the chorda tympani. This allows access to disease via the ear canal as well as via the mastoid. The combined approach tympanoplasty is the main canal wall up procedure. It has a high rate of recurrent cholesteatoma, but if performed skillfully it is suitable for patients who are available for long-term follow-up and second- and third-look surgery.

Complications of mastoidectomy

Injury to the anatomical structures of the temporal bone is the main danger for the patient. The facial nerve is always at risk and damage to it is the most obvious disaster that can occur. The dura and lateral sinus are also at risk, as is the otic capsule. Great care is necessary when removing disease from the lateral semicircular canal as a fistula can be opened and the resulting loss of perilymph may lead to a dead ear. Indeed it may be better to leave disease *in situ* on such occasions. The middle-ear part of a mastoidectomy needs equal care to avoid damage to undiseased ossicles.

Prior to mastoid surgery each patient should be warned about the risk to the VIIth cranial nerve, the risk of deterioration in hearing, the possibility of a dead ear and a chance of postoperative vertigo. It is important to document this consultation in the case history notes.

Further reading

Ear. In: Ballantyne JC and Morrison A (eds). *Rob and Smith's Operative Surgery*. London: Butterworths, 1986.

Related topics of interest

MENIÈRE'S DISEASE

Menière's disease has been recognized since the first description by Prosper Menière, in 1861, of a condition consisting of episodic vertigo, tinnitus and deafness.

Pathophysiology

Despite mountains of research the aetiology of this condition still remains unknown. Current theories of aetiology include labyrinthine ischaemia and an autoimmune response following a viral infection. Regardless of the primary cause, there follows expansion of the endolymphatic compartment, endolymphatic hydrops, which is thought to give rise to the classical symptoms. The increased endolymphatic pressure leads to an alteration in basilar membrane mobility, resulting in hearing loss and tinnitus. The same pressure increase leads to distortion of the ampullae of the semicircular canals with subsequent vestibular dysfunction. In severe cases rupture of Reissner's membrane may occur, leading to the delicate neural tissues being exposed to potassium-rich and neurotoxic endolymph with further provocation of symptoms.

Clinical features

Menière's disease accounts for between 10 and 20% of cases of true vertigo in a typical outpatient population. Patients are typically in their fifth decade at presentation with no gender bias. Episodic vertigo and hearing loss are the main complaints, although tinnitus and a sense of fullness in the affected ear are not infrequent. Attacks vary in frequency but typically last between 1 and 24 hours and are often associated with systemic upset in the form of nausea and vomiting. Movement may exacerbate the vertigo so the patient will lie as still as possible during an attack. Nystagmus is present but its direction is not indicative of the side of origin of the symptoms. In the early stages of the disease the hearing may return to normal after the attacks, but if the condition progresses and attacks recur deafness becomes established and more severe.

Patients are usually seen in the clinic between attacks, and consequently physical examination is normal. The condition is punctuated by frequent remissions and relapses over a time period of many years. There is no doubt that a large psychological component exists. In the long term (10 years) over 75% of patients' vertiginous symptoms will improve regardless of treatment type, although hearing in the affected ear invariably tends to deteriorate. Bilateral disease is thought to occur in about one-third of cases.

Investigations	An audiogram is essential and may show evidence of a sensorineural hearing loss. Classically this loss is described as low frequency, but in fact is flat in two-thirds of cases. A fluctuating sensorineural loss shown on consecutive audiograms over a period of time, with an appropriate history, is good evidence for the diagnosis.

An audiogram is essential and may show evidence of a sensorineural hearing loss. Classically this loss is described as low frequency, but in fact is flat in two-thirds of cases. A fluctuating sensorineural loss shown on consecutive audiograms over a period of time, with an appropriate history, is good evidence for the diagnosis.

Electrocochleography may show an enhanced negative summating potential indicative of altered cochlear function, and caloric tests may demonstrate impaired vestibular function.

The glycerol dehydration test works on the principle that dehydrating the cochlea and thus reducing the endolymphatic hydrops will produce an improvement in the audiogram and the ECochG; it can be used as a preoperative assessment of the potential response to conservative surgery, but is unpleasant for the patient as it causes nausea and headache.

The triad of symptoms of episodic vertigo, tinnitus and deafness is sometimes described as Menière's syndrome. There are causes of this other than Menière's disease. In those patients with an asymmetrical hearing loss, it is essential to exclude a cerebellopontine angle tumour (e.g. acoustic neuroma). Other causes of intermittent vertigo should also be excluded.

Management

It is important to bear in mind that Menière's disease is a condition that responds well to a supportive and sympathetic therapeutic approach, regardless of which treatment modality is ultimately used (i.e. strong placebo effect). Treatment can be either medical or surgical and can be regarded as a therapeutic ladder, climbing from the simple to the complicated.

1. Medical. Medical treatment starts with the manipulation of diet in an effort to reduce salt and fluid intake, and strong psychological reassurance. Betahistine 16 mg t.i.d., a labyrinthine vasodilator, has been shown to give significantly greater symptom control than placebo. Vestibular sedatives, such as prochlorperazine and cinnarizine, are without doubt useful in short-term symptom control and are best prescribed to be taken at the onset of any attack. Diuretics, thiazides in particular, are frequently prescribed but there is no good study to demonstrate any greater efficacy than placebo in this condition. Medical treatment should provide adequate symptom control in about 80% of patients.

2. *Surgical.* The simplest surgical procedure is the insertion of a grommet in the affected ear. This procedure is without any logical or scientific support and probably works by placebo effect alone. The mainstay of surgery for this condition is decompression of the endolymphatic sac with the aim of treating the underlying pathophysiological abnormality without destroying the function of the ear, particularly hearing. This is accomplished via a cortical mastoidectomy approach to the sac as it lies in the posterior cranial fossa. Decompression is achieved by exposing and opening the sac with or without the use of a shunt to provide prolonged drainage. Although 90% of patients report initial satisfactory symptom control, by 5 years this figure is down to 60%. The greatest controversy surrounding endolymphatic sac surgery concerns the Danish sham study in 1981, in which sac surgery was prospectively and randomly compared with simple cortical mastoidectomy. The study was blind and demonstrated no significant differences between the two surgical options. More radical surgery for this condition involves vestibular nerve section, which abolishes signals from the troublesome labyrinth while still preserving hearing. Control rates of 90%, maintained for up to 10 years, have been reported, although the morbidity is higher as a neurosurgical approach is required. The vestibular labyrinth may be selectively destroyed by the use of ultrasound, but this technique does also risk cochlear damage. Finally, in those ears with poor hearing a total labyrinthectomy may be the procedure of choice. This is usually achieved by destroying the labyrinth surgically but can also be performed by the local application of gentamicin.

Follow-up and aftercare　　By the very nature of the condition, these patients are often long-term attenders at an ENT department. However, with appropriate support and encouragement, they need not be frequent attenders.

Further reading

Ludman H. Menière's disease. *British Medical Journal*, 1990; **301**: 1232–3.
Ruckenstein, MJ, Rutka JA, Hawke M. The treatment of Menière's disease: Torok revisited. *Laryngoscope*, 1991; **101**: 211–8.

Related topics of interest

NASAL POLYPS

Aetiology

As part of the nasal inflammatory response there occurs swelling of the nasal and particularly ethmoid sinus mucosa. When this swelling becomes sufficiently pronounced, polyp formation may result. The initiator of this inflammatory response may be chronic infection, allergy or intrinsic rhinitis, but in the majority of cases the cause is unknown. Recent work suggests that most cases of nasal polypsis occur in patients with intrinsic rhinitis with eosinophilic secretion. Some cases may be associated with house dust mite allergy.

Pathology

Pathologically, polyps demonstrate marked oedema of the connective tissue stroma, which also contains a variety of inflammatory mediators such as histamine, prostaglandins and leukotrienes. There is a marked eosinophilic and histiocytic infiltrate and the epithelium displays goblet cell hyperplasia and in some areas a squamous cell metaplasia. A polyp forms when the oedematous stroma ruptures and herniates through the basement membrane. Nasal polyps are rare in childhood, and if they occur one should suspect cystic fibrosis or immune deficiency. Recurrence is common after surgical removal, although it may often be delayed for many years. It is more likely and tends to occur sooner in those patients with coexistent asthma and aspirin hypersensitivity.

Clinical features

Nasal polyps may be asymptomatic, but even when small most patients complain of a feeling of congestion or obstruction high in the nose. As the polyps enlarge there is associated worsening of nasal obstruction and usually a profuse watery nasal discharge causing rhinorrhoea or a postnasal space drip. At the same time patients frequently complain of loss of taste and smell. Headaches, pressure sensation in the face and sinusitis may occur. In severe cases the polyps may be visible at the external nares and widening of the intercanthal distance may occur. The polyps are insensitive. A history of epistaxis or contact bleeding should raise suspicion of the possibility of a neoplastic polyp.

Investigations

There are few essential investigations. It is worth performing skin tests or a plasma radioimmunosorbent test (PRIST) and radioallergosorbent (RAST) test to identify an allergic cause. Sinus radioographs may be helpful in demonstrating maxillary sinus involvement. In recurrent cases and those to be treated by functional endoscopic sinus surgery (FESS) a coronal CT scan of the sinuses is essential.

Following surgical removal the polyps should be sent for histological analysis, especially unilateral polyps or unusual-looking polyps.

Management

1. Medical. In patients with small polyps and following surgical removal it is worth trying medical therapy. This consists of intranasal steroids, as either drops or spray, with the addition of oral antihistamines if there is an allergic element. Short courses of low-dose oral steroids may be extremely useful in those patients with particularly aggressive polyposis.

2. Surgical. Large polyps are best removed by intranasal polypectomy under either local or general anaesthetic. In recurrent cases this may be combined with an ethmoidectomy, which can be performed by either an intranasal or external route. The intranasal approach should only be performed by an experienced surgeon. It is not popular because of the risk of damage to the orbit and to the floor of the anterior cranial fossa. External ethmoidectomy is safer and allows a more thorough clearance as there is better visual access. FESS can be used, but is sometimes difficult because of bleeding.

Follow-up and aftercare

In simple cases no follow-up is required and the patient can be asked to return should future problems arise. It is unlikely that intranasal steroids given long term make any difference to the recurrence rate. In severe cases intranasal and even oral steroids can be given following surgery. Periodic surveillance and follow-up are usually required.

Antrochoanal polyp

The antrochoanal polyp is uncommon. It is usually unilateral and commences as oedematous lining from the maxillary sinus. This lining prolapses through the ostium into the nasal cavity and enlarges towards the posterior choana and nasopharynx.

The patient, commonly a young adult, complains of unilateral nasal obstruction, which is worse on expiration owing to the ball valve-like effect of the polyp in the posterior choana. If sufficiently large, it may produce bilateral obstruction and cause otological symptoms as a result of blockage of the Eustachian tube orifice. Anterior rhinoscopy may look normal as only the thin stalk may present in the nose. The enlarged posterior end may be seen on posterior rhinoscopy.

Radiography of the maxillary sinus will show complete opacification of the affected antrum.

Treatment is by complete nasal avulsion with removal of the antral portion. Failure to remove the antral lining will result in a recurrence. An intranasal antrostomy is the usual approach. Functional endoscopic sinus surgery is an option. With recurrence a Caldwell–Luc procedure should be performed to clear the sinus

Further reading

Drake-Lee AB. Nasal polyps. In: Mackay IS, Bull TR (eds) *Scott-Brown's Otolaryngology*, 5th edn. London: Butterworths, 1987; 142–53.

Related topics of interest

Acute sinusitis (p. 5)
Allergic rhinitis (p. 16)
Chronic sinusitis (p. 47)
Functional endoscopic sinus surgery (p. 119)
Intrinsic rhinitis (p. 141)

NASAL TRAUMA

The commonest causes of nasal trauma are assault, road traffic accident and sports injuries. Nasal trauma does not imply only nasal fracture. Injury to the nose may result in one or a combination of soft-tissue injury, fracture of the nasal bones, fracture or dislocation of the septum, septal haematoma, cerebrospinal fluid (CSF) leak and facial bone fracture.

Classification of fracture of the nasal bones

An isolated nasal fracture is usually caused by low-velocity trauma. If the nose is fractured by high-velocity trauma then facial fractures are often an accompaniment. Nasal fractures are classified on a 1–3 scale depending on their severity and extent.

A class 1 fracture is usually due to a frontal or fronto-lateral blow and results in a vertical fracture of the septum (Chevallet fracture) with a depressed or displaced distal portion of the nasal bone. A class 2 fracture is nearly always due to lateral trauma and results in a horizontal (Jarjavay fracture) or C-shaped fracture of the septum involving the perpendicular plate of the ethmoid and the septal cartilage in combination with a fracture of the frontal process of the maxillae. A class 3 fracture indicates that the velocity of the trauma has been even greater and results in a nasal fracture which extends to include the ethmoid labyrinth. The perpendicular plate of the ethmoid rotates backwards and the septum collapses into the face, turning up the tip of the nose and revealing the nostrils. There is a marked depression of the nasal bones, which are pushed under the frontal bones, and there is an apparent widening of the space between the eyes (telecanthus).

Clinical features

Trauma to the nose may be part of a more extensive injury to the facial skeleton and base of skull. It should be remembered that the most important consideration in maxillofacial injuries is the maintenance of an airway. A history of trauma to the midface accompanied by epistaxis, a noticeable deformity and nasal airway obstruction are the usual complaints. Nasofrontoethmoid fractures may produce symptoms of diplopia and epiphora. It is important to carefully record the time and nature of the trauma, previous episodes of trauma and whether the nasal deformity is new or old. Remember to enquire about any trauma to the head and neck and any other injuries.

Tenderness, haematoma and swelling may make the assessment difficult. It is appropriate in uncomplicated cases to reassess the patient 5–7 days after the injury. The nasal swelling is often accompanied by periorbital and subconjunctival ecchymosis. Check the nasal airways and examine the septum; note any deformity and exclude a septal haematoma. Ocular movements should be tested and Vth nerve function (infraorbital sensation) and dental occlusion should be checked. All injuries should be carefully documented in the case notes supplemented with drawings and occasionally photographs. The elucidation and documentation of these clinical symptoms and signs should be standard medical practice. They are also important for medicolegal purposes.

Investigations

In the majority of simple uncomplicated fractures no investigations are required, but in more serious injuries radiographs are the most important investigation. They should include views of the skull, face and nasal bones depending on the extent and severity of the injury. They may be important for medicolegal purposes. A CT scan on bone setting may delineate maxillofacial fractures when there is uncertainty.

Management

1. Soft-tissue injury. Wounds are thoroughly cleaned and any foreign body removed. Appropriate antibiotic and antitetanus cover should be given. Abrasions are best left open. Small lacerations can be closed with Steristrips, but larger lacerations should be closed with fine monofilament sutures.

2. Nasal fracture. Treatment is not required in some patients because there is no fracture or bony deformity. These patients should be reassured and reviewed again when swelling has subsided. It is also inappropriate to try and manipulate a longstanding deformity as this will result in a failure to reduce. It is possible to reduce a simple class 1 fracture under local anaesthetic before any swelling appears if it is seen early enough. Disimpaction and realignment can usually be achieved with laterally applied digital pressure and Walsham's forceps, one blade in the nasal cavity and the other outside. If the fracture is seen later and there is much swelling, manipulation should be delayed for 5–7 days. Manipulation should never be delayed for more than 2 weeks post injury because the nasal bones will fix and reduction will be difficult if not impossible. Class 2 fractures have a propensity to redisplace owing to overlapping of the fractured ends of the septal cartilage and the perpendicular plate of the ethmoid. The manipulation of the nasal bone should be accompanied by an excision of the septal fracture and overlapping segments through a Killian incision. A class 3 fracture will require an open reduction. The depressed nasal bones need to be elevated out of the face and supported with wires via an incision over the nasofrontal angle. The septum is approached through a a Killian incision with the aim of pulling the rotated septal cartilage forwards and downwards. Malunion following nasal trauma will require treatment by a formal septorhinoplasty procedure.

3. Septal haematoma. This is due to a collection of blood beneath the mucoperichondrium of the nasal septum. It may follow nasal trauma, but it can also occur as a complication of septal surgery (e.g. submucosal resection (SMR)) and, rarely, blood dyscrasias. There is usually complete bilateral nasal obstruction caused by a soft swelling. If this is missed or not treated correctly, a septal abscess, cartilage necrosis and nasal saddle deformity may ensue. Aspiration may suffice if the haematoma is small, but incision and drainage with quilt suturing (to obliterate the dead space) is required if the collection reaccumulates. The patient should be given a course of antibiotics to reduce the risk of local and systemic infection.

4. Cerebrospinal fluid leaks. The presence of clear rhinorrhoea at any stage following nasal trauma should raise the suspicion of a CSF leak. The cribriform plate is extremely thin and is the commonest area of fracture. Confirmation of the diagnosis is obtained by checking the glucose content of the rhinorrhoea, which will approach that of serum levels, or alternatively β_2-transferrin assays (this is a protein present in perilymph and CSF) can be used. Fluorescein injected into the CSF via a lumbar puncture can be collected from the leak in the nose. High-resolution CT scan may delineate the fracture. Until the leak ceases the patient is at risk of pneumococcal meningitis and should be given oral penicillin and sulphadimidine as antibiotic prophylaxis. Many leaks will close spontaneously, but some will require surgical repair with temporalis fascia, fascia lata or a mucosal flap from the nasal septum. Repair can be approached by an external ethmoidectomy, a trans-septal route, by an intranasal endoscopic approach or by a frontal craniotomy and repair with reduction of the bony fragments.

Further reading

Maran AGD. The fractured nose. In: Mackay IS, Bull TR (eds) *Scott-Brown's Otolaryngology*, Vol. 4, 5th edn. London: Butterworths, 1987; 212–21.

Vuilleriun T, Imola M. Nasal and sinus trauma. *Current Opinion in Otolaryngology and Head and Neck Surgery*, 1994; **2**: 37–41.

Related topics of interest

Examination of the nose (p. 93)
Septal perforation (p. 278)

NASOPHARYNGEAL TUMOURS

There are four important groups.
(a) Nasopharyngeal squamous cell carcinoma.
(b) Other nasopharyngeal tumours.
(c) Angiofibroma.
(d) Adenoids (see p. 13).

Nasopharyngeal squamous cell carcinoma

Pathology

This probably comprises two distinct disease types, namely keratinizing squamous cell carcinoma, which is similar to other upper aerodigestive tract squamous carcinomas in which smoking and alcohol are risk factors, and non-keratinizing squamous cell carcinoma (nasopharyngeal carcinoma, NPC), which is of a poorly or undifferentiated type. The latter has a predilection for those of Southern Chinese or Hong Kong extraction, forming 20% of all malignancies in these people and 80% of their head and neck cancers.

Aetiology

The consensus view supports the proposal that in the genetically predisposed a carcinogen is triggered by an environmental co-factor to transform nasopharyngeal epithelial cells. The environmental factor most widely implicated is salted preserved fish, a staple diet of the Hong Kong boat people, the male population of which constitute the world's highest at-risk population group. Latent Epstein–Barr virus (EBV) infection is endemic in this group and the evidence for EBV being the carcinogen is compelling. In particular:
(a) Southern blot and polymerase chain reaction consistently detect DNA sequences of EBV in NPC cells.
(b) NPC cells consistently express two species of EBV proteins: EB nuclear antigen 1 and latent membrane protein, 1, detectable by immunofluorescence.
(c) Plasma antibodies to *viral capsid antigen* and to *early antigens* (one of which is an EBV DNase) are seen, titres of the latter being a significant predictor of tumour relapse after radiotherapy.

Genetic factors

The human leukocyte antigen allele A2 without BW46 or B17 is associated with long-term survival. The A2 BW46 allele combination is associated with intermediate-term survival, while the occurrence of B17 is associated with short-term survival.

| Clinical features | The majority of patients present with a history of epistaxis, nasal obstruction, a neck lump or referred otalgia. Seventy per cent of patients will have metastatic lymph node involvement at presentation, and in 20% this is the mode of presentation. NPC usually arises from the fossa of Rosenmuller and may spread by direct extension to involve: |

- Anteriorly the Eustachian tube causing a serous otitis media.
- Posterolaterally the pharyngobasilar fascia then through this to the parapharyngeal and retrostyloid space. Involvement of the former causes mandibular nerve paralysis with partial loss of facial, palatal and pharyngeal sensation and involvement of the pterygoid musculature causing trismus. Involvement of the latter, containing the cervical sympathetic trunk and the IXth to XIIth cranial nerves causes Horner's syndrome, vocal cord, pharyngeal, palatal, shoulder and tongue paralysis and pain.
- Superiorly through the foramen lacerum to cause paralysis of the IIIrd, IVth and upper two divisions of the Vth cranial nerves, causing diplopia, facial hypoaesthesia and headaches.

Investigations

The diagnosis is made from the history, examination and special investigations. NPC often spreads submucosally from the fossa of Rosenmuller so that no nasopharyngeal abnormality is visible, although there may be metastatic lymph node disease. Fibreoptic pharyngoscopy is probably the most reliable method of examining the nasopharynx and should be used if a biopsy of the fossa of Rosenmuller is to be obtained under a local anaesthetic. A blind biopsy is not recommended as the specimen obtained may be non-representative.

The polymerase chain reaction to EB virus genome has been used to diagnose NPC in patients with a malignant neck node with an occult primary. Computerized tomography is the investigation of choice to assess skull base and paranasal sinus involvement. MRI imaging including a STIR sequence to suppress fat clearly defines the tumour margins in soft tissue and will best define the presence and extent of metastatic neck disease. A chest radiograph, liver ultrasound and, if symptoms dictate, a bone scan are useful screening tools in the search for distant metastases.

Management	Radiotherapy using a field which includes the nasopharynx, skull base, the sphenoid and posterior ethmoid sinuses, and posterior orbit is the treatment of choice. The consensus view now is to irradiate the neck bilaterally to reduce the incidence of future neck node metastases. Some authorities advocate a radical neck dissection if there are mobile lymph node metastases larger than 3 cm, prior to radiotherapy. The alternative view proposes that because the undifferentiated NPC is highly radiosensitive surgery is not indicated.
Prevention	EBV infection of the nasopharynx is not a regular feature in healthy EBV virus carriers. In high-risk areas screening nasopharyngeal biopsies for viral genome is useful in determining high-risk individuals. Counselling this group on their diet and the need for frequent regular follow-up is recommended.
	A vaccine based on the EBV envelope glycoprotein gp340, a major target for the virus-neutralizing antibody response, is currently undergoing phase I trials.
Follow-up and aftercare	All patients with treated head and neck cancer must be reviewed monthly for the first year, bimonthly for the second year, every 3 months for the third year and 6-monthly for the fourth and fifth years post treatment. If they are disease free then for most cancers they may be considered cured (adenoid cystic carcinoma and malignant melanoma are notable exceptions). Most head and neck units will continue to follow patients annually for another 5 years because such patients are at significant risk of developing a second primary cancer.

Other EBV-associated disease

- Burkitt's lymphoma (a monoclonal B-cell, non-Hodgkin's lymphoma).
- T-cell lymphoma.
- Hodgkin's lymphoma.
- Infectious mononucleosis.

Other nasopharyngeal tumours

- Non-Hodgkin's lymphoma.
- Extramedullary plasmacytoma (predilection for the nasopharynx and paranasal sinuses).
- Paediatric nasopharyngeal tumours:
  Ectodermal – dermoids, teratomas.
  Neuroectodermal – encephalocele, meningocele.
  Dysontogenetic – craniopharyngioma, chordoma.

Angiofibroma

This histologically benign tumour comprising fibrous tissue with a variable proportion of vascular tissue, often with large endothelial spaces, arises from the posterolateral wall of the nasal cavity and the superolateral nasopharyngeal wall. The sphenopalatine foramen is always involved and may be the specific site of tumour origin. It occurs predominantly and perhaps exclusively in young adult males.

Clinical features

The tumour expands to erode or compress surrounding fissures, foramina and tissues. The commonest symptoms are epistaxis and nasal obstruction. It may expand laterally into the pterygopalatine fossa, through the pterygomaxillary fissure and into the infratemporal fossa, expanding superiorly to erode the pterygoid plates, the greater wing of the sphenoid and the skull base foramina. Anterosuperior expansion into the nasal cavity, paranasal sinuses, parasellar region, cavernous sinus and orbit may also occur. Presenting signs are similar to NPC except that there is a smooth mass filling the nasopharynx on endoscopic or mirror examination. A high index of suspicion for any nasopharyngeal mass is essential because angiofibroma should not as a rule be biopsied. In particular, it must not be confused with a large adenoid pad.

Investigations and treatment

An MRI scan with a STIR sequence is the investigation of choice to define the extent and vascularity of the tumour. Surgery is the treatment of choice for all but the smallest tumours as they may continue to expand and are typically poorly radiosensitive. Large vascular tumours require digital subtraction angiography to define the important feeding vessels. These should be embolized 1–2 days preoperatively. *Depending on tumour extent* a midfacial degloving or, if the cribriform plate is involved, a craniofacial approach is most widely advocated, and these procedures may need to be combined with an infratemporal approach. Other approaches include the Le Fort 1 and the transpalatal.

Further reading

Sam CK, Prasad U, Pathmanathan R. Serological markers in the diagnosis of histopathological types of nasopharyngeal carcinoma. *European Journal of Surgical Oncology*, 1989; **15**: 357–60

Related topic of interest

Adenoids (p. 13)

NECK DISSECTION

A primary carcinoma arising from the upper aerodigestive tract may ultimately drain into the lymph nodes of the neck, which form an efficient barrier to the further spread of the disease. The prognosis for the patient regardless of the site of the primary tumour is worse if there are cervical lymph nodes involved at presentation. Only 30–40% of such patients will survive longer than 5 years. The surgeon now has two effective treatment modalities for neck node metastases in radiotherapy and surgery. Broadly speaking, radiotherapy will only be effective in the curative treatment of cervical lymph node metastases if they are less than 2 cm in diameter. The advantage of using radiotherapy in these cases is that it precludes the need for surgery, which can be kept in reserve for the treatment of any recurrence. Patients who have larger nodes are less likely to be cured by radiotherapy and must be treated surgically. The operation may be required to remove the nodes alone, or it can be performed in continuity with removal of the primary tumour as an *en bloc* dissection.

Classification

The classification below is suggested by the American Academy's Committee for Head and Neck Surgery and Oncology. Radical neck dissection is considered to be the standard basic procedure, and all others represent one or more alterations to this procedure. Modified radical neck dissection involves the preservation of one or more non-lymphatic structures routinely removed in radical neck dissection. It is suggested that this term be used in preference to functional neck dissection, which should be abandoned. However, for the foreseeable future it is likely that both these terms will continue to be used. Selective neck dissection involves the preservation of one or more lymph node groups routinely removed in radical neck dissection. Extended radical neck dissection involves removal of additional lymph node groups or non-lymphatic structures relative to the radical neck dissection (i.e. a superior mediastinal dissection in patients with subglottic or cervical oesophageal tumours).

1. Radical neck dissection.
2. Modified radical neck dissection.
3. Selective neck dissection.
   (a) Supraomohyoid neck dissection.
   (b) Posterolateral neck dissection.
   (c) Lateral neck dissection.
   (d) Anterior compartment neck dissection.
4. Extended radical neck dissection.

Radical neck dissection

This operation refers to the removal of lymph nodes in the anterior and posterior triangles extending from the inferior border of the mandible superiorly to the clavicle inferiorly, the midline anteriorly and the anterior border of the trapezius muscle posteriorly. The cervical lymph node groups routinely removed are as follows: submental and submandibular; upper, middle and lower jugular (deep cervical); and the posterior triangle group. The submandibular gland, spinal accessory nerve, internal jugular vein and sternocleidomastoid muscle are also removed. Surgical technique will not be discussed.

Complications of radical neck dissection

1. Immediate.

- Haemorrhage (from either end of the internal jugular vein or other ligated vessel).
- Chyle leak (if the thoracic duct has been inadvertently damaged).
- Nerve palsies (phrenic, vagus, marginal mandibular branch of the facial, lingual, hypoglossal, sympathetic trunk, brachial plexus).

2. Intermediate.

- Facial oedema.
- Cerebral oedema (after a synchronous or staged bilateral neck dissection).
- Wound infection.
- Wound breakdown (poor surgical technique, previous radiotherapy, diabetes, poor nutritional status).
- Rupture of the carotid artery (may be a sequel to wound breakdown).

3. Late.

- Frozen shoulder (less likely to occur if the cervical nerve branches of C3 and C4 are preserved as they pass under the fascia of the floor of the posterior triangle).
- Recurrence in the glands or skin.

Bilateral neck dissection

The presence of bilateral neck nodes is not an independent poor prognostic sign, but univariate analysis demonstrates a reduced 5-year survival to around 5%. This is because when bilateral disease is present at least one set of nodes is usually of greater diameter than 6 cm and fixed. Surgery probably does not influence the natural history of the disease. Supraglottic carcinoma with bilateral glands is an exception and can still have a reasonable prognosis. Bilateral synchronous neck dissection carries a significant morbidity and a mortality of about 3%. Many of the complications can be reduced by either staging the procedure with an interval of 6 weeks or longer or performing a modified procedure on the opposite side to preserve the internal jugular vein. The most serious complication is that of raised intracranial pressure. Ligation of one internal jugular vein results in a threefold increase in the intracranial pressure, and when the second side is tied there is a fivefold increase in pressure. The patient should have a temporary tracheostomy, be nursed propped up in the bed, and may require an infusion of mannitol (500 ml of 10% mannitol over 4 hours). The most critical period is the first 12 hours postoperatively. Over the following 8–10 days after the operation, the intracranial pressure tends to fall, though it never returns to its normal level.

Further reading

Robbins TK. Neck dissection. *Current Opinion in Otolaryngology and Head and Neck Surgery*, 1993; **1**: 114–19.
Robbins TK *et al.* Standardising neck dissection terminology. *Archives of Otolaryngology and Head and Neck Surgery,* 1991; **117**: 601–5.

Related topics of interest

Hypopharygeal carcinoma (p. 133)
Laryngeal carcinoma (p. 148)
Oral cavity carcinoma (p. 198)
Oropharyngeal carcinoma (p. 204)

NECK SPACE INFECTION

Anatomy

Understanding neck space infections is straightforward but requires some anatomical knowledge.

The prevertebral fascia arises from the base of the skull in front of the atlas and inserts into the body of T3. An abscess behind this fascia cannot extend below this level unless the fascia is breached.

Immediately anterior to the prevertebral fascia is a potential space extending from the skull base to the diaphragm. That portion behind the pharynx is the retropharyngeal space. It should be emphasized that there is no anatomical barrier preventing an abscess tracking inferiorly into the superior and posterior mediastinum, although the inflammatory reaction usually localizes the abscess to the retropharyngeal space.

The parapharyngeal space is a potential space immediately lateral to the oropharynx and nasopharynx, the styloid process dividing it into an anterior or prestyloid and a posterior or poststyloid compartment. The latter contains the carotid sheath, which is firmly attached on its lateral aspect to the investing layer of deep fascia on the deep aspect of sternomastoid but has only loose areolar tissue lying medially and posteriorly. Infection may therefore spread from the prestyloid to the poststyloid compartment by passing medial to the carotid sheath or from the retropharyngeal space to the poststyloid compartment (and vice versa) by passing posterior to the carotid sheath. An abscess in the poststyloid compartment may track further laterally to a point just behind the posterior aspect of the sternomastoid. In the prestyloid compartment a collection may extend as far forward as the fascia surrounding the submandibular gland, just anterior to the sternomastoid but above the hyoid bone.

The infratemporal fossa lies beneath the base of skull between the side wall of the pharynx and the ascending ramus of the mandible. It is bounded posteriorly by the styloid process and the anterior wall of the carotid sheath, anteriorly by the posterior wall of the maxilla and superiorly by the infratemporal surface of the greater wing of the sphenoid. The infratemporal fossa is therefore equivalent to the prestyloid compartment of the parapharyngeal space.

The submandibular space is bound by the mucosa of the floor of the mouth superiorly and by the mylohyoid muscle and deep fascia investing the submandibular gland inferiorly.

Neck space infections

Citelli's abscess and Bezold's abscess, both complications of acute suppurative otitis media, have been previously described, as has peritonsillar abscess (see Related topics of interest).

Prevertebral abscess

This is rare today and occurs in adults from tuberculosis of the cervical spine. The attachment of the fascia limits the inferior extent to the vertebral body of T3. A progressively painful and tender neck with limitation of movement is the usual presentation. A lateral neck radiograph shows prevertebral soft-tissue shadowing and a rarified vertebral body which may be wedge shaped through collapse. Occasionally collapse will cause acute spinal cord compression, requiring urgent drainage of the abscess and cord decompression. Aspirating the abscess allows the diagnosis to be confirmed, after which antituberculous therapy is instigated.

Retropharyngeal abscess

The overwhelming majority of cases arise in children of less than 4 years old. Older children have fewer retropharyngeal nodes and adults have only the node of Rouviere. The condition occurs in adults when a prevertebral tuberculous abscess ruptures the prevertebral fascia. Suppuration of retropharyngeal nodes occurs after an upper respiratory tract infection from lymphatics draining infected tonsils, teeth, pharynx or paranasal sinuses, although occasionally the source is an unsuspected foreign body. The child becomes increasingly toxic and may dribble, have stertor or dysphagia. The neck is held rigidly and may become hyperextended. Symptoms mimic laryngotracheobronchitis and acute epiglottitis, although in the latter case the history is shorter. It is safer therefore not to examine the throat which, even with a correct diagnosis, might cause rupture of the abscess with inhalation or tracking of the abscess into the mediastinum.

Investigations

A lateral soft-tissue neck radiograph with the neck extended to prevent the retropharyngeal soft tissues causing a pseudomass will show the widened retropharyngeal space and narrow oropharyngeal airway.

Treatment

Treatment consists in incision and drainage in the tonsillectomy position under a general anaesthesia and intravenous antibiotics. The child will sometimes need to remain intubated on ICU for 24–48 hours, until the retropharyngeal soft tissue swelling settles.

Parapharyngeal abscess

Sixty per cent arise from tonsillitis or peritonsillitis and 30% from an abscess of the root of the lower third molar, which lies below the mylohyoid line. Mastoiditis or a pharyngeal foreign body are unusual causes.

Clinical features	These are similar to a peritonsillar abscess. There is trismus, soft palate oedema, and the tonsil is pushed medially. The main distinguishing feature is a neck swelling, which may be firm or fluctuant, and most commonly just behind the posterior aspect of the middle third of the sternomastoid because infection tends to drain from the prestyloid to the poststyloid compartment and thereafter laterally.
Treatment	Repeat fine-needle aspiration of the abscess and intravenous antibiotics, benzylpenicillin and metronidazole being the combination of choice, may obviate the need for formal incision and drainage.

Submandibular abscess (Ludwig's angina)

In over 80% of patients infection arises from a root abscess of the lower premolars or the first and second molars. There may be no history of dental pain if the root is close to the inner table of mandible, which gives way early. The remaining cases are secondary to tonsillitis. Anaerobic organisms are usually present.

Clinical features	Floor of mouth oedema secondary to cellulitis can progress rapidly to endanger the airway. The tongue is pushed posterosuperiorly and there is trismus and dribbling. The submandibular region is red, hot, swollen and tender.
Treatment	If the airway is not in immediate danger, fine-needle aspiration of the abscess and intravenous antibiotics with anaerobic cover are usually adequate. Incision and drainage is only necessary if the airway is becoming precarious, and this is usually preceded by the insertion of a nasopharyngeal airway to secure the airway.

Related topics of interest

Acute suppurative otitis media (p. 9)
Paediatric airway problems (p. 234)
Stridor and stertor (p. 301)
Tonsillitis (p. 320)

NOISE-INDUCED HEARING LOSS

Aetiology

The ear is a sound-sensitive organ but can be damaged by excessive noise levels. Excessive noise can arise from a variety of sources: occupational, such as factory machinery, building sites and high-impact tools; and recreational, such as shooting, discos and personal stereos. Occupational deafness is a compensatable disease and legislation exists to protect the employee (Health and Safety at Work Act). In the UK the current safe maximum is 90 dB for an 8 hour working day, but this is soon to be reduced to 85 dB in line with EC directives.

Pathology

Biological variability means that individuals are not affected equally by the same noise exposure, however with increasing noise levels above 90 dB a greater proportion of the exposed population will exhibit pathological changes. Initially noise exposure will lead to temporary threshold shift (TTS). There are no obvious pathological changes in TTS and the problem is felt to be due to metabolic exhaustion of the hair cells of the cochlea. With increasing and repeated noise exposure there is damage to the outer hair cells (OHCs) of row 1, and subsequently to the OHCs in rows 2 and 3 and the inner hair cells. Damage also occurs to the supporting pillar cells and the stria vascularis. The audiometric hearing loss tends to parallel the loss of hair cells. It has previously been stated (see Impedance audiometry, p. 137) that doubling sound intensity corresponds to an increase of only 3 dB, while a 10-fold increase in intensity corresponds to an increase of 10 dB. Therefore small increases in noise exposure recorded in dB expose the cochlea to large increases in sound energy.

Clinical features

TTS may produce ringing in the ears (tinnitus) following excessive noise exposure. Permanent threshold shift (PTS) is frequently asymptomatic and is often found on routine screening audiometry carried out in the workplace. Such screening is a requirement of any hearing protection programme. When PTS becomes symptomatic the first complaint is usually reduced understanding of speech, especially when there is background noise. As it becomes more severe the patient complains more of being hard of hearing and often has tinnitus.

Examination will reveal normal tympanic membranes (unless the patient has had previous middle-ear disease) and the audiogram will show a dip at around 4–6 kHz in the early stages. This may become exaggerated as exposure continues, eventually with flattening of the audiogram as sensorineural damage progresses.

Investigations

A good history is the keystone to diagnosis and is essential in medicolegal cases in order to provide apportionment of disability if more than one type of noise exposure has occurred. Cerebellopontine angle tumours may produce a unilateral asymmetrical, high-tone sensorineural hearing loss or intermittent tinnitus so that investigation to exclude this cause is necessary. A brainstem evoked response audiogram is the minimum requirement, or, if the 4-kHz threshold has declined to less than 60–70 dB so as not to allow a reliable trace, a gadolinium-enhanced MRI scan of the internal auditory meati.

Management

Damage to the cochlea caused by noise is cumulative so that, once diagnosed, further deterioration must be prevented by adequate protective measures. Counselling is necessary, preferably from a hearing therapist, regarding the hearing loss and tinnitus in order to minimize disability. Awareness of the potential hazards of noise will allow prophylactic measures to be taken both at work and recreationally, e.g. the use of earplugs and muffs. A hearing aid may be required.

Management: medicolegal

Occupational noise-induced hearing loss (NIHL) became a compensatable disorder in 1975, and as such a scheme exists to calculate the disability and hence the amount of compensation. In essence this involves averaging the hearing thresholds for each ear for the frequencies of 1, 2 and 3 kHz. Allowance is then made for any difference between the two ears, age, any conductive loss and the type of audiogram, and a figure for the disability is finally reached. Tables for:
(a) median age-associated hearing threshold levels for males and females,
(b) percentage disability as a function of better-ear hearing threshold level, and
(c) excess noise level above 84 dB and exposure duration in years to provide an 'equivalent continuous sound level' in dB
are available to calculate total disability and apportionment of disability to different sources of noise.

Follow-up and aftercare

Continuing advice and review by a hearing therapist is recommended to minimize disability.

Further reading

Berger EH, Lindgren FL. Current issues in hearing protection. In: Dancer A, Henderson D, Salvi R, Hamernik R (eds) *Noise Induced Hearing Loss.* St Louis: Mosby Year Book, 1992; 377–88.

King PF, Coles RRA, Lutman ME, Robinson DW. *Assessment of Hearing Disability. Guidelines for Medicolegal Practice.* London: Whurr, 1992.

Related topics of interest

Acoustic neuroma (p. 1)
Impedance audiometry (p. 137)
Non-organic hearing loss (p. 195)
Pure tone audiogram (p. 255)

NON-HEALING NASAL GRANULOMATA

A granulomatous reaction is a specific type of chronic inflammation characterized by the local accumulation of macrophages and their morphologically and functionally diverse derivatives. These comprise the epithelioid cell and multinucleate giant cell. Usually surrounding and interacting with these is a zone of lymphocytes.

Most nasal granulomata are formed as a result of specific chronic infections. The most important of these are tuberculosis, syphilis, leprosy and fungal infections. Non-specific granulomata occur when no infectious agent can be defined and comprises sarcoidosis and Wegener's granulomatosis (WG). The formerly and inappropriately named lethal midline granuloma is now recognized to be a high-grade T-cell lymphoma.

Wegener's granulomatosis

Wegener in 1939 described a granulomatous disease of unknown aetiology comprising destructive lesions of the upper and lower respiratory tracts and glomerulonephritis. Histological examination shows granuloma formation and necrotizing vasculitis. It is now accepted that only a single system may be affected by the disease or there may be multisystem involvement, affecting not only the three classical systems but also virtually every organ in the body including the ear. These are considered to be variations of WG, but no consensus view exists on the nomenclature in these situations.

Pathogenesis	Current knowledge suggests that an infection, usually viral, in susceptible individuals triggers an immunological response to produce the features of WG.
Clinical features	In the nose, active WG classically causes a sanguinous discharge, crust formation and friable ulcerated mucosa. Chest features comprise haemoptysis and dyspnoea. Oliguria and micro- or macroscopic haematuria suggest renal involvement. The patient feels weak and lethargic and experiences marked weight loss. Untreated there is a 93% 2-year mortality. WG may affect the external and middle ear, causing a serosanguinous discharge and a conductive hearing loss. Vestibulocochlear symptoms, a facial palsy and a secondary infection may occur. On examination the appearances are similar to a carcinoma and the diagnosis can only be made by a representative biopsy. Friable, ulcerative lesions in the mouth, oropharynx and larynx have also been described.
Investigations	A chest radiograph may show opacities compatible with areas of infarction or of cavity formation. Urinalysis may show red cells, protein and casts. Creatinine clearance

declines. In the acute phase 95% of cases have a raised titre of cytoplasmic anti-neutrophil cytoplasmic antibody (c-ANCA) and 20–40% raised titres of p (perinuclear) ANCA. These titres parallel changes in disease activity. The classical three-system involvement and a representative biopsy of an active area are both necessary and sufficient to make the diagnosis. Random biopsies of normal-looking upper respiratory mucosa in subjects suspected of having the disease provide a zero WG diagnostic yield and therefore the biopsy of an active area is stressed.

Treatment

Long-term, low-dose antibiotic therapy aimed at preventing an infectious trigger or immunosuppressive therapy aimed at dampening the immunological response is the current strategy. Low-dose cotrimoxazole has been shown to prevent relapse in many patients. Cotrimoxazole has been shown to increase host cytotoxicity and enhance intracellular killing. Cell-mediated immunity against viruses involves the intracellular killing of free virus particles and the killing of virus-infected cells by macrophages. Cotrimoxazole's mechanism of action may be to enhance virus killing sufficiently to prevent immune complex formation, which causes inflammation and granuloma formation when deposited in the microcirculation. Cyclophosphamide and prednisolone are the current immunosuppressive drugs of choice, the dose of which are adjusted so as to reduce side-effects to a minimum while maintaining remission.

High-grade T-cell lymphoma

This was often confused with WG, but with the advent of modern immunocytochemical techniques a representative biopsy will allow an accurate diagnosis.

Clinical features

The nasal features are similar to WG but there is little systemic disturbance and in particular no bronchial or renal disease. There is progressive destruction of the midfacial structures. Untreated the patient succumbs from secondary infection or cachexia.

Investigations

A representative biopsy will show huge numbers of small cells with a high incidence of mitoses. There may be zones of acute inflammatory cells if a secondary infection supervenes. Necrotizing vasculitis and granuloma formation are absent. As the small cells may represent a poorly differentiated squamous cell carcinoma, malignant melanoma, neuroblastoma or rhabdomyosarcoma immunocytochemical analysis is necessary to confirm the diagnosis. As with any lymphoma, full staging should be carried out.

Treatment
(a) Antibiotics to control secondary infection.
(b) Surgical debridement of necrotic tissue.
(c) Radical radiotherapy, usually 60–66 Gy in 30 fractions, followed by further debridement if indicated.
(d) Reconstructive surgery to the nose and midfacial regions as required.

Syphilis, tuberculosis and sarcoidosis

Only tertiary syphilis produces a granulomatous reaction, the pathological lesion being the gumma. This can invade mucous membrane, cartilage or bone, the bony septum being the site most commonly involved. The usual presentation is nasal swelling, putrid discharge, bleeding and crusting. A red nodular swelling which can be diffuse or localized may be visible. The treponema pallidum haemagglutination test (TPHA) and fluorescent treponemal antibody test (FTA) for syphilis are positive and a biopsy of the lesion shows perivascular cuffing of arterioles by chronic inflammatory cells and endarteritis. There may be a septal perforation, erosion of the nasal bridge with a saddle deformity, stenosis of the nares or atrophic rhinitis.

Tuberculosis and sarcoid affect mainly the cartilaginous septum. In tuberculosis there may be apple jelly nodules around the vestibular skin and signs of pulmonary involvement. Biopsy shows caseating granulatoma and acid-fast bacilli may show on a Ziehl–Neelsen stain or following culture. Biopsy of a sarcoid lesion shows non-caseating granulatoma, angiotensin-converting enzyme levels are usually raised, the Kveim test is positive and there may be evidence of multisystem involvement.

Further reading

Van der Woude FJ, Van Es LA, Daha MR. The role of the c-ANCA antigen in the pathogenesis of Wegener's granulomatosis. A hypothesis based on both humoral and cellular mechanisms. *Netherlands Journal of Medicine*, 1990; **36**: 169–71.

Related topic of interest

Sinonasal tumours (p. 280)

NON-ORGANIC HEARING LOSS

Non-organic hearing loss (NOHL) is a condition in which a patient consistently displays an apparent auditory deficit, when no true hearing loss exists, or exaggerates a real hearing loss.

This condition is usually encountered either in an adult in whom there is an ongoing claim for compensation as a result of ototrauma (hearing loss from noise exposure, ototoxic drugs or trauma) or in a child or young adult with psychological disturbance. In the former group the patient usually exaggerates an existing hearing loss in an effort to improve any compensatory payment. In the latter group this psychosomatic symptom represents a cry for help in response to some current stressful event, although it may not always be possible to identify the stressor. The underlying hearing is usually normal.

Clinical assessment

The diagnosis of NOHL depends primarily on a high index of clinical suspicion, particularly financial claims and in children without obvious pathology. The preliminary clinical investigation may reveal some inconsistencies which suggest the diagnosis. The patient appears to hear much better than the subsequent audiogram would suggest (but beware of lip readers). The pure tone audiogram itself may be performed in an erratic and hesitant fashion. Patients complaining of a unilateral hearing loss may deny any hearing of a tuning fork placed on the mastoid process of the affected side. A patient with a genuine unilateral hearing loss would perceive the bone-conducted stimulus in the normal cochlea and report the perception of sound. Those patients who have some degree of psychological upset often appear completely unconcerned about the hearing loss but are very often accompanied by an extremely concerned carer.

Unfortunately, in all patients who are pursuing a financial claim, a non-organic component must be excluded; it has been estimated to occur in up to 25% of cases.

Investigations

A plethora of tests exist to try and distinguish non-organic from organic hearing loss.

1. Tuning forks. These can be used as part of the clinical assessment in cases of apparent unilateral hearing loss, e.g. the Stenger test (see Clinical assessment of hearing, p. 58), which can also be performed using an audiometer.

2. Pure tone audiometry. In the truly deaf patient pure tone audiometry reveals consistent results. One should suspect a NOHL when pure tone responses are inconsistent or when the patient denies hearing, in the good ear, a sound over 70 dB above the threshold applied to the bad ear.

2. Impedance audiometry. The stapedius reflex threshold normally varies from 70 to 95 dB above the pure tone threshold. There may be recruitment, so this is not invariably the case. Even then there is usually at least 20 dB between the reflex threshold and the pure tone threshold. If the thresholds are within 20 dB or less then a NOHL is likely.

4. Speech audiometry. This is often useful in making the diagnosis. Patients often find it more difficult to exaggerate their impairment to the same extent in speech as in pure tone audiometry.

5. Delayed speech feedback. The patient is asked to read aloud from a book. The voice is recorded and played back into the bad ear via headphones, the recording being delayed by milliseconds. If there is a genuine deafness the patient will be able to read without pausing. If the patient is feigning deafness then the delayed speech feedback will alter the reading pattern causing the patient to stammer, slow down or shout.

6. Evoked response audiometry. If knowledge of the auditory thresholds is required with some precision, as in medicolegal cases, electric response audiometry will be required. Cortical responses are preferred to brainstem evoked responses as they provide precise threshold levels and establish integrity of the entire auditory pathway. Electrocochleography can be used, but this technique is invasive and gives no information about the central auditory pathways.

Management

The aims in management are first to recognize that there is a non-organic hearing loss and thereafter to ascertain the true, pure tone thresholds.

Patients pursuing a financial claim are well aware of their actions. Once it is indicated to a patient that the true thresholds are suspected, and an honourable escape route is provided, the NOHL will often disappear on repetition of testing. Any true hearing loss can then be treated on its merits, including the provision of a hearing aid if required, and compensated accordingly.

Fortunately, in the younger, disturbed, group the condition is usually short lived, rarely lasting more than a few weeks or months, as the stressing event disappears or the patient develops appropriate coping strategies. Confrontation is rarely, if ever, successful. Strong reassurance that there is nothing serious present and that the hearing will improve in time is usually all that is required. A hearing aid may be provided for its placebo effect when there is great distress on the part of the patient or carers.

Follow-up and aftercare   In severe or prolonged cases (up to 20%) appropriate psychiatric referral may be required.

Follow-up is only required to document the return of normal hearing.

Further reading

Alberti P. Non-organic hearing loss in adults. In: Beagley HA (ed.) *Audiology and Audiological Medicine*, Vol. 2. Oxford: Oxford University Press, 910–31.

Brooks DN, Geoghegan PM. Non-organic hearing loss in young persons: transient episode or indicator of deep-seated difficulty. *British Journal of Audiology*, 1992; **26**: 347–50.

Northern JL, Downs MP. *Hearing in Children,* 3rd edn. Baltimore: Williams & Wilkins, 1984.

Related topics of interest

ORAL CAVITY CARCINOMA

The oral cavity consists of the buccal mucosa, the upper and lower alveoli, the hard palate, the anterior two-thirds of the tongue and the floor of the mouth to the anterior tonsillar pillars. It does not include the posterior third of the tongue, soft palate or tonsils, which are in the oropharynx.

Pathology

Although benign tumours of epithelial, salivary gland and connective tissue origin occur in the oral cavity, the majority are malignant. Over 90% of the malignant tumours are squamous cell carcinoma. The remainder include adenoid cystic carcinoma, mucoepidermoid tumours, sarcomas and melanomas.

The incidence of squamous cell carcinoma of the oral cavity varies worldwide. In the UK it accounts for less than 2% of all malignancies, but in India it accounts for more than 40%. This is because of the common practice of chewing betel quid containing tobacco in India. Other aetiological factors include smoking tobacco, particularly in a pipe, and high alcohol consumption. There is also an increased incidence in patients with cirrhosis of the liver. Most patients are over the age of 40 years with a peak incidence in the sixth and seventh decades. The male to female ratio is 2:1.

The commonest sites are the lateral border of the tongue and the floor of the mouth. They usually present as an ulcer but may protrude as an exophytic-type lesion. Tumours of the anterior floor of mouth and alveoli tend to spread to the submandibular nodes, and those from the posterior oral cavity tend to metastasize to the jugulodigastric nodes. The tongue has a well-developed lymphatic drainage. Tongue tip tumours spread to the submental lymph nodes first, tumours of the lateral border of the tongue spread to the jugulodigastric nodes, but some anterior tumours may spread directly to the jugulo-omohyoid nodes. Second primary tumours occur in up to 30% of patients with oral cavity carcinoma. They are most commonly found in the oral cavity, but also occur in other sites in the head and neck, the oesophagus and in the lungs.

Clinical features

The patient may complain of a painful ulcer, a warty growth, halitosis and, later, difficulty in eating and speaking. Alveolar tumours may interfere with dentures. On examination the site, size and extent of the tumour should be assessed. Tongue mobility and dental hygiene should also be noted. The neck should be examined for nodal metastases, which are present in nearly a third of patients at the time of presentation.

Investigations

An orthopantomogram may demonstrate involvement of the lower alveolus by the appearance of a moth-eaten rim or an opacity of the normal lucent dental canal. A CT scan is also useful to delineate the extent and local spread of these tumours and an MRI scan is the most sensitive method of detecting invasion of the dental canal. A chest radiograph is mandatory to exclude lung metastases. All patients should have an examination under anaesthetic to obtain a biopsy, evaluate the tumour, exclude a second primary, check the neck for nodes and stage the disease. Therapy, including the feasibility and nature of a surgical resection, can then be planned.

TNM classification

Tis Carcinoma *in situ*.
T1 Tumour 2 cm or less in its greatest dimension.
T2 Tumour more than 2 cm but less than 4 cm in its greatest dimension.
T3 Tumour more than 4 cm in its greatest dimension.
T4 Tumour with extension to bone, muscle, skin, etc.

Management

The management of all patients depends on the site and size of their tumour, the extent of local and distant spread, the presence of any intercurrent disease and their general condition. The aim of surgery is to resect the disease while maintaining maximal function and cosmesis. It is important to remember that the surgery required can impair the functions of swallowing and speech besides its effect on the appearance of the patient.

1. Palliative treatment. Some patients who have a large tumour with advanced local spread or with distant metastases will not be suitable for curative treatment. In addition, it may be inappropriate to subject elderly, infirm patients who are in poor general condition, or who have severe intercurrent disease, to radical treatment. These patients should have supportive nursing care and when necessary adequate analgesisa for pain relief.

2. Radiotherapy. T1 and small T2 tumours in all sites of the oral cavity will respond to this treatment modality. A dose of 6500 cGy is given in fractions over a 4–5 week period.

Lesions of the lateral border of the tongue can be treated with interstitial implants to deliver a dose of 10 000 cGy to a precise area. A combination of external beam and implants can be used. The patient is spared the ordeal of surgery and maintains good oral function, but xerostomia, loss of taste and mucositis can be troublesome side-effects. Primary radiotherapy should not be used to treat tumours involving the mandible as later excision of the bone may lead to osteoradionecrosis. T3 and T4 lesions do badly when treated by radiotherapy alone.

3. Surgery. Surgery is as efficient as radiotherapy in the treatment of T1 and T2 tumours and offers an alternative option for these lesions. Small tumours can be resected transorally using a cutting diathermy or CO_2 or KTP laser with primary closure or closure with a quilted split-skin graft. Larger tumours of the tongue need a partial or total glossectomy. A partial glossectomy, removing up to half of the tongue, can be repaired with a radial forearm free flap. If more than half of the tongue is removed it should be reconstructed by a pectoralis major myocutaneous flap or a rectus abdominus free flap. Small tumours of the alveolar margin can be treated by a marginal mandibulectomy, preserving the outer cortex of the mandible, but a partial mandibulectomy may be required. If much of the anterior segment of the mandible is removed the soft-tissue and bony defect should be reconstructed with a composite osteocutaneous radial forearm free flap. Most surgeons advocate the use of postoperative radiotherapy, to be given within 6 weeks of surgery. This is effective in reducing primary recurrence and has been shown to improve survival.

4. Neck nodes. In some cases no nodes are palpable (N0), but in all cases of oral cancer (apart from the smallest tumours) treatment to the first echelon nodes should be given (levels I and II) either by radiotherapy or selective neck dissection. If the patient has palpable neck node metastases, surgical excision of the primary tumour and radical neck dissection is the treatment of choice. If the patient has bilateral neck node disease, the prognosis is poor. Irradiation to both sides of the neck or bilateral neck dissections with preservation of one internal jugular vein are possible, but the decision to treat other than for palliation should be carefully considered.

Follow-up and aftercare The highest mortality is in the first 2 years after diagnosis. If there is going to be a recurrence it is likely to be in the first year. Patients should have a monthly outpatient review for the first year and 2 monthly for the second year. The oral cavity and neck should be carefully examined for signs of recurrent disease. The risk of a second primary tumour should be remembered. The donor sites of grafts and flaps should be checked until they have healed. The nutritional status and weight of the patient should be monitored, and speech therapy may be appropriate in some cases. Intense prosthodontic rehabilitation should be given where appropriate.

Further reading

Mackenzie IJ. The mouth. In: Stell PM (ed.) *Scott-Brown's Otolaryngology*, Vol. 5, 5th edn. London: Butterworths, 1987.

UICC, Hermanek P, Sabin CH, eds. *TNM Classification of Malignant Tumours,* 4th edn. Berlin: Springer Verlag, 1992.

Wildt J *et al.* Squamous cell carcinoma of the oral cavity: a retrospective analysis of treatment and prognosis. *Clinical Otolaryngology*, 1989; **14**: 10–13.

Zaretsky L, Shindo ML. Soft tissue reconstruction of the oral cavity and pharynx. *Current Opinion in Otolaryngology and Head and Neck Surgery,* 1994; **2**: 343–7.

Related topics of interest

OROANTRAL FISTULA

Definition

A fistula is an abnormal communication between two epithelium-lined surfaces. An oroantral fistula is a communication between the oral cavity and maxillary antrum. Its incidence is probably higher than is recognized because many fistulae escape diagnosis following dental extraction and heal spontaneously without complications.

Aetiology

1. Dental extraction. The fistula forms through the tooth socket following a dental extraction, particularly of the first upper molar and second premolar teeth, the roots of which may penetrate the floor of the antrum. A fistula may also follow the search for retained root fragments after a tooth has been broken.

2. Caldwell–Luc operation. The incision line fails to heal.

3. Trauma. Fractures of the maxilla or penetrating wounds such as a gunshot injury of the hard palate.

4. Neoplasm. Malignant disease of the antrum may occasionally cause erosion into the oral cavity.

Clinical features

The patient may complain of symptoms of chronic maxillary sinusitis. Purulent discharge may collect in the nose or mouth and has a foul smell or taste. A patient who has previously had inferior meatal antrostomies may notice that air or fluid and food particles can be sucked through the fistula into the nose. The diagnosis can be established by passing a probe through the fistula into the antrum.

Investigations

Radiological examination by sinus radiography and orthopantomogram may show retained root fragments, foreign bodies, signs of erosion by neoplastic disease or infections of the maxillary sinus. The injection of a contrast medium into the defect is helpful in confirming the presence of a fistula in doubtful cases. Biopsy is needed if neoplastic disease is suspected.

Treatment

The important factors determining treatment are the length of time the fistula has been present and the presence or absence of infection.

For those following dental extraction the most satisfactory treatment is immediate suture at the time of the dental treatment. If there is a retained root, this must be removed or treatment will be unsuccessful. When a fistula is discovered later there will nearly always be friable granulation tissue in the tract and possibly an antral infection. The infection should be treated first. Pus should be sent for culture and sensitivity and a 2×1 cm inferior meatal antrostomy carried out under antibiotic cover in order to aerate the sinus and allow drainage of pus or secretions. The patient should be reviewed 4 weeks later. If the fistula has not healed it will need formal surgical closure.

Any foreign body must be removed and the bony edges of the alveolus reduced. The fistula tract is incised circumferentially around the margins of the fistula and turned inwards. The bare area is then covered by a mucoperiosteal flap. The adjacent buccal mucosa or a palatal flap based on the greater palatine artery may be used. If adjacent teeth cause a problem in closure they should be removed. The patient should give consent for this. If there is evidence of chronic sinus infection an antrostomy, if not present, should be fashioned at the same time as the fistula closure.

Follow-up and aftercare Decongestant nose drops and a broad-spectrum antibiotic should be prescribed for the first postoperative week and the choice revised according to culture results. The patient should be reviewed in the outpatient department monthly until healing is complete.

Further reading

Snow GB, Van Der Waal. Diseases of the oral cavity. In: Maran AGD, Stell PM (eds) *Clinical Otolaryngology*. Oxford: Blackwell Scientific Publications, 1979; 363–5.

Related topic of interest

Pharyngocutaneous fistula (p. 249)

OROPHARYNGEAL CARCINOMA

The oropharynx is a junctional area between the purely respiratory nasopharynx and larynx, and the alimentary oral cavity and hypopharynx.

Boundaries
- Roof: oral surface of the soft palate.
- Posterior wall: from the level of the hard palate to the level of the aryepiglottic folds.
- Lateral wall: anterior and posterior tonsillar pillars and the palatine tonsil.
- Anterior wall: posterior third of tongue, vallecula and lingual surface of epiglottis.

Pathology

85%: squamous cell carcinoma (SCC).
10%: non-Hodgkin's lymphoma (NHL).
2%: minor salivary gland carcinoma (MSGC).
3%: others, e.g. rhabdomyosarcoma.

Ninety-five per cent of oropharyngeal NHLs involve the palatine or lingual tonsil. Most MSGC arises from the lateral wall; of these 50% are adenoid cystic carcinomas. Most soft palate minor salivary gland tumours are pleomorphic adenomas. Thirty per cent of SCC patients will either have a synchronous second primary or will develop a metachronous second primary within 10 years of presentation. There is a male–female ratio of 5:1 for SCC. Chewing tobacco, smoking and in smokers alcohol (not proven to be a risk factor alone) are risk factors. Leucoplakia and erythroplakia are premalignant conditions.

Staging summary

Tx Tumour cannot be assessed.
Tis Carcinoma *in situ.*
T0 No primary tumour evident.
T1 Carcinoma < 2 cm at largest dimension.
T2 Carcinoma > 2 but < 4 cm at largest dimension.
T3 Carcinoma > 4 cm at largest dimension.
T4 Carcinoma extending beyond oropharynx, e.g. into the pterygoid muscles or neck skin.

Clinical features

Twenty per cent of patients present with a neck lump as the only symptom. Sore throat, referred otalgia, odynophagia and muffled speech are common. Trismus is a late symptom and suggests pterygoid involvement. A full head and neck examination is mandatory because of the high incidence of a second primary carcinoma. SCC is either exophytic or ulcerative, but with NHL the tonsil is either large and vascular or small and shrivelled, looking abnormal compared with its paired counterpart. Palpating the tumour and the neck is important to assess the extent of infiltration of the primary and to assess the size, level, number and fixation of any palpable neck lump(s). NHL requires assessment by an oncologist to stage the disease properly.

Investigations

1. An MRI scan with a STIR sequence will help to define the extent of soft-tissue invasion and neck node involvement. It is preferred to CT scanning. A chest radiograph and liver ultrasound scan are required as lung and then liver are the commonest sites for distant metastases.

2. Fine-needle aspiration cytology (FNAC) of any palpable neck lump.

3. If a neck lump is not palpable but is defined on MRI or CT imaging FNAC should be performed under either ultrasound or preferably CT guidance.

4. A panendoscopy under general anaesthesia is necessary to properly assess the nasopharynx, oral cavity, hypopharynx, oesophagus, trachea and bronchi for synchronous disease. If disease is thought to be limited to the tonsil, a tonsillectomy is performed in an effort to obtain macroscopic clearance. Suspicious tongue base lesions always require a deep biopsy as the cancer may be submucosal.

Management

Most oncologists treat medium and high grade NHL as a disseminated disease and the CHOP [cyclophosphamide, hydroxydaunorubicin, oncovine (vincristine) and prednisolone] regime is the most commonly favoured. VAPEL-B is a more recent regime favoured by some oncologists (vincristine, adreomycin, prednisolone, etopside, cyclophophosphamide and bleomycin). Low grade lymphoma may be treated with chlorambucil or not treated at all. In the relatively unusual event that the lymphoma is very localized, radiotherapy may be used.

MSGC and SCC require a macroscopic margin of 1–2 cm, and clearance should be confirmed by frozen section. T1 and small T2 stage SCC is treated with radiotherapy, as is N1 neck disease. Large T2 and T3 stage disease is treated with surgery. With many T4 tumours macroscopic clearance is not possible. Chemotherapy or radiotherapy may reduce tumour size for clearance to be attempted, but this will depend on the patient's age, fitness and wishes.

To obtain adequate exposure of the lateral oropharynx, a stepped paramedian mandibulotomy is necessary in order to preserve the inferior dental nerve. The exact site is determined after assessing an orthopantogram as the incisor and canine roots are often not parallel. One canine and an incisor often need to be extracted at mandibulotomy to ensure that the plating screws do not impinge on a root, thereby predisposing to a root abscess, osteomyelitis and non-union of the plated mandible. If involvement up to and including the mandibular periosteum has occurred, an inner table mandibulectomy is performed. Should the dental canal be involved a partial mandibulectomy is performed with reconstruction using a composite radial forearm free flap (if less than 10 cm of mandible is taken), a composite fibial or a composite deep circumflex iliac microvascular free flap. T2 tongue base SCC may be excised after a paramedian mandibulotomy by a midline tongue split or via a lateral pharyngotomy after exposing the structures in the poststyloid compartment of the parapharyngeal space. The pre-epiglottic space in large tongue base cancer is almost certain to be invaded so that the only oncologically safe procedure is a total glosso-laryngectomy with oral and pharyngeal reconstruction with a pectoralis major myocutaneous flap.

Soft palate oropharyngeal cancer should be irradiated if small, but larger tumours may require a partial soft palatectomy with reconstruction using a radial forearm fasciocutaneous microvascular free flap which gives the best result in terms of function and cosmesis. T1 and small T2 posterior wall SCCs can be irradiated. If a recurrence occurs, excision with at least a 1-cm margin may allow reconstruction of the posterior wall with a radial forearm fasciocutaneous microvascular free flap, allowing the patient to keep the larynx. Large posterior wall SCC is rare and is probably best treated by a total laryngopharyngo-oesophagectomy and reconstruction with a stomach transposition.

Follow-up and aftercare

Swallowing is frequently seriously impaired after surgery. Swallowing rehabilitation should be instituted by a speech therapist with a special interest in swallowing as soon as nourishment is allowed by mouth, normally on around the 10th postoperative day. Rehabilitation so that sufficient fluid and nourishment can be swallowed to maintain homeostasis can take many weeks, and in this case a percutaneous gastrostomy is preferable to nasogastric feeding. Strictures at the anastomosic line in those who have had a stomach transposition are unusual but may require repeated dilation. Any mucosal irregularity in this region must be biopsied in case there is underlying recurrent disease. The regularity of follow-up is the same for any head and neck cancer and is outlined elsewhere (see Laryngeal carcinoma (p. 148) and Sinonasal tumours (p. 280)).

Further reading

Hermanek P, Sobin LH. *TNM Classification of Malignant Tumours,* 4th edn. Lyon: UICC, 1987.
Million RR, Cassisi NJ. Oropharynx. In: Million RR, Cassisi NJ (eds) *Management of Head and Neck Cancer,* 2nd edn. Philadelphia: JB Lippincott, 1994; 401–31.

OTALGIA

Otalgia is pain in the ear. It is a symptom not a diagnosis. It may be primary (or otological in origin) or secondary (referred).

Anatomy

The sensory nerve supply of the external and middle ears arises from many sources. The lower half of the pinna receives its sensory supply from the great auricular nerve via the cervical plexus, predominantly C2 and C3. The upper half receives its supply from the lesser occipital nerve (C2) medially and the auriculotemporal nerve laterally (mandibular branch of Vth cranal nerve). The external auditory meatus and lateral tympanic membrane receive their supply from the auriculotemporal nerve and branches of the facial and vagus nerves (Arnolds nerve). The medial aspect of the tympanic membrane and middle ear is supplied through the tympanic plexus by the facial and glossopharyngeal nerves (Jacobsens nerve).

Pathophysiology

Primary otalgia may arise as a result of direct stimulation of these otological sensory nerves from primary otological pathology. In this regard acute inflammatory processes are particularly effective in producing pain and include acute otitis externa, furuncles, shingles and acute otitis media. Malignant otitis externa and tumours, by virtue of involving bone, may also produce severe pain.

Referred otalgia may arise from disease in any peripheral territory supplied by these nerves. Finally, otalgia, in theory, may arise from a primary neuralgia of any of these nerves, although it is most common in the glossopharyngeal nerve. This condition gives rise to severe lancinating pain arising in the tonsillar fossa or tongue base and radiating deeply in the ear, often induced by talking or swallowing. Less commonly the pain may be centred in the external auditory meatus and not be induced by throat movement.

Causes

A brief list and system of classification for the commoner causes of referred otalgia is given below.

1. Second and third cervical nerves.

- Arthritis/cervical spondylosis.
- Soft tissue injury.

2. Trigeminal nerve.

- Dental disease such as tooth impaction, caries and abscess, particularly of posterior teeth, and

temporomandibular joint dysfunction are probably the commonest non-otological causes of otalgia.
- Nasopharyngeal disease such as viral infection, tumour or post adenoidectomy.
- Sinonasal disease and salivary gland disease are uncommon causes of referred otalgia.

3. Glossopharyngeal nerve and vagus.

- Almost any oropharyngeal infective process may lead to otalgia, such as pharyngitis, tonsillitis and quinsy. Otalgia is common following tonsillectomy.
- Tumours of the tongue base or pyriform fossae are potent causes of otalgia.

Management

A full history and examination will normally direct attention to the offending part of the head and neck. Particularly thorough attention should be paid to the tongue base and pyriform fossae as pathology here can be catastrophic if overlooked. Appropriate treatment should then be directed at the underlying cause.

Occasionally no abnormality can be found even after a thorough examination and further investigation, except perhaps some mild clunking of the temporomandibular joint. It is certainly not uncommon to find a small group of patients with otalgia shuttling back and forth between ENT and oral surgeons, with both claiming the symptom is in the other's department. In such cases, and in those in whom there are absolutely no abnormal findings, it is worth considering glossopharyngeal neuralgia. A trial of carbamazepine may benefit the patient. This condition may be successfully treated by tympanotomy and section of the tympanic plexus.

Follow-up and aftercare

This is usually as dictated by the underlying causative condition.

Further reading

Cook JA, Irving RM. Role of tympanic neurectomy in otalgia. *Journal of Laryngology and Otology*, 1990; **104:** 114–17.

Related topics of interest

Acute suppurative otitis media (p. 9)
Facial pain (p. 107)
Otitis externa (p. 210)

OTITIS EXTERNA

Definition

Otitis externa is an inflammation of the skin of the external auditory meatus (EAM).

The skin of the EAM comprises in the outer third an epithelial layer containing hair follicles, ceruminous glands and sebaceous glands, lying on a thin dermal bed containing sweat glands. The skin of the bony ear canal lacks appendages and migrates outwards from within. The secretions of the sebaceous glands keep the stratum corneum watertight and supple. Sweat gland secretions keep the secretion at a pH between 3 and 5, which is lethal for most human pathogens. Usually the EAM is sterile or contains *Staphylococcus albus* commensals. *Staphylococcus aureus* and non-haemolytic streptococci are unusual.

Pathology

In the acute phase of otitis externa there are dilated dermal blood vessels of increased permeability which cause signs of a red, hot, oedematous and tender ear canal. The epithelial reaction consists of vesication, parakeratosis and spongeosis.

Predisposing factors

(a) Heat, humidity, bathing, swimming.
(b) Trauma, especially from dirty fingernails, cotton buds and hairgrips.
(c) Inherited: narrow ear canals and non-atopic eczema.

Classification

1. Infective.
(a) Bacterial Diffuse otitis externa commonly caused by *Pseudomonas aeruginosa*, *S. aureus* and *Proteus*.
Furunculosis, usually caused by *S. aureus*.
Malignant otitis externa, usually caused by *P. aeruginosa*.
Erysipelas caused by *Streptococcus pyogenes*.
Perichondritis, usually caused by *S. aureus* and *S. pyogenes*.
Impetigo, an infection of the superficial layers of the epidermis, usually caused by *S. aureus* or occasionally by *S. pyogenes*.
Secondary to an acute or chronic otitis media.
(b) Fungal *Aspergillus niger*.
Aspergillus fumigatus.
Candida albicans.
(c) Viral Herpes simplex.
Herpes zoster.
Presumptive in otitis externa haemorrhagica.

2. *Reactive*	Eczema.
	Seborrhoeic dermatitis.
	Neurodermatitis.
	Keratitis obturans.
	Psoriasis.

Clinical features

Otitis externa may be confined to the meatus (localized) or involve other areas of skin (generalized). Localized infection can be circumscribed or diffuse, while generalized infection can be either primarily otological or primarily dermatological.

Enquiries regarding direct trauma to the ear canal, swimming habits, atopic tendency and previous otological problems should be made. Symptoms of infection elsewhere in the head and neck, for example tonsillitis and sinusitis, and preceding symptoms of otitis media should be sought. Conditions affecting the ear canal are limited and a diagnosis can usually be made on examination. Although the history may provide a pointer towards the diagnosis, severe itching suggests eczema, neurodermatitis or mycotic infection. Otalgia occurs with furunculosis, diffuse otitis externa and herpes infections.

On examination erythema is a feature of eczema, seborrhoeic dermatitis, mycosis or acute trauma. Vesication occurs in eczema and herpetic infection, excess squamous debris suggests chronic eczema or mycosis and hypertrophic meatal skin suggests chronic disease.

It is not uncommon to find the ear canal occluded by oedema in a patient with acute otalgia. Careful examination will usually distinguish furunculosis (common) from acute mastoiditis (now much less common). In the former there is postauricular tenderness localized to a palpable lymph node. Exceptionally this node may break down to cause diffuse tenderness and oedema, which may displace the pinna slightly forwards. There is always pain on moving the pinna. A patient with acute mastoiditis will have a more marked postauricular swelling which may be fluctuant, displacing the pinna, down as well as forwards. There is no pain on moving the pinna, and there will be a preceding history of acute suppurative otitis media. Plain lateral oblique and Towne's projection mastoid radiographs may show mastoid air cell coalescence in acute mastoiditis, but in this and furunculosis the mastoid air cells may be cloudy on the lateral view. In furunculosis this is because postauricular oedema is superimposed on the plate.

Investigations	A cultural swab should be taken for microbiological culture, including fungal culture and antibiotic/antimycotic sensitivity.
Management	(a) Meticulous and regular aural toilet paying particular attention to the anteroinferior meatal recess.
	(b) Splinting the meatus. The two recommended choices are 12-mm ribbon gauze, impregnated with 10% ichthammol in glycerine, the hygroscopic action of which reduces meatal swelling, or a pope's sponge ear wick onto which eardrops containing an antibiotic and steroid mixture are applied. Splinting will be necessary when there is EAM oedema preventing an adequate view of the tympanic membrane on otoscopy, implying that ear drops will not reach the deeper recesses of the ear canal. The dressing should be changed at least every 48 hours until the canal swelling has settled sufficiently to allow any applied drops to reach the anteroinferior recess directly.
	(c) The ears should be kept scrupulously dry until resolution. Swimming is inadvisable and precautions should be taken when bathing to prevent water entering the ear canal.
	In most reactive conditions the above regime is also recommended in order to prevent secondary infection of a raw ear canal surface.
Follow-up and aftercare	Treatment should continue for at least 1 week after resolution because of the tendency to recurrence, particularly in otomycosis. Itchy reactive conditions may benefit from a course of beclomethasone ear drops, and an 8% solution of aluminium acetate is recommended in patients with chronic otitis externa after the acute infection has been eradicated.

Malignant otitis externa

This condition describes an otitis externa which progresses to an osteomyelitis initially of the tympanic plate, which then may spread to involve the skull base and petrous portion of the temporal bone. It is most common after middle age and in diabetics and is usually caused by *P. aeruginosa*. The overwhelming symptom is a constant deep otalgia and it may cause nerve palsies of cranial nerves VII to XII, meningitis, sigmoid sinus thrombosis, brain abscess and death.

The condition should be suspected in a patient with granulation tissue deep in the external meatus which does not settle with the usual treatment. The diagnosis is often not considered until a cranial nerve palsy has developed. When such a patient develops a facial nerve palsy the differential diagnosis is between ASOM (almost always secondary to an dehiscent horizontal portion of the facial nerve), CSOM, malignancy of the EAM or middle ear and malignant otitis externa. Histological and microbiological examination of granulation tissue, and a high-definition CT scan of the petrous temporal bone are required to make a diagnosis.

Treatment   Appropriate intravenous antibiotics as gleaned from the culture and sensitivity results should be commenced. The dose and duration of treatment is decided after discussion with a senior microbiologist and by monitoring clinical response, but often therapy has to be continued for 6 weeks or more. Even with aggressive treatment there is still a significant mortality. Opiate analgesia may be required to control the deep-seated otalgia.

Further reading

Morrison AW, Mackay IS. The aetiology of otitis externa – a new concept. *Journal of Laryngology and Otology,* 1976; **15:** 495–7.

Related topics of interest

Acute suppurative otitis media (p. 9)
Chronic suppurative otitis media (p. 51)
Chronic suppurative otitis media – complications (p. 55)

OTITIS MEDIA WITH EFFUSION

Aetiology

The fundamental pathology is Eustachian tube dysfunction. The exact cause for this remains in doubt, but there are associations with recurrent upper respiratory tract infections and reduced overall nasopharyngeal dimensions and airway size owing to the presence of hypertrophied adenoids in a relatively smaller nasopharynx. The adenoid is recognized as an important contributor to otitis media with effusion (OME) because it is a source of pathological bacteria, and not because it mechanically obstructs the orifice of the Eustachian tube. There is no difference in effusion rates between those children who have large versus small adenoids.

Pathology

The prevalence of OME is highest in young children (40% at 2 years) and decreases with age so that it is uncommon in teenagers (1% at 11 years). The prevalence is also higher in the winter months, in boys, in children with cleft palate or Down's syndrome, in those with allergy and in the children of parents who smoke. The underlying Eustachian tube dysfunction leads to a chronic reduction in middle-ear pressure. This ultimately causes an inflammatory response in the middle-ear mucosa and the production of glue: thick, tenacious mucus rich in glyco- and mucoproteins and containing inflammatory cells which fill the middle-ear cleft. In most cases (90%) spontaneous resolution is the rule, punctuated by numerous remissions and relapses. In a small number of persistent and severe cases there is progressive atrophy and retraction of the tympanic membrane. Sequalae such as retraction pockets and even cholesteatoma may ultimately develop.

Clinical features

The presence of fluid in the middle-ear cleft leads to a conductive hearing loss of variable severity and is responsible for most of the clinical features. Hearing impairment, whether persistent or intermittent, noticed by parents, relatives or teachers or picked up at routine screening is the presenting symptom in over 80% of cases. Learning difficulties and speech delay account for the bulk of the remainder, and recurrent infections and otalgia are uncommon features of this condition (1–2%) although they are common complaints in childhood. Most cases present between the age of 3 and 6 years, with the more severe cases tending to present earlier. Examination may or may not reveal a middle-ear effusion depending on the activity of the process at consultation. The otoscopic appearance of the effusion varies. The tympanic membrane can look dull red, grey or an amber yellow colour. It can bulge forward or be retracted. Attic and posterior retraction pockets may occur, but bony erosion is relatively unusual. Air bubbles or a fluid level can occasionally be seen.

Investigations

An audiogram appropriate to age and impedance audiometry are all that is required. Pure tone audiometry if feasible will show a conductive hearing loss. Impedance audiometry will show a flat tympanogram (type b) which is typical of otitis media with effusion and helps distinguish the disease from Eustachian tube dysfunction and otosclerosis.

Management

Management should be appropriate to the severity of the symptoms and should always take account of the natural history of the condition towards spontaneous resolution. For many children explanation and reassurance to the parents are all that is required. A review visit after 3 months is useful to establish the persistent nature of the patient's condition, in particular a persistent hearing loss.

Medical treatment has little role to play in this condition, although some people have used long-term low-dose antibiotics. Autoinflation of the Eustachian tube using the Otovent device has been shown to give useful results but is significantly less effective than grommets.

In the more severe cases the insertion of ventilation tubes improves hearing and shortens the overall duration of the condition. The benefits of ventilation tubes may be augmented by combination with adenoidectomy. The benefits of this are greatest between the ages of 4 and 8 years. Tonsillectomy does not seem to influence the condition. Grommets should be used rather than T-tubes, which are associated with an unacceptably high rate of residual perforation (50%). The main complications of grommets are infections and the development of tympanosclerosis (which is found in 30–40% of children 1 year after grommet insertion). Tympanosclerosis is associated with multiple episodes of grommet insertion and intratympanic bleeding at myringotomy. The use of mini-grommets seems to cause fewer problems. Infections should be treated by aural toilet and antibiotic/steroid ear drops in the first instance, but grommet removal may be required if the condition fails to settle.

Follow-up and aftercare   Grommets require little aftercare. There is no good evidence that swimming with unoccluded ears increases the risk of infection, although some form of ear plug should be worn when shampooing (because soap reduces the surface tension of the water). Grommets extrude after 3–12 months after which some form of review is required to recheck the hearing. A sizeable proportion of affected children (25%) will require further subsequent grommet insertion.

Further reading

Maw AR, Bawden R. Spontaneous resolution of severe chronic glue ear in children and the effect of adenoidectomy, tonsillectomy and insertion of ventilation tubes (grommets). *British Medical Journal*, 1993; **306**: 756–60.

Maw AR, Tiwari RS. Children with glue ear: how do they present? *Clinical Otolaryngology*, 1988; **13**: 171–7.

Related topics of interest

Impedance audiometry (p. 137)
Paediatric hearing assessment (p. 241)
Tympanosclerosis (p. 331)

OTOACOUSTIC EMISSIONS

Using modern computing technology and signal averaging techniques, outer hair cell vibrations can be detected in the external auditory meatus as otoacoustic emissions (OAEs). They were first described by David Kemp in 1978 and represent an objective measure of cochlear function. Acoustically evoked OAEs are almost never found in ears with a hearing level worse than 40 dB.

Physiology

The cochlea provides an elegant mechanism for transforming the physical properties of sound into electrical neural impulses. Sound vibrations pass from the environment through the external and middle-ear systems to cause vibrations of the cochlear perilymph. These vibrations produce travelling waves in the basilar membrane. As a result of the gradient of width, thickness and consequently stiffness of the basilar membrane, these travelling waves reach maximal amplitude at specific points along the cochlea. High frequencies are represented at the basal turn and low frequencies at the apical portion. These vibrations are detected as a result of shearing forces on two separate hair cell systems in the organ of Corti: the inner (IHCs) and outer (OHCs) hair cells. The inner hair cells are purely sensory and are responsible for detecting these vibrations and producing neural impulses to allow them to be perceived by the central nervous system as sound. The outer hair cells also detect these vibrations but, in contrast, have a motor function. The outer hair cells at the region of maximal travelling wave amplitude vibrate in synchrony with the stimulating signal while the OHCs on either side of this region suppress vibration of the basilar membrane. This mechanism allows the fine tuning found in the healthy cochlea. These outer hair cell vibrations can be detected in the external auditory meatus as otoacoustic emissions.

Types of otoacoustic emissions

Four classes of OAE exist:

1. Spontaneous OAEs (SOAEs). These are low-level signals which occur without external acoustic stimulation in about 40–50% of the normal hearing population. Although they are relatively constant in frequency, they vary in terms of occurrence and intensity and consequently have little use in clinical monitoring.

2. Stimulus-frequency OAEs. These are recorded at the frequency of a stimulating pure tone. They appear to have little clinical or research use.

3. Transient evoked OAEs (TEOAEs). These signals, usually between 0.7 and 4 kHz, occur in response to short-lasting stimulatory acoustic signals (usually clicks or tone bursts). The signal is very different for each individual but remains fairly constant for any given ear. TEOAEs occur in almost all human ears with hearing levels better than 40 dB, but are of greater amplitude and wider frequency range in children. As they are relatively quick and easy to measure, they are finding increasing use for clinical screening and research.

4. Distortion-product OAE (DPOAE). Stimulation with two pure tones of specific frequency and intensity ratios gives rise to DPOAEs. They are nearly always present in normal hearing ears and can be measured in the 6–8 kHz range. These characteristics make them an ideal tool for investigating frequency-specific cochlear function.

Measurement of otoacoustic emissions

An OAE analyser consists of a mobile probe which contains a sound emitter and microphone for recording. Unlike a tympanometer, an airtight seal is not required. The acoustic stimulus on currently available OAE analysers are broadband clicks, at a maximal rate of 50/s. The measured signals are then fed to a signal processor where, by the use of appropriate frequency filters and time window averaging, OAEs can be demonstrated on either a visual or print-out display. Research is still being undertaken into the optimal method of producing and subsequently analysing OAEs.

Clinical uses

Although still primarily a research tool for the investigation of cochlear function, the use of evoked OAEs has now found a place in clinical practice in the screening of neonates and high-risk infants for hearing loss. Evoked OAEs are quick, easy to test and do not require an anaesthetic, in contrast to electrical evoked response audiometry. The sensitivity and specificity of the test is sufficiently good that in the United States it is recommended that all newborn infants are screened for hearing loss by OAE prior to discharge from hospital.

Further reading

3rd International symposium on cochlear mechanisms and otoacoustic emissions, 1992. *British Journal of Audiology*, 1993; **27** (2): 71–159.

Related topics of interest

Evoked response audiometry (p. 85)
Paediatric hearing assessment (p. 241)

OTOLOGICAL ASPECTS OF HEAD INJURY

A blow to the side of the head by a blunt or sharp instrument may cause injury to the external, middle or inner ear in isolation or in combination. There may be a fracture of the temporal bone and other skull base fractures. Conditions caused by such trauma are described below.

External ear
(a) Subperichondrial haematoma.
(b) Perichondritis.
(c) Loss of pinna tissue.
(d) Otitis externa.
(e) External auditory meatus stenosis.
(f) Occlusion of the external canal by clot.

Middle ear
(a) Tympanic membrane haematoma and petechiae.
(b) Tympanic membrane rupture with or without the deposition of squamous epithelium within the middle ear.
(c) Ossicular chain discontinuity.
(d) Facial nerve injury.
(e) Haemotympanum and acute non-suppurative otitis media.
(f) Acute suppurative otitis media.

Inner ear
(a) Perilymph fistula from either a round window rupture or from the oval window.
(b) Serous or a purulent labyrinthitis.
(c) Intracranial complications: lateral sinus thrombosis, meningitis, extradural, subdural, intracerebral (cerebellar and temporal lobe) abscess and otitic hydrocephalus.

Temporal bone fractures
These are classified into longitudinal, transverse and mixed, depending on the orientation of the fracture line to the long axis of the petrous temporal bone. Occasionally with a fracture of the squamous temporal bone, a type of longitudinal fracture, the only sign will be bruising of the postauricular skin (Battle's sign).

1. Longitudinal fractures. These constitute 80% of temporal bone fractures and usually arise from a lateral blow to the skull. The fracture extends from the squamous temporal bone in the roof of the bony external auditory meatus to the tympanic membrane and the roof of the middle ear before turning anterior to the labyrinth where it may involve the carotid canal.

2. Transverse fractures. These constitute 20% of temporal bone fractures and usually arise from a blow to the front or back of the skull. The fracture extends across the long axis of the petrous bone through the labyrinthine capsule and is demonstrated with plain temporal bone radiographs in 50% of cases.

Clinical features

Longitudinal fractures tear the skin of the external auditory meatus and tympanic membrane to cause swelling of the canal skin and bleeding from the ear. These findings should be presumed to indicate such a fracture following a head injury. A haemotympanum and ruptured tympanic membrane will occur if the fracture line extends to the middle-ear cleft. This usually heals without residual conductive deafness if infection is prevented. A sensorineural hearing loss is usually secondary to inner ear concussion and therefore temporary. Facial nerve injuries are uncommon, although CSF otorrhoea is more common with this fracture. The latter is suspected when there is a persisting serosanguinous aural discharge.

In a pure *transverse fracture* there is a haemotympanum but no bleeding from the ear because the tympanic membrane remains intact. Facial nerve injury occurs immediately in half of these fractures. Labyrinthine capsule disruption causes an irreversible sensory hearing loss, usually a dead ear, severe vertigo, nystagmus to the opposite ear, IXth to XIIth cranial nerve injury, and perhaps focal neurological signs. These fractures occur with a more severe head injury so otological symptoms may not become apparent until recovery from the acute head injury. Symptoms of secondary endolympatic hydrops may be caused by involvement of the vestibular aqueduct in the fracture line.

Temporal bone fractures usually have a mixed longitudinal and transverse component, and this will be suspected from combined clinical features.

Management

The general management of the head injury takes precedence, but it is important to avoid introducing infection into the ear so prophylactic antibiotics are indicated. In the absence of a facial palsy leave the ear untouched in the early postinjury period. Sequelae are unusual in longitudinal fractures and a conductive hearing loss is unlikely to be due to a traumatic ossicular discontinuity. It should resolve when the ear canal skin and tympanic membrane heal. A facial nerve palsy, if present immediately following injury, should be investigated by a high definition CT scan of the temporal bone on bone setting. If there is CT evidence of nerve disruption of the tympanomastoid segment of the nerve, then this portion should be explored and decompressed.

If tympanomastoid exploration is negative an expert otoneurosurgeon may feel that exploration of the labyrinthine segment is indicated. If the scan showed no fracture of the temporal bone, evoked electromyography will provide an indication of severity of injury and prognosis. If the summating potential is more than 10% of normal after 14 days the prognosis is good, with about 90% recovery to House and Brackmann grade I or II. If it is less than 10% after 14 days then many otoneurosurgeons advocate exploration of the temporal bone, exposing the nerve from the internal auditory meatus to the stylomastoid foramen. A facial palsy occurring hours after injury will be secondary to a neuropraxia and a conservative policy should be observed. The same follows for CSF otorrhoea, confirmed by the presence of glucose and β_2-transferrin. A policy of bed rest but sitting up to reduce intracranial CSF pressure and antibiotic cover to prevent intracranial infection allow resolution to occur after about 10 days. Should the leak persist, a CT scan using intrathecal Omnopaque 500 may identify the site of the leak, usually from the middle fossa, and allow exploration. Traumatic perilymph fistula is discussed on p. 244.

Further reading

Bassiouny M, Hirsch BE, Kelly RH, Kamerer DB, Cass SP. Beta2 transferrin application in otology. *American Journal of Otolaryngology*, 1992; **13**: 552–5.

Related topic of interest

Perilymph fistula (p. 244)

OTORRHOEA

Definition

Otorrhoea is the discharge of material from the external auditory meatus. It is both a symptom and a sign. It is not a diagnosis.

Clinical features

The character of the discharge depends on and therefore gives clues as to its source.

1. External ear. There are no mucinous glands in the external canal. Acute inflammatory conditions of the external meatus therefore tend to produce a watery, serous exudate or transudate. In addition, they tend to provoke a hyperkeratosis. This combination generally leads to soggy white debris collecting in the canal and a thin white watery discharge from the ear. The external canal may also be the subject of trauma, which may lead to bleeding from the ear.

2. Middle ear. The middle-ear cleft is well endowed with mucous glands. Thus, if there is a mucoid component to the discharge it must arise from the middle ear via a perforation of the tympanic membrane. Trapped keratin is offensive; if a cholesteatoma should become infected the discharge tends to be particularly unpleasant and once smelt is never forgotten. As the cholesteatoma exists in a retraction pocket there will only be a mucoid component to the discharge if there is a communication with the middle-ear cleft. A serosanguinous discharge is common with chronic otitis media when the middle-ear mucosa has become granular and polypoid; there is glandular hyperplasia and the mucosa bleeds easily.

3. Cerebrospinal fluid. CSF rarely discharges from the ears spontaneously but may do so following skull base surgery or more commonly trauma, when it will develop in about 5% of cases. In both cases the fluid may initially be mixed with blood and may be recognized by the halo sign in which there is a clear ring of moisture surrounding the blood after absorption on to blotting paper. This is due to the faster diffusion of the less viscous CSF. Differentiation of CSF from thin serous discharge from a middle-ear cavity may be more difficult but can be done by estimation of the glucose content or by confirming the presence of β_2-transferrin in CSF. If the tympanic membrane is intact CSF may still leak from the ear should there be a fracture in the roof of the ear canal. Otherwise it may pass down the Eustachian tube and become evident as rhinorrhoea or postnasal drip.

Management

Optimum management depends on making an accurate diagnosis. Although the history will give many clues, the diagnosis is usually not made until the tympanic membrane has been visualized. This may not be possible at the initial consultation owing to swelling and debris in the external auditory meatus, and treatment should therefore commence on the basis of a best guess diagnosis. This will invariably require treatment of the primary or secondary otitis externa by thorough aural toilet and the insertion of a wick. At the time of definitive diagnosis more appropriate treatment can be continued. Treatment of the otitis externa will be sufficient if this is the diagnosis. Middle-ear disease will demand treatment on its own merits.

All CSF otorrhoea should be initially covered with prophylactic antibiotics to reduce the risk of meningitis. Post-traumatic leaks usually resolve spontaneously within a short period, but surgical repair will be required if they continue beyond 5 days. Iatrogenic leaks should hopefully be recognized and repaired at the time of surgery. If this is not the case, conservative management is reasonable for the first few postoperative days but surgical repair will be required if the leak fails to settle.

Conservative management includes sitting upright in bed and avoidance of manoeuvres that raise intracranial pressure (e.g. coughing, straining, etc.) Prior to any surgical exploration a thorough radiological assessment of the temporal bone should be undertaken to try to establish the site of the leak. This is best achieved with high-resolution CT scanning and the subarachnoid injection of Omnopaque 500. Fluorescein injected by lumbar puncture may be helpful in finding the site of the leak at the time of surgery.

The type and method of repair employed will depend on the site and cause of the leak and to some extent the state of the middle ear and the patient's hearing; it would be inappropriate to obliterate the middle ear of an individual with normal hearing, for instance.

Further reading

Applebaum EL, Chow JM. CSF Leaks. In: Cummings CW *et al.* (eds) *Otolaryngology, Head and Neck Surgery,* 2nd edn. Vol. 1. St. Louis: Mosby, 1993; 965–74.

Related topics of interest

OTOSCLEROSIS

Definition

This is an autosomal dominant disease of incomplete penetrance affecting bone derived from the otic capsule in which mature lamellar bone is replaced by woven bone of greater cellularity and vascularity featuring large Haversian canals, lacunae, canaliculi and marrow spaces.

Otosclerotic foci are most commonly located just anterior to the oval window in the region of the fissula ante fenestram. Symptoms occur when these foci fix the stapedial footplate and encroach upon the labyrinth. It is uncertain whether cochleovestibular symptoms arise directly from this encroachment, from factors released by the plaque or from both. Foci have also been noted in the region of the fissula post fenestram, the semicircular canals, the round window, the base of the styloid process, the petrosquamous suture and in the cochlea.

The three main theories of pathogenesis are:

1. It is an expression of a genetic mutation in collagen metabolism which is only phenotypically expressed in bone derived from the otic capsule.
2. It is an expression of humoral autoimmunity to type II collagen.
3. It is an expression of persistent measles virus infection of the otic capsule-derived bone.

Prevalence and incidence

The clinical disease has been estimated to affect 0.5–2% of the population (the prevalence) and the subclinical disease affects about 10% of the population. The incidence of clinical disease (number of new cases per year) is much lower. A recent study by Zeitoun showed that the typical consultant/trainee team perform on average eight stapedectomies per year (range 0–30), making an incidence of stapedectomy in the average 150 000 population catchment area of 0.005%. The incidence of otosclerosis is higher, perhaps 0.05%, as we would not expect all subjects with clinical otosclerosis to have a stapedectomy, but will nowhere near approach the 1% incidence that is often quoted in major texts. Eighty-five per cent of patients with otosclerosis have bilateral disease.

Otosclerosis is more common in Caucasians. A female–male ratio of 2:1 has been noted, perhaps because women are more likely to seek advice because pregnancy, menstruation and the menopause may cause the disease to progress rapidly. Women are more likely to have bilateral clinical disease.

Clinical features

The main symptoms are:

1. Deafness. Noticed in most cases before the age of 30. Hearing better in noisy surroundings is often described (paracusis Willisi).

2. Tinnitus. Present in 75% of patients, especially when there is a cochlear element to the deafness.

3. Vertigo. Mild and usually transient. Symptoms may mimic benign paroxysmal positional vertigo.

Ten per cent of ears display Schwartz's sign, a pink tinge of the tympanic membrane imparted from dilated blood vessels on the mucous membrane of the promontory. There are no other otoscopic signs. Rinne's test usually suggests a conductive hearing loss. The Weber test may be referred to either ear, depending on whether disease is unilateral or bilateral, and on the cochlear reserve.

Investigations

1. Pure tone audiometry. In addition to a conductive hearing loss there may be cochlear impairment. Masked air conduction typically shows a loss which is greater at low frequencies when there is minimal cochlear impairment, but the frequency–response curve flattens and then shows a predominantly high-frequency loss as cochlear impairment progresses. The masked bone conduction curve typically shows a dip at 2000 Hz, and may be small or exaggerated. It occurs typically when there is no or a slight cochlear loss (Carhart's notch). The curve shows a predominantly high-tone loss when there is more severe cochlear impairment.

2. Speech audiometry. With amplification the score approaches 100 with normal cochlear function, but the score falls according to the severity of the cochlear loss.

3. Impedance audiometry. Unreliable as a diagnostic aid although it may be useful in selecting the more suitable ear for surgery in bilateral otosclerosis with a symmetrical PTA by suggesting the more rigid stapes.

Differential diagnosis

- Fibro-osseous footplate fixation.
- Congenital footplate fixation.

- Ossicular discontinuity.
- Fixed malleus–incus syndrome.
- Crural atrophy.
- Congenital cholesteatoma.
- Paget's disease (usually produces a mixed hearing loss).
- Osteogenesis imperfecta.

Management

1. Sodium fluoride. No major randomized, prospective, double-blind trial has been performed to assess its effectiveness. Its use remains controversial.

2. A hearing aid.

3. Stapedectomy. The minimum requirements are at least a 15 dB conductive hearing loss with 60% speech discrimination. The ear, including the external ear canal, should be dry. It is contraindicated in pregnancy. If both ears are suitable for surgery in bilateral disease, the poorer hearing ear should be chosen. Second ear stapedectomy is still controversial but is advocated by many who perform the small fenestra procedure.

Preoperative counselling

- A hearing aid is an alternative method of treatment.
- A dead ear may occur with stapedectomy. The incidence reported by expert otologists varies from less than 1% to 4%, and a further 10% may have no better or worse hearing than preoperatively.
- Tinnitus may not improve and may be more intense after surgery.
- Vertigo may be present immediately postoperatively, and in a minority there may be a permanent sense of imbalance.
- Taste may alter or be lost on one side of the tongue.
- There is a very small chance that the facial nerve will run an anomalous course, either splitting around or coursing inferior to the oval window, and may be injured.

Postoperative advice

- Avoid diving when swimming, lifting heavy objects and aggressive nose blowing.
- Open the mouth on coughing or sneezing.
- Avoid flying for the first 3 weeks postoperatively.

Technique

1. Small fenestra. A microdrill, a stapedotomy needle, or an argon or KTP laser may be used to create the fenestra in the stapes footplate. The smaller the fenestra, the smaller the risk of a high-tone cochlear hearing loss. A 0.6-mm fenestra drillpiece and 0.4-mm prosthesis are popular. The Causse technique comprises a 0.8-mm fenestra, over which a vein graft is placed, and a 0.4-mm prosthesis.

2. *Large fenestra.* A portion of the footplate is removed with picks and fine right-angle hooks. An attempt is usually made to seal the oval window with a vein or fat graft prior to prosthesis insertion.

The otologist aims to achieve complete or overclosure of the air–bone gap. Overclosure is possible because of the Carhart effect and is greatest at 2000 Hz (see Related topics of interest).

Complications of stapedectomy

1. *Peroperative.*
(a) Tympanic membrane tear.
(b) Chorda tympani injury.
(c) Overhanging facial nerve.
(d) Persistent stapedial artery.
(e) Tympanosclerosis arthrodesing the incudostapedial joint.
(f) Perilymph flooding.
(g) Floating footplate.
(h) Depressed footplate.
(i) Injury to the saccule. This lies as close as 0.4 mm beneath the footplate and is easily disturbed when performing the stapedotomy or inserting the prosthesis. It may be the cause of a dead ear from an apparently uncomplicated procedure.

An immediate dead ear may arise from (f)–(i) above.

2. *Early.*
(a) Detachment of prosthesis from incus.
(b) Displacement of prosthesis from oval window.
(c) Loose attachment of incus and prosthesis.
(d) Footplate granuloma.
(e) Persisting primary perilymph fistula.

3. *Late.*
(a) Secondary perilymph fistula.
(b) Necrosis of the long process of the incus.
(c) (a)–(c) above.

Cochlear otosclerosis

Consider when there is a family history of otosclerosis and progressive sensorineural hearing loss in early adult life of no apparent cause. Look for Schwartze's sign on otoscopy. A high-definition CT scan may detect an otosclerotic plaque.

Further reading

Altermatt HJ, Gerber HA, Gaeng D, Muller C, Arnold W. Immunohistochemical findings in otosclerotic lesions. *HNO,* 1992; **40**: 476–9.

Browning GG, Gatehouse S. The prevalence of middle ear disease in the adult British population. *Clinical Otolaryngology,* 1992; **17**: 317–21.

Roald B, Storvald G, Mair IWS, Mjoen S. Respiratory tract viruses in otosclerotic lesions. *Acta Otolaryngologica*, 1992; **112**: 334–8.

Zeitoun H, Porter MJ, Brookes G.B. Current practice of stapedectomy in Great Britain. *Clinical Otolaryngology,* 1993; **18**: 392–5.

Related topics of interest

OTOTOXICITY

Ototoxicity is the partial or total reduction in cochleovestibular function caused by the interaction of chemicals, commonly therapeutic agents, with the vestibule, cochlea or the vestibulocochlear nerve.

There are over 200 ototoxic substances, but only a small group of drugs in common therapeutic use are regularly associated with ototoxicity.

Aminoglycosides

All aminoglycoside antibiotics have a tendency to be predominantly either cochleotoxic (e.g. neomycin and kanamycin) or vestibulotoxic (e.g. gentamicin and tobramycin). The former relates to the number of free amino groups ($-NH_2$), the latter to the number of free methylamine groups ($-NHCH_3$).

Mechanism of action

Current opinion holds that secretion of aminoglycoside from the stria vascularis into the endolymph and perhaps from the vessels of the spiral ligament into the perilymph occurs with active uptake of antibiotic from the perilymph into the endolymph. Resorption by the stria clears the endolymph of aminoglycoside. The concentration in the endolymph therefore depends on the ratio of secretion to resorption, which in turn depends on the drug's serum concentration.

Light microscopy shows destruction of the sensory cells of the organ of Corti, the ampullary cristae and the maculae of the saccule and utricle. Electron microscopy confirms that injury to the first row of the outer hair cells, particularly at the basal turn of the cochlea, occurs with cochleotoxicity.

It is important to note that damage to the vestibular and cochlear sensory cells is greatly enhanced by the simultaneous use of a loop diuretic.

Aminoglycosides are excreted by the kidney and the administered dose must be reduced in renal failure. A pyrexia, a large total dose (in the case of gentamicin >1 g) and a subject aged over 60 all increase the chances of ototoxicity.

Clinical features

1. *Tinnitus* may occur during or after withdrawing treatment. It may become more intense and persistent in spite of drug withdrawal.

2. *Hearing loss* is principally high frequency and sensorineural, presenting some days into treatment and progressing. Withdrawing therapy may prevent further significant deterioration provided renal function is adequate.

3. Vertigo is characteristically a bobbing oscillopsia whereby distant objects appear to jump about on head movement. Nystagmus may not be demonstrable but caloric testing shows a bilateral decline in labyrinthine function.

Investigations

Monitoring of patients taking these antibiotics by regular enquiry about otological symptoms and by the regular measurement of serum peak and trough levels is necessary to reduce the incidence of ototoxicity and to allow early withdrawal of therapy should symptoms arise.

Loop diuretics

Frusemide, bumetamide and ethacrynic acid in high doses may produce a reversible high-tone sensorineural hearing loss. Light microscopy shows the stria vascularis to be grossly oedematous, but the organ of Corti remains essentially normal. A permanent hearing loss is unusual but has been described in renal dialysis and transplant patients. Since 5% of this group become deaf purely as a result of their disease, the contribution of the diuretic to the deafness is, in many cases, uncertain.

Cytotoxic agents

Cisplatin is the most important drug in this group as for many oncologists it is the drug of choice in palliating head and neck cancer. Cisplatin is unusual in causing greatest injury to the inner hair cells. Pre- and postdose audiometry is necessary to monitor cochleotoxicity, which may be partially reversible on withdrawal of treatment.

Beta-blockers

A mixed deafness has been described, the conductive element being secondary to a middle-ear effusion. The pathogenesis of both the cochleotoxicity and the effusion is unknown. The cochleotoxic effects are generally mild and reversible.

Salicylates

Aspirin in overdose may induce tinnitus and a flat pure tone sensorineural hearing loss of up to 60 dB. This is usually reversible on withdrawing the drug. The vestibular apparatus is undisturbed, and recent work has suggested a direct effect of salicylates on the outer hair cells of the cochlea. Aspirin is cleared rapidly by the kidney so that treatment comprises adequate hydration and the use of an H_2-antagonist, e.g. cimetidine, or a proton pump inhibitor, e.g. omeprazole, to prevent upper gastrointestinal tract complications.

Quinine

Formerly used in the treatment of malaria and still used today to control night leg cramps, quinine has cochleotoxic effects similar to aspirin except that hearing loss may progress after withdrawing therapy and is more likely to be permanent. In a minority, hypersensitivity occurs whereby cochleotoxicity develops at therapeutic plasma levels. As most of the drug is bound to plasma proteins, plasmapheresis is an effective therapy in massive overdose.

Anticonvulsants

Vestibulotoxicity has been described with phenytoin and ethosuximide. The vertigo may be either acute and reversible on withdrawing treatment or more commonly chronic. In those in whom phenytoin must be used to control the disorder, careful monitoring of the serum levels is necessary.

Follow-up and aftercare

Cochleotoxic symptoms require regular pure tone audiometric monitoring until thresholds are stable or improve (temporary threshold shift) in order to quantify the disability. Vestibulotoxic recovery can be symptomatically monitored by outpatient assessment and if necessary quantified by ENG or caloric measurements. Vestibulosedative medication and rehabilitation exercises, e.g. Cooksey–Cawthorne exercises, minimize morbidity and may accelerate symptomatic recovery.

Further reading

Black FO, Pesznecker SC. Vestibular ototoxicity. *Otolaryngology Clinics of North America,* 1993; **26:** 713–36.
Campbell KCM, Durrant J. Audiologic monitoring for ototoxicity. *Otolaryngology Clinics of North America,* 1993; **76:** 903–14.

Related topics of interest

Caloric tests (p. 35)
Sudden hearing loss (p. 304)
Tinnitus (p. 313)
Vertigo (p. 334)
Vestibular function tests (p. 338)

PAEDIATRIC AIRWAY PROBLEMS

Introduction

Paediatric airway problems are different from adult problems because congenital abnormalities manifest themselves early in life and the airway is significantly narrower. Any factor which reduces the size of the lumen will therefore have a greater effect in the neonate and child. There are many diseases which can cause paediatric airway problems, but this topic confines itself to the following conditions:

- Laryngotracheobronchitis.
- Laryngomalacia.
- Vocal fold paralysis.
- Subglottic stenosis.
- Vascular ring.
- Miscellaneous conditions (papillomata, cysts, webs, etc.).

Problems will nearly always produce noisy breathing or affect the voice, and individual conditions are best discussed through these symptoms.

Stridor

Abnormal noise during breathing may emanate from the chest, the neck or the mouth and nose. Noisy breathing from the chest is usually expiratory, is known as wheezing and is the result of an asthma-like condition. Noise from the neck region is known as stridor and is caused by narrowing of the respiratory lumen in the upper trachea or larynx. It may be expiratory or inspiratory and if associated with a harsh cough and pyrexia is known as croup. A laryngeal lesion is usually characterized by inspiratory stridor and a tracheal lesion by expiratory stridor. Wheezing is the province of the respiratory physician and will not be discussed here.

Stertor is noise originating from the back of the mouth or nose. Bilateral choanal atresia can cause such symptoms but there are other more serious problems in this condition and surgical relief is provided as a matter of urgency. Choanal stenosis, enlarged adenoids (or tonsils), rhinitis and muscular incoordination can all be responsible and each condition should be treated on its merits. Children with Down's syndrome and cerebral palsy are particularly prone to trouble. The insertion of a nasopharyngeal tube which projects just beyond the soft palate is helpful in most refractory cases.

Hoarseness

Hoarseness indicates an abnormality of the vocal cord. It is temporary in laryngitis and is the presenting symptom with papillomata. The commonest cause of persistent hoarseness is the presence of vocal nodules. These are unlikely to be caused by misuse of the voice as they have been described in the neonate, but they do respond to speech therapy. Removal with the laser is only indicated when they are large. Unilateral vocal cord palsy can also produce a weak or hoarse voice and is seen following cardiac operations.

Laryngotracheo-bronchitis

This is the commonest cause of stridor, and most of the milder cases will not reach the hospital. The inspiratory stridor accompanied by a harsh cough will usually follow a throat infection. Infective oedema will narrow the lumen, particularly in the subglottic area, where the airway in the child is narrowest and the submucosal tissue lax. Since the diameter of the subglottis in the normal population follows a normal distribution curve, it is self-evident that those who have a small glottis initially will be more affected. The condition follows a self-limiting course, and many patients can be treated at home with antibiotics and humidity in the form of steam. If the symptoms get worse, admission to hospital, preferably to an intensive therapy unit, becomes necessary. The child is closely observed after treatment with humidity, antibiotics, oxygen, dexamethasone and sometimes an adrenaline nebulizer.

If further deterioration occurs, intubation is carried out. This is best done by a paediatric intensivist or anaesthetist and as small a tube as possible is used. As the condition improves a leak appears around the tube and the child is extubated. On those unusual occasions when extubation is not possible a tracheostomy will be necessary.

Endoscopy should be avoided in the acute period (as it increases oedema) but should be done to identify an underlying abnormality if attacks recur. The usual finding is a relatively narrow subglottis which will widen with growth. Allergic oedema produces similar symptoms, and they appear more quickly and clear equally rapidly. Epiglottitis produces more severe symptoms which are discussed elsewhere.

Laryngomalacia (floppy supraglottis)

This condition may appear within an hour or two of birth and is characterized by an intermittent stridulous squeak of varying severity. It is due to an indrawing of floppy supraglottic structures (particularly the arytenoids and aryepiglottic folds) during inspiration. It may only be slight and present in certain positions, but at worst there would be recession of the chest and suprasternal region and interference with feeding. If slight and parental anxiety is absent, nothing need to be done apart from a 3-monthly follow-up with advice to return in the interim if symptoms worsen. If severe or if there is parental anxiety, a direct laryngoscopy is carried out. The diagnosis is confirmed and, if symptoms are marked, the surplus lax mucosa can be excised from the superior border of the aryepiglottic fold under the microscope. The symptoms gradually improve with time but may take several years to stop.

Tracheostomy is virtually unknown for laryngomalacia and, if considered, an associated vocal cord palsy should be suspected and excluded.

Vocal cord paralysis

A unilateral vocal cord paralysis will usually produce no symptoms apart from some weakness of the voice, but a bilateral vocal cord paralysis produces a stridor which is very similar to that found with laryngomalacia. However, with vocal cord paralysis the symptoms and signs become worse with time as the baby makes stronger inspiratory effort. The cry is usually normal as adduction is not affected. The diagnosis is made by laryngoscopy and it is sometimes possible to see the larynx in the awake patient with a transnasal fibreoptic endoscope. More commonly it is necessary to perform direct laryngoscopy with the baby anaesthetized but maintaining vocal cord function. In order to exclude the diagnosis, wide abduction of the cords must be seen.

Adduction and passive movements of the cords with respiration can easily be mistaken for normal function and there are occasions when a diagnosis cannot be made with certainty. It is useful to reach a consensus by inviting the anaesthetist and any available surgeon present to make an assessment as there is a considerable subjective element.

In many cases the cause is unknown, although a significant number have other abnormalities.

An attempt should be made to treat the condition conservatively, as most will recover within 2–3 years. The baby should be seen at regular intervals and the movement reassessed every 6 months. The parents will require support and must have easy access to the hospital if they are worried. In some cases the stridor is so bad and indrawing so severe that tracheostomy is the only treatment. This should obviously be closed as soon as normal function returns. The decision to treat the vocal cord surgically should be left for several years and should be made only after thorough informed consultation with the child and parents.

Subglottis stenosis

The subglottis is the narrowest portion of the paediatric airway, and any additional narrowing due to oedema or scar tissue will tend to cause stridor. The stridor of laryngo-tracheitis is due to temporary oedematous stenosis and a relatively small cricoid ring may first manifest itself with these symptoms. The most severe cases, however, follow trauma, and in the neonate prolonged intubation associated with prematurity is the usual cause. It may be impossible to extubate the infant; sometimes a progressive stridor develops weeks or months after extubation. A large tube predisposes to stenosis, but a constitutional tendency to fibrosis is the only explanation for those who develop stenosis after only 2 or 3 days of small tube intubation.

If extubation is impossible, the cricoid can be split in the neonate and a temporary stent inserted. More often, however, a tracheostomy becomes necessary. The size of the subglottis is then assessed under general anaesthesia every few months by passing endotracheal tubes until a snug fit is obtained. If the lumen is obviously enlarging, the child can be left until there is an adequate airway and then decannulated. If there is total stenosis or if a pin-hole lumen persists, surgery is necessary, although this is best left until the age of 2 years.

Splitting of the cricoid and upper trachea with insertion of costal cartilage into the split is the standard surgical approach. More severe cases will require an anterior and posterior split, but an anterior split will suffice in milder cases. A stent is usually introduced for a few weeks, but this is not mandatory. This operation, known as laryngotracheoplasty, may need to be repeated before an adequate airway and decannulation is achieved.

Vascular ring

Abnormal blood vessels in the chest may compress the trachea and oesophagus and classically produce an inspiratory and expiratory stridor associated with feeding difficulties. Every neonate with no obvious cause for the stridor should therefore have a barium swallow, which will demonstrate the oesophageal narrowing.

Endoscopy will show a pulsatile narrowing of the trachea and correction is carried out by the chest surgeons. Even after correction there may still be narrowing due to tracheomalacia, which is believed to be caused by softening of the tracheal rings by the pulsatile vessel. There is little to be gained from consideration of the vascular abnormalities as these are complex and often confusing to the chest surgeons themselves.

Miscellaneous

Numerous lesions in the laryngeal region will encroach upon the airway and cause stridor.

Papillomata are viral warts which vary greatly in virulence. They usually disappear when immunity develops, but in the interim laser removal is required and certain individuals do not develop immunity. If very virulent and florid, a tracheostomy may become necessary. Hoarseness and airway problems occur as a result of scarring and can require reconstructive surgery.

Cysts, haemangiomata and lymphangiomata can occur in the subglottis and less often in the glottis and supraglottis. A conservative approach can often be taken, but the laser has made early removal possible. Cysts can also be aspirated and sometimes removed.

Laryngeal webs may be congenital or acquired. If they are small and only produce minimal symptoms they are best left alone. Larger webs may be opened with the laser, but reconstructive surgery with stenting can be necessary.

Micrognathia or a large tongue can narrow the upper airway, as in the Pierre–Robin syndrome. Nursing in the prone position is helpful, but even a tracheostomy is considered in the worse cases. Where there is no obvious anatomical cause for stridor, reflux oesophagitis needs to be exluded by investigation.

Related topics of interest

PAEDIATRIC ENDOSCOPY

Endoscopy of the respiratory tract is commonly carried out by the otolaryngologist, although subsequent treatment is often the province of the chest surgeon, physician or anaesthetist. Paediatric oesophagoscopy is commonly performed by the paediatric surgeons.

Fibreoptic examination of the nose, postnasal space and larynx can be done in the child or infant, but it can be difficult owing to lack of cooperation in the awake patient. The fibreoptic endoscope can be passed through the nose or through a laryngeal mask and the latter procedure is very useful in the diagnosis of vocal cord paralysis.

In most cases, paediatric endoscopy involves the use of a rigid laryngoscope or bronchoscope (with a telescope incorporated). This gives a better view and suction is available. Endoscopy is best avoided within a week following infection and oedema should first be allowed to subside. Essentially, paediatric endoscopy is indicated to provide a diagnosis in the presence of hoarseness and stridor.

Laryngoscopy

Adult laryngoscopes such as the Kleinsasser range can be safely used for children, and the smaller ones can even be used for neonates. As large a size as possible is advantageous in order to obtain the widest view of the larynx. It is important that the lower lip is not pinched between the instrument and the teeth (or gums) and the upper teeth should be protected. An endotracheal tube is in place for the induction of anaesthesia, but this is withdrawn into the hypopharynx during laryngoscopy and the patient breathes spontaneously.

For the purpose of identifying a lesion in the glottis or subglottis, the tip of the laryngoscope is passed posteriorly to the epiglottis as this structure may obstruct the view. If vocal cord movement or laryngomalacia is being assessed the tip of the laryngoscope is best placed in the vallecula to avoid fixation of the glottic and supraglottic structures. When a tracheoscopy or bronchoscopy is also to be done, it is best to watch glottic and supraglottic movement at the end of the procedure while the patient is regaining consciousness and producing more movement.

Laryngomalacia is easily distinguished by the indrawing of the arytenoids, but normal vocal cord movement is more difficult to identify. A wide abduction of the cords must be seen before normal cord movement is diagnosed.

Subglottic stenosis is identified on laryngoscopy if the vocal cords are not in spasm. Where a full examination of the respiratory tract is required, the hypopharynx, oropharynx and mouth are examined with the laryngoscope at the same time and both oesophagoscopy and examination under anaesthetic of the nose may be indicated.

Tracheoscopy

A rigid telescope and bronchoscope of suitable size is introduced into the larynx with the help of McGill's anaesthetic laryngoscope. The vocal cords are examined before passing the instrument gently through the glottis, and anaesthesia is then administered via the laryngoscope. This may not be possible if there is a high subglottic stenosis.

In the normal patient the carina can be seen as soon as the instrument passes through the glottis. An inability to see the carina when the lumen is apparently clear should raise suspicions of a vascular ring, tracheomalacia or some other source of extrinsic pressure.

The bronchoscope is passed down to the carina with examination of the walls to exclude a tracheo-oesophageal fistula. The main bronchus should be entered, but more extensive investigation of the bronchial tree is necessary if a foreign body is suspected. If there is a tracheostomy present, suprastomal granulations will nearly always be seen, but it is often possible to pass the bronchoscope past the tube. If not, the tube is removed. During the removal of the endoscope the surgeon should continue to visualize the respiratory tract as damage is avoided and rarely a lesion is seen which had previously been missed.

Related topics of interest

PAEDIATRIC HEARING ASSESSMENT

The assessment of hearing in children demands a variety of approaches which will vary with the age of the child. The choice of test will depend on the child's age, intellect and motor abilities. Screening tests, subjective hearing tests and objective tests are all available. Nearly all subjective testing will require two testers. The best results are achieved in multidisciplinary paediatric assessment centres where the environment and organization are geared for children. A thorough history from the parent or regular carer and a clinical examination are essential parts of the assessment.

Screening tests

Hearing is important for normal speech development, and it is important that moderate and severe hearing losses are diagnosed early. This will allow the provision of suitable support and aid, which will help facilitate the development of speech and communication. In an effort to achieve this aim, children are subject to regular screening tests, at 7 months, 2–4 years and again shortly after school entry. Any child who persistently fails a screening test will be referred for a full assessment. In addition, children may be referred for assessment from other sources because of concern about their hearing, e.g. parental concern, post meningitis, family history, intensive care units, etc. Most health authorities maintain an at-risk register of families in whom possible prenatal and perinatal causes exist. Listed below are the current screening methods of choice for the three age groups at which testing occurs.

- 7 months: distraction test (see below).
- 2–4 years: distraction tests or conditioned response audiometry.
- 5 years and over: pure tone audiometry.

Subjective hearing tests

1. Behavioural techniques (0–6 months). This method is based on the presentation of a loud sound and observation of the baby's response. Some experience is needed in interpreting the variety of possible responses, which include startle, blinking, crying or the cessation of activity. A positive response is one in which there is a significant alteration in activity.

2. Distraction techniques (6–18 months). With the child sitting comfortably on his or her mother's lap, an assistant attracts the attention of the child. The tester then distracts the child by making sounds of various intensity, behind and to one side of the child, without giving any visual cues. A positive response is when the child turns to the sound. The procedure is repeated on both sides. Test sounds include conversational voice for low frequency, sibilant s for higher frequency or a high-frequency rattle in younger children. A hand-held audiometer may be used with older children.

3. *Visual reinforcement audiometry (9–36 months).* This technique is relatively uncommon in the UK but more frequently used in USA and Australia. In essence it is a free field audiogram. The child sits in an acoustic room at a table (usually with a parent) and is allowed to play with some toys. Sounds (warbles or pure tones) are produced from one of two loudspeakers placed at 30° either side of the child. If the child turns to the correct speaker at signal presentation a visual (reinforcing) stimulus is presented adjacent to the speaker (e.g. a flashing light) to reinforce the turning response. The tester sits outside the test room and observes the procedure through a one-way mirror. In this way a reasonably accurate free field audiogram may be obtained.

4. *Conditioned reflex (performance testing) audiology (24–60 months).* This technique involves training the child to perform a specific task such as putting a marble in a cup, or giving a toy to the mother, after hearing a specific auditory stimulus. The stimulus may be the spoken word or a tone produced by a hand-held audiometer. With this method it is important to avoid any visual cues. This technique may also be used with older children to obtain a pure tone audiogram.

5. *Speech discrimination tests (24–60 months).* These tests involve asking the child to point to or handle a variety of toys. The toys are selected so that their names cover a range of speech patterns. In the McCormick toy test there are seven pairs with names that are acoustically very similar, e.g. cup/duck, key/tree. Only those toys that are recognized by the child are used and the aim is to establish the speech level that gives an 80% correct response rate.

6. *Pure tone audiogram (60 months+).* This technique is discussed in detail elsewhere (pure tone audiometry). Most children of around 5 years can with a little encouragement be persuaded to perform an audiogram, even if only at three frequencies in each ear.

Objective hearing tests

1. Auditory response cradle (0–6 months). This device monitors four behavioural responses to the production of sound. Head turning, startle responses and body movements are recorded by pressure transducers in the head rest and mattress. Respiratory changes are monitored by a transducer in a band around the baby's chest. The stimulus is 5-second bursts of 85 dB sound pressure level (SPL) sound made into earphones. A microprocessor analyses the responses to the sound stimuli, taking account of the baby's overall level of arousal, and makes an objective verdict of pass or fail.

2. Otoacoustic emissions (0–12 months). Much of the recent work with otoacoustic emissions is related to their feasibility as a screening tool for sensory hearing loss. Distortion-product otoacoustic emissions have been shown to be particularly effective at 4 and 8 kHz.

3. Evoked response audiometry. This is indicated if there is any difficulty or uncertainty in the results of conventional distraction techniques, or if the child is too young for conventional testing and there are doubts as to the child's hearing ability.

Further reading

McCormick B. *Paediatric Audiology 0–5 Years*. London: Whurr, 1992.

Related topics of interest

Evoked response audiometry (p. 85)
Impedance audiometry (p. 137)
Otoacoustic emissions (p. 217)
Pure tone audiogram (p. 255)

PERILYMPH FISTULA

Definition

A perilymph fistula is a perilymph leak into the middle ear arising from a defect of the oval and/or round window. It should not be confused with a labyrinthine fistula, which is a fistula in the cortical labyrinthine bone secondary to CSOM. This may or may not erode through the endosteum to cause a perilymph leak.

Aetiology

1. Congenital middle and inner ear deformities, in particular Mondini's dysplasia or when there is a malformed stapes superstructure.

2. Head injury.

3. Barotrauma.

4. Iatrogenic, in particular following stapedectomy.

Clinical features

A congenital perilymph fistula (PLF) should be suspected in children with an unexplained fluctuating or progressive sensorineural hearing loss with or without vertiginous symptoms. An external ear deformity may occur with the middle- and inner-ear malformation. A similar history following a head injury, barotrauma or middle-ear surgery should be regarded as secondary to a PLF until proven otherwise. Shea's series of iatrogenic poststapedectomy PLFs presented with a mild mixed hearing loss and occasional dizzy spells, but in over 36 000 otological operations he has not seen a spontaneous PLF. Schuknecht has never seen temporal bone evidence of a spontaneous PLF including the review of the temporal bones of patients reported by Kohut as having a spontaneous PLF. The current consensus view now holds that a spontaneous PLF does not occur in an otherwise normal ear without the above risk factors.

Investigations

A high-definition CT scan of the petrous temporal bone is mandatory in suspected congenital PLF. Many subjects demonstrate a minor or major aplasia (see Congenital hearing disorders), in particular an enlarged vestibular aqueduct or Mondini's dysplasia. Eighty-five per cent of congenital PLFs will have anomalies of the stapes superstructure, incus, promontory or round window demonstrable on CT. It has recently been shown that β_2-transferrin is found in all human CSF and perilymph, but in the serum of only 1 in 100 subjects. In those in whom a PLF is suspected from the history but not confirmed by a tympanotomy, washings of the middle ear for β_2-transferrin can be made. Difficulty arises in deciding whether CSF or perilymph is the responsible agent in head injury patients with a positive β_2-transferrin test. It has been suggested that positioning a patient with suspected PLF with the affected ear uppermost often improves hearing thresholds, presumably because little perilymph escapes as a result of gravity.

Management

The diagnosis of PLF can only be made at tympanotomy. Sixty per cent arise from the oval window, 20% from the round window and 20% are bilateral. The oval or round window should be plugged with fat, a graft of temporalis fascia or vein. This is held in position in oval window PLF with a stapes prosthesis provided the incus superstructure is not malformed. Fibrin glue and more recently the KTP laser have been suggested as means of properly anchoring an oval or round window graft in position. Temporalis muscle may be used to splint a round window graft reinforced by fibrin glue.

Follow-up and aftercare

Bed rest in the sitting up position for 2–6 weeks is recommended, as is avoiding straining or flying for 3 months. Diving is contraindicated. The patient is advised to cough or sneeze with the mouth open to reduce the chance of air entering the Eustachian tube and displacing the graft. One week antibiotic cover is recommended.

Further reading

Bassiouny M, Hirsch BE, Kelly RH, Kamerer DB, Cass SP. Beta$_2$ transferrin application in otology. *American Journal of Otolaryngology*, 1992; **13**: 552–5.

Kohut RI, Hinojosa R, Ryu JH. Perilymphatic fistulae: a single-blind clinical histopathologic study. *Advances in Otorhinolaryngology*, 1988; **42**: 148–52.

Schuknecht HF. Myths in neurotology. *American Journal of Otolaryngology*, 1992; **13**: 124–6.

Shea JJ. The myth of spontaneous perilymph fistual (editorial). *Otolaryngology and Head and Neck Surgery*, 1992; **107**: 613–16.

Related topics of interest

PHARYNGEAL POUCH

Diverticula of the pharynx are uncommon. The term pharyngeal pouch refers to a posterior pharyngeal pulsion (Zenker's) diverticulum, and this has an incidence of approximately 1 case per 200 000 population per year. Other diverticula are very rare but include congenital lateral diverticulae, pharyngoceles and posterolateral pharyngeal diverticula.

Aetiology and pathogenesis

The cause of pulsion diverticulae is unknown. They arise posteriorly by herniation of the pharyngeal mucosa through a relatively unsupported part of the posterior pharyngeal wall known as Killian's dehiscence. This weak area is at the lower part of the inferior constrictor muscle and is bound superiorly by the thyropharyngeal fibres and inferiorly by the cricopharyngeal fibres of this muscle. The pathogenesis is probably multifactorial, in part the result of a weakness at Killian's dehiscence, incoordination of the pharyngeal phase of swallowing and cricopharyngeal spasm causing high intrapharyngeal pressure. A hiatus hernia and gastro-oesophageal reflux are sometimes present. Once a pouch is formed, food enters it and stretches it even more so that it enlarges. It may remain static for many years or slowly increase in size until it eventually passes into the posterior mediastinum. When the pouch reaches a moderate size it lies in line with the oesophagus and food may enter it preferentially. Pressure from the pouch may then be exerted on the oesophagus from behind to cause dysphagia.

Clinical features

Pharyngeal pouches are usually only seen in the elderly. They cause a sensation of a lump in the throat, long-standing dysphagia, regurgitation of undigested food, halitosis, weight loss and recurrent chest infections due to aspiration. Hoarseness is unusual, but may occur as a result of irritation of the vocal cords from repeated aspiration or more rarely as a result of involvement of the recurrent laryngeal nerve by a carcinoma arising in the pouch. Approximately 0.5–1% of all pouches have an invasive squamous cell carcinoma in their wall. Swelling in the neck may be present and is nearly always on the left side. It may gurgle and empty on external pressure.

Investigations

1. Radiology. A lateral plain film of the neck may reveal an air bubble in the pouch, but the definitive investigation is a barium swallow, which demonstrates the pouch.

2. Endoscopy. Oesophagoscopy should be carried out to exclude the presence of carcinoma. The instrument usually enters the pouch and an anterior bar may be seen separating it from the oesophagus. This investigation is often performed immediately prior to surgical excision of the pouch. In such instances a nasogastric tube is passed and the pouch is packed with proflavine gauze after any debris has been sucked clear. This will aid identification of the pouch during surgery.

Management

1. No treatment. Each case must be judged on its individual merits, with the patient being fully aware of the possible complications and potential benefits of operation. No treatment is indicated for a diverticulum which is causing few symptoms or in patients who are old, infirm and in poor general condition.

2. Endoscopic dilatation of the cricopharyngeal sphincter with bougies is only temporarily effective in relieving symptoms. It does not remove the diverticulum, which results in an eventual recurrence, and there is a risk of perforating the sac.

3. Endoscopic diathermy (Dohlman's procedure) of the bar between the pouch and the oesophagus is a quick procedure and a reasonable treatment for the frail and the elderly. The procedure does not remove the pouch, but it relieves the symptoms and restores swallowing by dividing the cricopharyngeus and widening the mouth of the diverticulum. The major risks are haemorrhage, mediastinitis, surgical emphysema and later stenosis.

4. Pouch inversion. In this procedure a cricopharyngeal myotomy is performed and the pouch is mobilized, and then invaginated into the oesophagus and its neck oversewn with vicryl sutures. This operation avoids the risks of opening the sac, has a low complication rate and requires only a short hospital stay. This is the treatment of choice in all but very large pouches.

5. Diverticulectomy. Excision of the diverticulum combined with a cricopharyngeal myotomy has remained the treatment of choice for many years. The operation is performed in two stages, the first of which is the oesophagoscopy and the second the external approach to excise the pouch.

Nasogastric feeding is continued for 5–7 days postoperatively, after which fluids are given. If there are no problems the tube is removed and a soft diet can be commenced the next day.

Complications

1. Immediate.

- Primary haemorrhage.
- Surgical emphysema (mucosal tear or incomplete suture line).
- Pneumothorax.

2. Intermediate.

- Secondary haemorrhage (infection).
- Hoarseness (recurrent laryngeal nerve damage).
- Wound infection.
- Fistula (usually the result of infection).
- Mediastinitis (leak tracking downwards).

3. Late.

- Persistent hoarseness (recurrent laryngeal nerve divided).
- Stricture (too much mucosa excised when dividing the neck of the sac).
- Recurrence (endoscopic diathermy 7%, diverticulectomy 2–3%).

Further reading

Bowdler DA. Pharyngeal pouches. In: Stell PM (ed.) *Scott-Brown's Otolaryngology*, Vol. 5, 5th edn. London: Butterworths, 1987; 264–82.

Parker AJ, Hawthorne MR. Endoscopic diverticulotomy versus external diverticulotomy in the treatment of pharyngeal pouch. *Journal of the Royal College Of Surgeons of Edinburgh*, 1988; **33**: 62–4.

Related topics of interest

Globus pharyngeus (p. 122)
Hypopharyngeal carcinoma (p. 133)

PHARYNGOCUTANEOUS FISTULA

Definition

A fistula is an abnormal communication between two epithelial-lined surfaces. A pharyngocutaneous fistula is an abnormal tract joining the pharynx to the skin of the neck.

Pathology

Fistulae are unlikely after closed pharyngeal surgery but may occur following open surgery to the head and neck in which the pharynx has been opened. Consequently, laryngectomy is the most commonly associated procedure, but it may occur after pharyngeal pouch surgery, partial pharyngectomy or major oropharyngeal procedures (e.g. commando operation). Risk factors are:

- Previous radiotherapy.
- Infection (a persistent cough from a chest infection will put strain on the repair, and infection of the operated site will cause necrosis of the affected tissue with a leak through this defect).
- Postoperative haematoma/chylous fistula/seroma.
- Residual disease.
- Poor nutritional status.
- Poor surgical technique.

Clinical features

The patient most commonly develops a pyrexia 3 or 4 days postoperatively, associated with cellulitis of the neck wound. A swinging pyrexia and abscess formation may ensue. Typically on the seventh day the collection will rupture and a fistula will form. At this stage there will be a discharge of mucopus and the patient's general condition will improve. In time, the discharge will become more mucoid than purulent and ultimately saliva alone is discharged. In many cases spontaneous resolution will occur, usually within 6 weeks. In persistent cases, especially in those having residual tumour or previous radiotherapy, there is the uncommon but ever present spectre of a carotid blow-out.

Investigation

The diagnosis will be strongly suspected from the clinical features, especially from a red fluctuant swelling in the neck. After rupture, if the tract is small, the diagnosis may be confirmed by a gastrograffin swallow. With persistent and profuse discharge from a fistula, the urea, electrolytes and serum proteins should be checked regularly and the haemoglobin kept above 10 g/dl. Occasionally a fistula occurs several days after commencing oral feeding in patients who have had an apparently uncomplicated postoperative course. A gastrograffin swallow performed on the 10th to 12th postoperative day will show an anterior sinus in about 15% of patients, and it is this group who are at a significantly higher risk of developing such a fistula. It is suggested that nasogastric feeding be continued in this group for a further week and the gastrograffin swallow thereafter repeated. In most cases the sinus will have resolved, but if not the process is repeated until healing.

Management

A pharyngocutaneous fistula is initially managed conservatively. Nasogastic feeding continues until the fistula has healed. The wound should be cleaned regularly and absorbent dressings used to avoid maceration of the surrounding skin until all necrotic tissue has separated and healing has started, this initial stage taking 2 or 3 weeks. The size of the external opening of the fistula should thereafter be measured weekly. The fistula may take many weeks to close spontaneously, and if personal and home circumstances are suitable the patient can be allowed home to be reviewed weekly in outpatients. Provided that the fistula continues to reduce in size, no surgical intervention is necessary, although granulation tissue should be biopsied to exclude recurrent disease in cancer patients. If the size does not reduce over any 2-week period after the initial separation stage, a prudent plan would be to endoscope the patient under a general anaesthetic to exclude recurrent disease then to proceed with a repair. If the fistula opening is less than 1 cm diameter, a local rotation skin flap should be considered in the first instance. These often fail, however, because local tissue is relatively ischaemic either as a result of previous radiotherapy or because of scar tissue formation during healing. If a local flap fails or the defect is too large to consider this, the repair method of choice is, depending on the surgeon's experience and microvascular training, a choice of two out of a pectoralis major myocutaneous flap, a deltopectoral flap or a radial forearm fasciocutaneous microvascular flap (see p. 269). Two flaps are needed because it is important to line the mucosal and cutaneous surfaces with skin.

Follow-up and aftercare

Patients who have had surgery for head and neck cancer are followed up at the same interval as those who did not develop a fistula, although they are at a higher risk of developing a stenosis at the level of the fistula. This may settle after several dilations, but occasionally the stenosis recurs persistently and frequently so that excision of the affected segment with reconstruction is indicated. The repair method of choice is a microvascular jejunal loop because of its low morbidity and mortality compared with a gastric transposition. Those who have had surgery for benign disease are unlikely to develop a stenosis, but follow-up for a year to exclude a late onset would seem sensible.

Further reading

Stringer, SP. Flaps and grafts for reconstruction. In: Million RR, Cassisi NJ (eds). *Management of Head and Neck Cancer*, 2nd edn. Philadelphia: J.B. Lippincott, 1994; 157–69.

Reconstruction. In: Maran AGD (ed.). *Stell & Maran's Head and Neck Surgery*, 3rd edn. London: Heinemann, 1993; 42–57.

McCombe AW, Jones AS. Radiotherapy and complications of laryngectomy. *Journal of Laryngology and Otology*, 1993; **107**: 130–2.

Related topics of interest

PRESBYACUSIS

As with all sensory systems in the human body, there is a progressive degeneration in the auditory system with ageing, which leads to hearing impairment in the affected individual. Presbyacusis is defined as the lessening of the acuteness of hearing that characterizes old age.

Pathophysiology

Both the sensory peripheral (cochlea) and central (neural) components of the auditory system are affected and the deterioration appears to become more rapid with increasing age. Peripheral degeneration is reported to be responsible for at least two-thirds of the clinical features of presbyacusis. A variety of possible mechanisms exist. Cellular degeneration gives rise to a reduction in the numbers of inner and outer hair cells, particularly at the basal end of the cochlea. This can lead to secondary neural degeneration in the spiral ganglion. Circulatory changes such as arteriosclerosis, atrophy of the stria vascularis and microangiopathy can lead to metabolic upset and further cell death. This leads to an elevation of hearing thresholds and a loss of frequency selectivity. Degeneration in the central pathways leads to a reduction in performance in terms of signal processing. The end result in most instances will be a combined sensorineural, rather than a sensory or neural, impairment.

Clinical features

Moderate hearing impairment (45 dB hearing level averaged over 0.5, 1, 2 and 4 kHz) occurs in 4% of the age group 51–60 but in 18% of those aged 71–80. Men and women are both affected, although the men's hearing loss tends to be slightly worse for the same age group. Patients typically complain of difficulty in hearing which is worse in the presence of background noise, so that they find conversations difficult to follow. Recruitment is a frequent problem and adds to the distortion. Many patients eventually become socially isolated and even depressed. In the absence of any other otological pathology the clinical examination is normal bar the hearing loss.

Investigations

In the presence of an appropriate history and a symmetrical sensorineural hearing loss on pure tone audiometry, little further investigation is required. Hearing loss in a young patient, asymmetry on a pure tone audiogram, unilateral tinnitus or a conductive component to the audiogram will require investigation in its own right. An evoked reponse audiogram may be necessary to exclude an acoustic neuroma in patients thought to be at risk. Although several different audiological patterns of hearing loss have been described, depending on the predominant histological changes, in general a sloping high-frequency loss is the commonest pattern found.

Management

As there is no curative treatment for deafness associated with ageing, the main aim in management is to assess the degree of disability and to provide a hearing aid and rehabilitation.

1. Hearing aids. Although about 75% of hearing aid users are over the age of 60, only 18% of the elderly with hearing loss have and use hearing aids. There are several reasons for this, including denial of hearing impairment, vanity, acoustic feedback and difficulty with manipulating the aid. In those with neural presbyacusis poor speech discrimination may limit the beneficial results. Some patients have minimal handicap from their hearing difficulty despite a significant loss and therefore do not present themselves to medical services. Obtaining a hearing aid has become less of a problem for many patients since the introduction of direct referral schemes from general practice.

2. Rehabilitation. Some patients may be helped by rehabilitation in the form of speech reading or auditory training. The role of rehabilitation and its benefits for the average hearing-impaired individual are not proven.

3. Accessory aids. An induction coil fitted to the telephone or television may help some patients. The sound is transmitted by induction from a special attachment and is picked up by the patient's aid when it is switched to the T position. This system is now available in many public places such as churches, concert halls and lecture theatres.

Follow-up and aftercare

Audiological support is initially required to familiarize and rehabilitate the user with the aid. In some centres patients provided with a hearing aid are not seen again. The ENT surgeon or audiologist therefore has no idea if the patient has benefited from the treatment. Many hearing aids dispensed are not used, perhaps because the patient experiences some of the difficulties outlined above. Follow-up of all patients issued with a hearing aid should be mandatory. Any difficulties the patient might have can then be identified and dealt with. In the longer term, access is required for repairs and replacements, which may be dictated by further hearing deterioration with the passage of time.

Further reading

Browning GG, Davis A. Clinical characterisation of the hearing of the adult British population. *Advances in Oto-rhino-laryngology,* 1983; **31:** 217–23.
Salomon, G. Hearing in the aged. The European Concerted Action Project. *Acta Otolaryngologica*, 1991, Suppl. 476.

Related topics of interest

Evoked response audiometry (p. 85)
Hearing aids (p. 126)
Noise-induced hearing loss (p. 189)
Pure tone audiogram (p. 255)

PURE TONE AUDIOGRAM

The pure tone audiogram is probably the cornerstone of clinical auditory assessment. It is a psychoacoustical test which aims to establish the subject's pure tone hearing threshold, that is the minimum sound level at which a specific response can be obtained.

The decibel

The sensation of sound loudness is related to the intensity of applied sound energy. The range of sound intensities met with in clinical practice is extremely large, and the values obtained in testing encompass large numbers. An easier way is needed to handle the numbers involved. The solution that has been adopted is to use logarithms of numbers. Sound pressure levels are expressed in terms of the logarithm of the ratio between the level being measured and a reference level. The *Bel* is defined as a ratio of intensity (energy flux per unit area). The intensities of two sources, I_1 and I_2, differ by n Bels, where

$$n = \log_{10} I_1/I_2$$

Since the bel is, in practice, a rather large unit, the *decibel* (dB) is usually used instead, where 1 dB (decibel) = 10 B (bels).

Decibel scales

1. Sound pressure level scale. In terms of pressure, the threshold of hearing corresponds to a sound pressure level (dB SPL) of 20×10^{-6} pascals and the threshold of pain to a level of 200 pascals. The auditory system is less efficient at detecting sounds at the upper and lower ends of the frequency spectrum than in the middle regions. The detection of sounds in decibels of sound pressure level (dB SPL) produces a pure tone audiogram which in normal circumstances would not be flat. It was considered that the use of a dB SPL scale in pure tone audiometry would make abnormalities difficult to identify.

2. Hearing level scale. A decibel scale of human hearing was designed so that 0 dB hearing level (HL) would be the expected threshold of detection of a pure tone irrespective of its frequency. The amount of energy at 0 dB HL at each frequency is not the same. It is measured in relative terms (dB ISO), where the reference zero is an internationally agreed standard. This standard represents the thresholds at each test frequency for a group of presumed otologically normal young adults. In the dB HL scale normal hearing individuals would be expected to have a flat audiogram, the mean level being 0 dB HL. The clinical audiogram therefore gives an estimate of the subject's hearing relative to normal.

3. The dB A scale. At low sound levels, low-frequency components contribute little to the total loudness of complex sounds, and so an A weighting is used, which reduces the contribution of low frequencies to the meter reading. This dB A scale is used in industrial noise measurements.

Background

Pure tones of several frequencies are tested, usually 250, 500, 1000, 2000, 4000 and 8000 Hz for air conduction (although 3000 and 6000 Hz will be required for noise-induced hearing loss claims) and 250, 500, 1000, 2000 and 4000 Hz for bone conduction. The results of bone conduction become unreliable above 4000 Hz and at 250 Hz are often not representative as they may be felt rather than heard.

Bone conduction is taken to give an indication of cochlea function, but because a variety of routes for the transmission of sound to the cochlea exist for bone conduction, it is not an absolute representation of inner ear threshold. When the skull is set in vibration by a bone conduction vibrator, the sounds reach the inner ear by the direct osseous route or via transmission across the middle ear. This causes an artificial depression of the bone conduction thresholds whenever a conductive defect is present. If the middle-ear defect is corrected, then the bone conduction thresholds will appear to improve because of the addition of the middle-ear component. This has become known as the 'Carhart effect' after he described it in patients who had successful fenestration surgery for otosclerosis.

Method

The subject is seated in a soundproof room and the procedure is explained by the examiner. Earphones are used for air conduction and the subject is asked to signal by pressing a small hand-held button as soon as the tone is heard. Pure tones are produced by a calibrated audiometer and are first presented to the subject's better ear.

Thresholds are ascertained using a psychophysical method of limits. Tones are first presented at an intensity above the patient's suspected threshold. The intensity is reduced in 10 dB steps until no sound is heard. The signal is then increased in 5 dB steps until half of the tone pips are consistently heard. This continues in the following order:

1000, 2000, 4000, 8000, 500 and 250 Hz. Finally 1000 Hz is tested again to check on subject accuracy and should be within 10 dB of the first result. The second ear is then tested in identical fashion. The timing and duration of signal presentation should be varied and no visual clues should be offered.

With any psychoacoustic test there is a variation in the results obtained in any test–retest situation, with a standard error of 3–5 dB. For this reason 5 dB steps are used for clinical audiometry. Smaller steps could be used (e.g. 2 dB) but the procedure would be markedly prolonged without significantly improving accuracy.

Masking

Masking is the phenomenon by which one sound impairs the perception of another. In the context of pure tone audiometry, masking is used to raise the threshold in the non-test ear using air-conducted sound. This overcomes any cross-hearing (the interaural attenuation for air conduction is of the order of 40–60 dB when wearing headphones) and allows an accurate assessment of the true threshold of the test ear for either air or bone conduction. As masking is most effective when the frequency of the masking noise overlaps the test tone, narrow band noise with a central frequency identical to the test tone is used. The masking level in the non-test ear is determined by shadow masking and recording the thresholds on a masking chart. The masking noise is delivered by an ear insert for bone conduction and headphones for air conduction.

There are three scenarios when masking is required:

(a) Masking must be applied to the better ear when testing air conduction in the deafer ear if the difference in unmasked thresholds is found to be 40 dB or more (to prevent interaural attenuation).

(b) Air conduction studies whenever the unmasked bone conduction is 40 dB or more better than the worse air conduction.

(c) Bone conduction testing whenever the unmasked bone conduction is 10 dB or more better than the worse air conduction

Variations

1. *Computerized pure tone audiometry.* In essence this is identical to the above but a microprocessor presents the tones and analyses the responses against predetermined values. It is useful as a screening test and in very busy clinics, but if the result is unusual it will require manual confirmation.

2. *Bekesy audiometry*. This variant uses a special audiometer which automatically sweeps from low to high frequencies while presenting continuous or pulsed tones. The subject alters the intensity of the tone by pressing a button if the tone is heard which lowers the intensity of the signal. When the signal cannot be perceived the button is released which increases the intensity again. Thus a zig-zag printout is obtained from which thresholds at each frequency can be estimated. As the test can be self-administered and provides an automatic printout, it is ideal for workforce screening. By varying the test technique (e.g. forward/backward sweeps, continuous/pulsed tones, etc.) additional diagnostic information about adaptation, recruitment and non-organic hearing loss can be provided. Although still used for screening industrial hearing loss, the method has fallen into disuse for most other problems because it is too unreliable.

Further reading

British Society of Audiology/British Association of Otolaryngologists. Recommended procedures for pure-tone audiometry using a manually operated instrument. *British Journal of Audiology*, 1981; **15**: 213–16.

Browning GG. Audiometric tests. In: *Clinical Otology and Audiology*. London: Butterworths, 1986; 38–47.

Leijon A. Quantization error in clinical pure-tone audiometry. *Scandinavian Audiology*, 1992; **21**: 103–8.

Related topics of interest

Noise-induced hearing loss (p. 189)
Non-organic hearing loss (p. 195)

RADIOLOGY IN ENT

Plain films

Plain radiography has undergone a dramatic decline recently. Complex projections and conventional tomography are now rarely indicated. A full series of plain views of an area is now rarely performed, in part to reduce radiation exposure but mainly because of the advent of CT and MRI. It should be noted that techniques and nomenclature often differ between departments.

1. Sinus disease. The basic facial/sinus view is the occipitomental (OM), which projects the maxillary antra clear of the petrous bones and may demonstrate the sphenoid sinus if taken with the mouth open. It is often the only view taken for sinusitis and should be taken erect to demonstrate any fluid levels. Other signs include mucosal thickening (should be 3 mm) and opacification. Opacification is best assessed by comparison with the orbit and zygoma. Density similar to the orbit is probably normal, but probably pathological if similar to the zygoma. Many rhinologists no longer use plain sinus radiographs, preferring antroscopy or CT scanning.

2. Acoustic neuroma. The occipitofrontal (perorbital) view affords the best view of the internal auditory meati but is rarely used for this now.

3. Ear disease. Views of the mastoid bones may demonstrate pathology or the anatomy prior to surgery but are rarely used since the advent of CT. The lateral oblique is the standard mastoid view.

4. Neck radiographs. No more than a single film of the cervical spine is required to demonstrate degenerative spondylosis in the context of vertebrobasilar insufficiency, and even this is arguable since symptoms correlate poorly with visible changes. A less penetrated, soft-tissue lateral is used to search for impacted foreign bodies, but interpretation is often difficult due to variable radio-opacity of the frontal bone and overlying calcification of cervical structures. Air in the retropharyngeal tissues is indicative of a mucosal tear.

Barium swallow

Barium swallow is indicated for the investigation of dysphagia and motility problems. Structural lesions (webs, strictures, tumours, pouches) are imaged with rapid sequencing (usually 100 mm film, one per second for 6 seconds) in three planes (lateral, oblique and anteroposterior). Functional motility disorders are best assessed with continuous imaging by a video swallow.

Ultrasound

Ultrasound can be used for the assessment and follow-up of masses in and around the neck, in particular parotid gland lesions, cervical abscesses and lymph nodes. A high-frequency probe is used (5–7.5 MHz), and guided aspiration may be performed simultaneously.

Sialography

Cannulation of the parotid or submandibular duct and injection of contrast media can demonstrate calculi, strictures and sialectasis. This has been used in conjunction with CT in the assessment of salivary gland masses with variable results; MRI seems better. Traditional contrast agents are being increasingly abandoned in favour of water-soluble agents (e.g. Omnopaque 500), which cause fewer problems when extravasated yet afford equally good images.

Computerized tomography (CT)

Most solid tumours are best imaged by MRI, but CT is still useful where MRI is contraindicated, less useful, for example in nasal, sinus and petrous temporal bone involvement, or unavailable. Thick (4–8 mm), contiguous axial slices are obtained through the region of interest and the relevant lymph node drainage. Infusion of water-soluble contrast may help to outline blood vessels, vascular and inflamed areas. Soft-tissue and bone settings should be obtained.

Disadvantages of CT include the radiation dose to the patient, artefact arising from high-density steps (especially dental amalgam) and the limitation of obtaining only one plane at a time. Reconstruction of different planes often produces disappointing results. Soft-tissue contrast and identification of blood vessels is good when compared with plain films but poor when compared with MRI.

1. Cerebellopontine angle tumours. High-resolution (2 mm) axial scans through the internal auditory meati after contrast on bone and soft-tissue settings is used to investigate acoustic neuromas. It has been superseded by MRI but will remain useful for patients who cannot undergo MRI. Air meatography is now obsolete.

2. Larynx. Thin (2 mm) sections are also used for carcinoma of the larynx. Irregular cartilage ossification may cause difficulties in assessment and both wide and soft-tissue settings should be obtained. MRI is to be preferred.

3. Paranasal sinus disease. In the assessment of sinusitis the patient should be scanned in the true coronal plane, preferably prone to take secretions and debris away from the sinus ostia. Most centres advocate aggressive medical pretreatment for similar reasons. Limitations may occur with patient tolerance, difficulties in neck extension and gantry angulation. Contiguous 4 mm slices should be obtained on extended bone settings to avoid any artefact from dental amalgam. Narrower (2 mm) slices are often obtained through the ostiomeatal complex. Axial scans may be helpful in assessing ethmoid disease that extends into the orbit (ethmoid mucocele, orbital cellulitis), in displaying the path of the optic nerves and the position of the internal carotid artery. Where intracranial complications are suspected, scanning should follow i.v. contrast or MRI may be preferred.

4. Ear disease. High-resolution CT on bone settings in coronal and axial planes is used for the assessment of cholesteatoma and developmental anomalies of the ear.

At all times care should be taken to avoid overirradiating the patient, especially when young or when repeated scanning is required.

Magnetic resonance imaging (MRI)

In MRI the patient is placed within a powerful magnetic field (0.15–1.5 Tesla). This causes the spinning protons of the patient's hydrogen nuclei (which behave like bar magnets) to adopt a predominant alignment along the axis of the magnetic field. Radiofrequency pulses deflect the axis of the spinning protons. The MR signal is emitted as the proton relaxes to the original position (spin lattice relaxation) and as the spins dephase with respect to each other (spin–spin relaxation). The pulse sequence can be selected to use predominantly the former (T1 weighted) or latter (T2 weighted) component. Various sequences (and acronyms) have been developed, including fat suppression by short tau inversion recovery (STIR), fast scanning (FLASH, FISP) and angiographic techniques.

Like CT, MRI produces cross-sectional images but is able to scan in any plane without altering patient position. It demonstrates better soft-tissue contrast than CT, and the signal void from flowing blood means excellent demonstration of blood vessels. It is therefore ideal for evaluation of head and neck tumours, for staging and assessment of recurrence/response as well as differentiating tumour from other pathology (inflammatory lesions, radiotherapy changes, retained secretions, etc.). Tumour infiltration of cranial nerves, skull base and foramina is best assessed with MRI following i.v. paramagnetic contrast (gadolinium), which enhances areas of involvement. Intracranial and neural spread is thus well delineated. This modality has completely altered the investigation of suspected acoustic neuroma.

A small minority of patients will find MRI too claustrophobic. Metallic implants and foreign bodies have been regarded as contraindications because of the danger of dislodgement in the magnetic field, especially from sensitive sites: aneurysm clips, intraocular implants and foreign bodies, prosthetic cardiac valves, pacemakers and otological implants. At least one patient has died following avulsion of an intracranial aneurysm clip. Many implants and foreign bodies, including most otological implants, are of non-ferromagnetic material and should be safe. If the nature of the implant is known, it may still be possible to scan the patient.

Further reading

Grainger RG, Allison DJ. *Diagnostic Radiology*. Edinburgh: Churchill Livingstone, 1992.
Mafee MF. Imaging of the paranasal sinuses and oro-maxillo-facial region. *Radiological Clinics of North America*, 1993; **31**: 1.
Rao VJ, Flanders AE, Tom BM. *MRI and CT Atlas of Correlative Imaging in Otolaryngology*. London: Martin Dunitz, 1992.
Shellock FG. MRI of metallic implants and materials: a compilation of the literature. *American Journal of Radiology*, 1988; **151**: 811–14.

Related topics of interest

RADIOTHERAPY

Definition

Radiotherapy is treatment with ionizing radiation. This may consist of high-energy electromagnetic radiation such as X-rays and gamma rays or particulate radiation such as electrons (beta particles) or neutrons.

Electromagnetic radiation

X-rays

X-rays have a smaller wavelength (10^{-15} m to 10^{-18} m) than ultraviolet light (between 4×10^{-12} and 10^{-13} m) and have high energy, from kilovolts (kV) to megavolts (MeV). The greater the energy, the greater its tissue penetration. They are produced when high-speed electrons expelled by thermionic emission from an electrically heated tungsten filament are arrested by a target anode of high atomic number, usually tungsten, converting their kinetic energy into heat and photons. The photon is simply a quantum or bundle of electromagnetic radiation.

Megavoltage linear acceleration of the electrons produces X-rays in the energy range of 4–20 MeV. Orthovoltage machines produce X-rays with energy of about 300 kV. For the treatment of head and neck cancer, energy in the region of 4–6 MeV is used.

Gamma rays

Radioactive atoms disintegrate to form a more stable atom, releasing energy, which may be particulate (usually electrons) or uncharged electromagnetic radiation called gamma rays, having the same wavelength and energy as X-rays.

The amount of energy of a photon beam is described by the roentgen (R), while the gray (Gy) is the unit of absorbed dose by the tissues and has replaced the rad (1 gray = 100 rad).

Mechanism of action

The attenuation of a photon beam passing through tissue occurs by the absorption and scatter of its energy by atoms in cells of that tissue with the ejection of electrons, leaving the atom ionized and able to enter into chemical reactions. Oxygen is the most important atom involved. If DNA is the structure damaged, this may be lethal for the cell. DNA is most susceptible to lethal injury when the cell is dividing and is not able to repair DNA damage. Malignant cells have a greater proportion of actively dividing cells at any point in time (a larger growth fraction) and so a greater percentage of cells will die.

Resting cells may also sustain DNA damage. Normal cells are able to synthesize factors such as p53 protein, which prolong the S-phase (synthesis of DNA phase) of the cell cycle, allowing repair of damaged DNA before the next cell division. Resting malignant cells have much less capability to arrest in S-phase, have a shorter cell cycle, are less likely to repair damaged DNA and therefore more likely to undergo apoptosis before entering mitosis. A higher proportion of malignant cells will therefore die from radiotherapy.

Scattering of low-energy photons may be in any direction, including backwards, but with high-energy photons scatter is in a forward direction, continuing the intensity of the beam. The corollary of this is that an orthovoltage beam produces a maximum dose on the skin, with a rapid fall-off in dose with depth, whereas a megavoltage beam is skin sparing with a maximum dose of 4 MeV at 1 cm and a lower fall-off in dose with depth.

The predominantly forward scatter of a high-energy beam allows a more precisely focused beam (or a narrower penumbra), whereas an orthovoltage beam produces a poorly focused beam as a result of side scatter (wide penumbra). Finally, much greater absorption occurs when orthovoltage radiation passes through tissue of a high atomic number such as bone, compared with megavoltage photons, which is relatively bone sparing.

Particulate radiation

These are principally electrons and neutrons.

Electrons (beta particles) External beam electrons produced by thermionic emission from an electrically heated tungsten filament in a linear accelerator can be used as an alternative to electromagnetic radiation. They give a uniform dose up to a certain depth which varies depending on the energy of the beam, with a rapid fall-off in dose beyond this. They are used in particular to boost the dose to a neck lump lying in close approximation to the spinal cord. The technique is more skin sparing than orthovoltage radiotherapy and is the treatment of choice for irradiating the nose and pinna.

These are produced by bombarding stable nuclei with electrons in a cyclotron. Unfortunately the maximum dose delivered is to the skin, there is a relatively slow fall-off in dose with depth, there is significant scatter and the dose is more difficult to map precisely. Its role in head and neck cancer has yet to be defined. It may find a place in the treatment of sinonasal and advanced salivary tumours.

Methods of application in the head and neck

1. External beam radiotherapy (teletherapy).

2. Interstitial or brachytherapy, for example iridium wires mounted on flexible silastic tubing; gold grains which can be left permanently *in situ* as their half-life is only 2.7 days.

3. Systemic radioactive isotopes, in particular iodine-131 for thyroid malignancy.

Radiotherapy should be defined in terms of type, method of application, number of fractions, fraction size, interval between fractions and volume treated.

The principle is to provide a sufficient dose to the tumour to effect a cure or adequate palliation but provide a minimal dose to the surrounding normal tissue in order to minimize complications. Each tissue has its own tolerance level beyond which radiation toxicity will occur, so that a small increase in dose may greatly increase tissue injury. Omission of one or two fractions of radiotherapy, perhaps because of acute side-effects, can significantly reduce the chances of cure.

Fractionation

The dose of radiation which may be given by a single treatment is limited by the tolerance of the surrounding tissues. If this dose is fractionated or divided into several treatments, then recovery of normal tissue may occur between fractions by repopulation, reducing complications. However, malignant cells are also able to recover between fractions and so the overall dose must be increased to effect a cure. As an example a single dose of 20 Gy to a cheek basal cell carcinoma may be curative but cause marked permanent peritumour scarring. Altering the regime to 60 Gy given in 30 fractions of 2 Gy over 6 weeks will also effect a cure but cause no residual scarring.

The treatment volume is defined by examination and CT or MR scanning. A variable margin around the tumour is included to allow for microscopic involvement. Accurate targeting is essential because of the close proximity of vital but radiation-sensitive structures such as the cervical spinal cord, eye and pharynx. To ensure this the patient is immobilized in an individually made plastic head and neck shell. On a simulator (an X-ray machine with an image intensifier) the field is chosen and lead alloy blocks used to protect vulnerable structures. These blocks are marked on the shell. Two or more beams from different angles may be needed to obtain an adequate radiation dose to the tumour volume while maintaining surrounding tissue tolerance. This is helped by the use of wedges which attenuate a beam's dose differentially across its width. A computer maps out a plan of the dose applied to the tumour and surrounding structures by calculating the summation of the contributions of the applied beams modified by wedges, blocks and compensators. Verification radiographs are taken during the first fraction dose and compared with the simulation films to ensure that the field is correctly positioned.

Side-effects

1. General. Tiredness, lassitude and anorexia are common, nausea and vomiting less so.

2. Local. These depend on the type of radiotherapy, volume treated, the total dose, the number of fractions and the total treatment time.
- Skin: erythema, dry or moist desquamation, epilation, atrophy of sweat glands and other skin appendages.
- Mucous membranes: mucositis, comprising erythema, a false membrane of slough, candidiasis and reduced saliva production from major and in particular minor salivary gland atrophy.
- Cartilage: perichondritis of the larynx, ear and nose, and atrophy (leading to a cauliflower ear or a nasal saddle deformity).
- Brain and spinal cord: transverse myelitis, localized cortical radionecrosis.
- Bone: osteoradionecrosis.

Related topics of interest

RECONSTRUCTIVE SURGERY

The advent of antibiotics and more refined anaesthesia have allowed more major head and neck resection procedures to be developed. Although skin cover could be achieved by staged transposition of tubed pedicled fasciocutaneous flaps from distant sites, cosmesis, retention of function and quality of life were usually poor. In addition some procedures took over a year to complete. The development of one-stage pedicled myocutaneous flaps and microvascular free tissue transfer over the last 15 years has largely removed these criticisms with the consequential enormous improvement in the quality of life for head and neck cancer patients.

Split skin grafts

Split skin grafts should be harvested using an electric dermatome set at 3 or 4 on the circular scale corresponding to a thickness of 0.3–0.4 mm. This will consist of epidermis and a thin layer of dermis, but leave the troughs of the rete pegs and epithelium lining the hair follicles *in situ* to allow re-epithelialization of the donor site. The graft has no blood supply and so needs a vascular bed. It will not take on raw bone, cartilage or tendon. It should be noted that the dermatome scale acts as a guide only: other factors such as angle of the dermatome to the skin and skin tension will alter the graft thickness. A thicker graft of 0.5 mm is recommended for covering within the oral cavity.

Indications

(a) To cover donor sites, for example radial forearm free flaps and deltopectoral flaps. It is recommended that, after taking the graft at operation, it be placed keratin side down on tulle gras, which is rolled, placed in a sterile pot and refrigerated at 4°C. Unroll the graft onto the donor site after 3–5 days when all bleeding and serous ooze from the raw bed has stopped and vascular granulated tissue has started to form.

(b) To cover excised conchal bowl skin and cartilage defect after the excision of a basal cell carcinoma.

(c) To line cavities, for example the inner layer of a maxillectomy cheek flap, to line the orbital cavity after exenteration or as a cover for a floor of mouth or tongue raw surface. Immediate grafting with quilt suturing and cross-hatching of the graft is recommended so that blood and serum can escape and do not lift the graft from its bed.

The donor site should be hairless and inconspicuous. The inner aspect of the upper arm or thigh is therefore recommended.

Full-thickness skin graft (Wolfe graft)

Indications

(a) Nasal tip and conchal bowl defects.

(b) A full-thickness graft with all adipose tissue excised is ideal when performing a septodermaplasty. The postauricular donor site is preferred because primary closure is easy and leaves an inconspicuous scar.

Pedicled skin flaps

These are skin flaps that remain attached at their base to provide a blood supply and lymphatic drainage. They can be classified into random, axial and myocutaneous.

Random

Examples of random skin flaps are Z-plasty, rhomboid and advancement rotation flaps. Although these flaps may be raised anywhere and run in any direction, careful planning is necessary to obtain optimal cosmesis. Where possible, the use of relaxed skin tension lines should be used. The length of the flap should not exceed the width of the base otherwise the distal portion of the flap may become ischaemic.

Axial flap

Examples include deltopectoral and nasolabial flaps. These are fasciocutaneous flaps with a named blood supply running superficial to the deep fascia supplying the overlying skin. The length of the flap corresponds to the area supplied by these vessels. The pectoralis major myocutaneous flap has replaced many of the indications for the deltopectoral flap, which may still occasionally be used to replace lateral neck skin and peristomal skin. The main disadvantage of these flaps is that the patient must submit to a two-stage procedure, the second to return the pedicle to its original site after the distal portion has gained an adequate blood supply at its new site; this normally takes 3–4 weeks. Between stages the patient must endure moist dressings to an unsightly granulating bed from which the flap has been lifted.

Musculocutaneous

A pectoralis major flap is an example. Although a large number of head and neck musculocutaneous flaps have been described, the pectoralis major flap is now by far the most popular. This is a flap of skin, deep fascia and muscle based on the acromiothoracic artery, a branch of the first part of the axillary artery. It runs in a layer between the deep aspect of the muscle and its underlying fascia. The vessels perforate the muscle to supply the overlying skin. Its advantages are that it is straightforward to raise, provides good bulk and is reliable. Its main disadvantage is that its bulk may compromise function, and for this reason the radial forearm fasciocutaneous free flap has taken over much of its previous work.

Two important points in technique in raising the flap are:

(a) Suture the muscle edge to the subcutaneous edge as the flap is raised to prevent shearing of the perforating vessels.

(b) After measuring the flap allow an extra 1–2 cm of pedicle length as the flap retracts on raising; it is important that the pedicle is not under tension when suturing the flap into position.

Free tissue transfer

These flaps provide the gold standard in terms of cosmesis and preservation of function. Good results require sound microvascular training and meticulous attention to detail. Raising the flap and preparing both the donor and recipient vessels and their subsequent anastomosis are critical areas in which small errors may cause the graft to fail. Good results come from expert training in a centre with an interest in such reconstructive surgery and cannot be learned from a book. A take rate of at least 90% should be obtained. Common free tissue transfer flaps in head and neck reconstruction with their main indications are:

1. Radial forearm fasciocutaneous free flap. Reconstruction of the floor of mouth, tongue, lateral oropharyngeal wall, soft palate and the repair of a pharyngocutaneous fistula.

2. Jejunal free flap. Reconstruction of a neopharynx after pharyngolaryngectomy.

3. Composite osteocutanous radial forearm free flap. Reconstruction of the floor of mouth and mandible after a mandibulectomy of less than about 8–10 cm. The length available depends on the interval between the insertions of pronator teres and pronator quadratus. One should aim to take no more than 40% of the diameter of the radius in the composite flap in order to reduce the risk of a subsequent radial fracture.

4. Rectus abdominis myocutaneous free flap. Reconstruction following total glossectomy and reconstructing the lateral skull base after petrosectomy. This flap is based on the inferior epigastric vessels.

5. *Iliac crest osteocutaneous free flap based on the deep circumflex iliac vessels.* Reconstruction of mandibulectomy greater than 8–10 cm, in particular a hemimandibulectomy with or without floor of mouth reconstruction. The osseous portion of this free flap is very reliable but the skin less so.

Further reading

Shaheen OH. The repair of defects. In: Shaheen OH (ed.) *Problems in Head and Neck Surgery.* London: Baillière Tindall, 1984; 70–91.

Related topics of interest

Hypopharyngeal carcinoma (p. 133)
Oral cavity carcinoma (p. 198)
Oropharyngeal carcinoma (p. 204)

SALIVARY GLAND DISEASES

There are four main salivary glands – two parotids and two submandibular glands – and multiple minor salivary glands which occur throughout the upper respiratory tract, notably in the oral cavity and oropharynx. Patients with enlargement of these glands or sialomegaly can pose an interesting diagnostic dilemma.

Pathology

1. Infection. (a) Viral: mumps virus, coxsackievirus, echovirus, human immunodeficiency virus (HIV). (b) Bacterial: staphylococcal, actinomycosis, tuberculosis, leprosy.

2. Neoplasm. (a) Benign: pleomorphic adenoma, adenolymphoma. (b) Malignant: adenoid cystic carcinoma, adenocarcinoma, squamous cell carcinoma. (c) Variable: mucoepidermoid carcinoma, acinic cell tumour. (d) Non-epithelial: haemangioma, lymphangioma, neurofibroma, lymphoma.

3. Inflammatory. Sjögren's syndrome is an autoimmune disease which is characterized by periductal lymphocytes in multiple organs. The salivary glands are affected in approximately 40% of all cases. In one in six patients the disease will progress to a lymphoma. Sjögren originally described xerostomia, keratoconjunctivitis sicca and rheumatoid arthritis, with no mention of salivary gland swelling. Now the disease can be classified into: (a) primary Sjögren's syndrome (or sicca complex) consisting of xerostomia and xerophthalmia with no connective tissue component, and (b) secondary Sjögren's syndrome, which consists of xerostomia, xerophthalmia and a connective tissue disorder, usually rheumatoid arthritis.

4. Metabolic. Myxoedema, diabetes, Cushing's disease, cirrhosis, gout, bulimia, alcoholism.

5. Drug induced. Coproxamol (dextropropoxyphene and paracetamol), oral contraceptive pill, thiouracil, phenylbutazone, isoprenaline.

6. Sialectasis. Progressive destruction of the alveoli and parenchyma of the gland accompanied by duct stenosis and cyst formation. Many cases are thought to be congenital. Epithelial debris or calculi may be found in the main ducts.

7. Pseudoparotomegaly. These disorders should be kept in mind as they may mimic sialomegaly: hypertrophic masseter, winged mandible, mandible tumours, dental cyst, branchial cyst, preauricular lymph node, sebaceous cyst, lipoma and neuroma of the facial nerve.

History

The diagnosis is often obvious from the clinical findings. The history should include the age of the patient (think of mumps or congenital sialectasis), the number of glands affected (tumours are unilateral apart from Warthin's on rare occasions), whether the swelling is exacerbated by eating (calculus disease secondary to sialectasis), duration of symptoms (benign tumours grow slowly and malignant ones fairly rapidly) and any related pain (infection, calculus or adenoid cystic carcinoma). There should be a thorough review of systemic symptoms (metabolic causes), and any medication the patient is taking should be noted. The social history including alcohol intake and risk of HIV infection may be relevant in some cases.

Examination

Inspect the enlarged gland and then all the other salivary glands. Inflamed skin over the swelling should make one consider an infection or skin involvement from a malignant lesion. The facial nerve should be tested as facial weakness also raises the suspicion of a malignant lesion. Before palpating the lesion be sure to ask if it is tender; this is kind to the patient and a good habit in clinical medicine – it is essential in an examination! Palpation should determine whether the lesion is local or diffuse, solid or cystic, mobile or fixed and whether or not other glands are affected. Inspect the oral cavity and palpate all of the glands bimanually. In the floor of the mouth a submandibular calculus may be felt or pressure on a parotid gland may express pus from the parotid duct. Then examine the pharynx to look for a parapharyngeal lesion (in particular one arising from the deep lobe of the parotid), which may push the tonsil medially. Complete the ENT examination and perform a general examination if systemic or disseminated neoplastic disease is suspected.

Investigations

1. Blood tests. A full blood count and ESR investigation should be done in all cases. Rheumatoid factor, antinuclear factor and abnormal electrophoresis are sometimes found in Sjögren's syndrome. Specific Sjögren's antibodies are usually also present (SSrho and SSla). Tests for the relevant endocrine disorders may be appropriate.

2. Radiography. A plain film is useful as it may reveal a radiopaque submandibular calculus. Most submandibular gland calculi are radiopaque, but most parotid calculi are radiolucent. A sialogram is probably the most useful investigation of benign salivary gland disease. Duct stenosis, calculi and sialectasis can all be diagnosed if sialography is possible. CT or MRI scanning is usually the preferred investigation in neoplastic disease to delineate any potential deep lobe involvement and to assess the tumour's relationship to the facial nerve.

3. Biopsy. Incisional and Trucut biopsy should not be performed as there is a risk of seeding neoplastic disease. Fine-needle aspiration biopsy is safe and often useful, but the results have to be interpreted in conjunction with clinical suspicion as incorrect reports are not uncommon, especially with cystic lesions. A parapharyngeal mass should never be biopsied through the pharynx because there may be uncontrollable bleeding if the patient has a vascular lesion. Sublabial biopsy is the definitive investigation to confirm the diagnosis in Sjögren's syndrome.

Management The management and specific treatment of the patient depends on the cause of the salivary gland swelling.

Further reading

Maran AGD. Non-neoplastic salivary gland disease. In: Stell PM (ed.) *Scott-Brown's Otolaryngology*, Vol. 5, 5th edn. London: Butterworths, 1987; 340–50.

Related topic of interest

Salivary gland neoplasms (p. 274)

SALIVARY GLAND NEOPLASMS

Pathology

Neoplastic lesions are divided into benign or malignant, and malignant lesions can be primary or secondary. In addition, if one can remember the epithelial and the non-epithelial histology of the organ, an excellent framework for working practice is easily established. Salivary gland tumours are no exception in this respect, except that some such neoplasms have variable biological behaviour. The World Health Organization histological classification of salivary tumours now includes over 35 variants and also includes tumour-like lesions (e.g. salivary gland cysts). A simplified classification is presented below:

1. Benign.
Pleiomorphic adenoma.
Myoepithelioma (myoepithelial adenoma).
Warthin's tumour (adenolymphoma).
Oncocytic adenoma.
Ductal papilloma.
Papillary cystadenoma.

2. Malignant.
Adenoid cystic carcinoma.
Adenocarcinoma.
Squamous cell carcinoma.
Undifferentiated carcinoma.
Carcinoma in pleomorphic adenoma.

3. Variable.
Mucoepidermoid carcinoma.
Acinic cell carcinoma.

4. Non-epithelial.
Haemangioma, lymphangioma, neurofibroma, lymphoma.

A good approximation to remember is that 80% of all salivary tumours are in the parotid, 80% of parotid tumours are benign and 80% of the benign tumours that arise in the parotid are pleomorphic adenoma. One in three tumours arising in the submandibular gland and one in two tumours that arise in the minor salivary glands are malignant.

Staging

With malignant tumours of the parotid gland, a significant correlation exists between tumour stage and survival. The stage of the disease has been shown to be a more important prognostic parameter than its histological grade. The AJC system is summarized below:

T0   No clinical evidence of tumour.
T1   < 2 cm in diameter, without significant local extension.
T2   2–4 cm in diameter, without significant local extension.
T3   4–6 cm in diameter, without significant local extension.
T4a > 6 cm in diameter, without significant local extension.
T4b A tumour of any size with significant local extension.

Investigations

1. Radiography. CT scanning of a parotid tumour is useful in the assessment and delineation of anatomical structures, extension to the deep lobe and relation to the facial nerve. MRI has significant advantages. Using short tau inversion recovery (STIR) sequencing appears to add to the sensitivity in detecting lesions of the parotid gland, delineating the facial nerve and in identifying the tumour edge.

2. Fine-needle aspiration biopsy (FNA). The role of FNA in the diagnosis of benign and malignant salivary gland disease is a controversial issue. Proponents of the technique argue that FNA provides diagnostic information which may allay a patient's anxiety and aid in preoperative counselling and planning of surgery. However, those against the routine use of FNA argue that one cannot rely on the sensitivity or specificity of the procedure. This is particularly true in patients with cystic lesions of the parotid, in whom the aspirates often yield straw-coloured fluid, which is almost invariably hypocellular or acellular, and thus non-diagnostic. FNA is a relatively painless procedure, has few complications (seeding of the tumour does not appear to occur) and may prevent an ill-advised and often ill-fated incisional or excisional biopsy of a parotid mass. If the result of FNA is at variance with other findings then clinical judgement should prevail.

Benign tumours

Pleomorphic adenoma is the commonest benign salivary tumour. The sex distribution is equal and the peak age incidence is in the fifth decade. It has a pseudocapsule of compressed parotid tissue into which the tumour usually has many protuberances. It arises from intercalated duct cells and myoepithelial cells. Microscopically it comprises epithelial and mesodermal elements with a mucopolysaccharide stroma giving rise to a characteristic mixed staining pattern. If the capsule is ruptured during removal, then tumour may implant, causing recurrence.

They are therefore excised with as large a margin as possible to reduce the risk of capsule rupture. Superficial parotidectomy or hemisuperficial parotidectomy when the lesion is small is now the preferred procedure. Management of recurrent tumour is difficult as the facial nerve may be involved and its sheath may need to be stripped. The facial nerve should if at all feasible not be sacrificed; rarely radical surgery is needed with resection of the facial nerve. Many surgeons advocate adjuvant postoperative radiotherapy in these situations.

The adenomas include *adenolymphoma* (Warthin's tumour), *oncocytomas* and *papillary cystadenoma*. Adenolymphomas are benign tumours usually seen in elderly men. The peak incidence is the seventh decade and the male–female ratio is 7:1. They are soft and cystic tumours which are thought to arise from heterotopic parotid tissue in the lymph nodes within the parotid gland. Ten per cent are bilateral, but rarely synchronously. Treatment is by excision and, unlike pleomorphic adenoma, recurrence almost never occurs. Oncocytoma is a benign eosinophilic tumour (also called oxyphil adenoma) that arises from intralobular ducts or acini. It can undergo malignant change and treatment is by excision.

Malignant tumours

Adenoid cystic carcinoma is the commonest malignant tumour and may arise from any salivary tissue, but is more common in minor than in major salivary glands. The sex incidence is equal and they are seen most often in patients in their sixth decade. The tumour is slow-growing and tends to spread along nerve sheaths. The patients often complain of facial pain and may present with a facial paresis. The incidence of lymph node metastases is low and distant metastases occur late. Treatment is usually by radical excision and adjuvant radiotherapy. If the facial nerve is free of tumour it may be dissected out and left intact. However, it is often involved, and in this situation it needs wide excision and anastomosis with a nerve graft. The sural nerve is preferred as the greater auricular nerve may be involved and should also be excised. Postoperative radiotherapy will not affect the graft. Radiotherapy in the curative and palliative treatment of patients with adenoid cystic carcinoma of salivary gland origin is useful in some cases, but is still being assessed.

Adenocarcinoma accounts for about 3% of parotid tumours and 10% of submandibular and minor salivary gland tumours. Some pathologists doubt the existence of squamous cell carcinoma, regarding them as high-grade mucoepidermoid tumours, and true malignant pleomorphic adenomas are rare.

Tumours of variable malignancy

Mucoepidermoid tumours arise in any salivary tissue but predominantly the parotid gland. It is the commonest salivary neoplasm in children. Low-grade or well-differentiated tumours usually behave in a benign fashion, intermediate ones are more aggressive and high-grade or undifferentiated tumours metastasize early and carry a poor prognosis. However, the behaviour is not always accurately predicted by the histological appearance. *Acinic* cell tumours are similarly difficult to classify. They are, however, much more benign than mucoepidermoid tumours.

Further reading

Medina JE. Salivary gland tumours. *Current Opinion in Otolaryngology and Head and Neck Surgery,* 1993; **1**: 91–6.
Roland NJ *et al.* Fine needle aspiration cytology of salivary gland lesions reported immediately in a head and neck clinic. *Journal of Laryngology and Otology,* 1993; **107**: 1025–8.

Related topic of interest

Salivary gland diseases (p. 271)

SEPTAL PERFORATION

Perforation of the nasal septum is most common in the anterior cartilaginous part except for that caused by syphilis, which normally involves the bony septum. Most perforations are iatrogenic in origin, usually as a complication of septal surgery, particularly when the Killian incision is used. Many septal perforations that were previously considered to be idiopathic are now thought to be secondary to nose picking. Septal perforations are usually preceded by ulceration except when following a septal haematoma or septal abscess.

Aetiology

1. Trauma.
Iatrogenic (SMR, septoplasty, nasal cautery).
Self-inflicted (nose picking).
Injury (assault, road accident, sport injury).

2. Infection (syphilis, tuberculosis).

3. Neoplasm (squamous cell carcinoma, adenocarcinoma, basal cell carcinoma, T-cell lymphoma).

4. Inflammatory (Wegener's granulomatosis, periarteritis nodosa, systemic lupus).

5. Inhalation of irritants (occupational, hexavalent, chrome, arsenic, alkaline dusts; drugs, cocaine, snuff).

6. Idiopathic.

Clinical features

The majority of perforations are asymptomatic. The main complaints are recurrent epistaxis, dryness in the nose, crusting and nasal obstruction. The severity of the symptoms depends on the position and the size of the perforation. The larger the perforation and the more anterior its position, the worse the symptoms. A very small perforation may cause whistling on nasal breathing.

Investigations

The history will very often give the diagnosis. In any patient where there is uncertainty about the cause, the following tests should be performed:

- Blood tests should include a full blood count and an ESR.
- A chest radiograph may show lesions in tuberculosis, Wegener's granulomatosis or metastases.
- Urinalysis (haematuria or proteinuria may result from nephritis in Wegener's granulomatosis or polyarteritis)
- Fluorescent *Treponema* antibody (FTA) test for syphilis.

- A biopsy from the edge of the perforation if there is suggestion of a neoplasm or granuloma.

Treatment

The first objective is to cure the causative disease process before specific treatment of the perforation. Medical treatment with 25% glucose in glycerol drops will loosen and help clear crusts. Silver nitrate cautery can be applied to bleeding granulations. Surgical closure of the perforation is difficult to achieve. A variety of operations including the use of split-skin grafts, septal mucoperichondrial flaps, composite grafts from the pinna and moving septal cartilage to fill the hole have all been described. If the perforation continues to trouble the patient it is worth trying to plug the hole with a silastic septal button.

Follow-up and aftercare

This will depend on the cause of the perforation, the severity of the symptoms and the particular treatment the patient has been given. A patient with a silastic button should be seen at regular 4- to 6-monthly intervals to decrust and clean the prosthesis.

Further reading

Brain D. The nasal septum. In: Mackay IS, Bull TR (eds) *Scott-Brown's Otolaryngology*, Vol. 4, 5th edn. London: Butterworths, 1987; 154–79.

Related topic of interest

Nasal trauma (p. 175)

SINONASAL TUMOURS

Tumours of the sinonasal region comprise a diverse group of benign and malignant neoplasms. The latter constitute a considerable challenge to the head and neck surgeon in view of the often late presentation. The low incidence and the lack of a consensus regarding staging has made comparison of treatment regimes between centres difficult.

Pathology

About 10% of head and neck cancer is sinonasal with a prevalence in the UK and North America of about 10 per million. It is about double this in Arabs, the Japanese and Africans. The male–female ratio in series varies between 1:2 and 1:5. Half of sinonasal cancer arises from the upper jaw, a quarter from the ethmoids and a quarter from the nasal cavity. Histologically 50% are squamous cell carcinoma, 15% anaplastic, 10% lymphomas and about 4% adenocarcinomas. The remainder comprise a large and diverse group of cancers. Immunocytochemical analysis (in particular neurone-specific enolase) of the small cell cancers will reveal a proportion to be olfactory neuroblastomas. The association between ethmoidal adenocarcinoma and hardwood workers is well documented. Those involved in nickel refining or handling chromate salts are at an increased risk of nasal malignancy. Chronic nasal pathology, including sepsis and Wegener's granulomatosis, and smoking cigarettes have recently been implicated as causing an increased risk of squamous cell carcinoma. Human papillomavirus genome has been implicated as an aetiological agent in non-dysplastic and dysplastic inverted papilloma and squamous cell carcinoma.

Classification

Both benign and malignant groups can be classified into epithelial, non-epithelial, odontogenic and fibro-osseous tumours.

Benign

Epithelial	Papilloma, adenoma and inverted papilloma
Non-epithelial	Fibroma, haemangioma, nasal glioma, schwannoma, chondroma, haemangiopericytoma, chordoma, meningioma and osteoma.

Malignant

Epithelial	Squamous cell carcinoma, adenocarcinoma, anaplastic carcinoma, transitional cell

carcinoma, malignant melanoma, salivary gland malignancy, in particular adenoid cystic carcinoma and olfactory neuroblastoma.

Non-epithelial Lymphoma, fibrosarcoma, angiosarcoma, chondrosarcoma, rhabdomyosarcoma and osteogenic sarcomas.

Important benign sinonasal tumours

Inverted papilloma, originally described by Ringertz, is the most important of this group, forming about 5% of all nasal tumours. Macroscopically there is usually a papilliferous exophytic mass, while microscopically there are deep invaginations of epithelium into the stroma, with microcyst formation, the epithelium retaining its basement membrane. Probably less than 2% undergo malignant change, although there may be a synchronous sinonasal squamous cell carcinoma in up to a further 10%, emphasizing the need for careful nasendoscopic follow-up.

Osteomas most commonly arise from the frontal region where they may expand medially to block the frontal recess predisposing to a secondary mucocele or frontal sinusitis, inferiorly to displace the orbit, superiorly where they may erode the cribriform plate or posteriorly to erode the posterior wall of the frontal sinus and impinge on frontal lobe dura. They consist of hard cortical bone and require excision if symptomatic or enlarging.

Haemangiopericytomas may arise anywhere in the sinonasal region and have a spectrum of aggression with a propensity to recur many years after apparent cure.

Malignant sinonasal tumours

Squamous cell carcinoma and adenocarcinoma both usually present at an advanced stage because their presenting symptoms of epistaxis, nasal obstruction and headaches occur only with a significant tumour mass. Further delays may arise because these symptoms are not usually associated with carcinoma by primary care physicians. Cheek swelling occurs only when the tumour has breached the anterior antral wall to impinge on periosteum. It is usually impossible to define a site of origin of the carcinoma because of its diffuse extent, which may include the ethmoids, maxilla, orbit, nasal cavity and anterior cranial fossa. Five per cent of subjects will have a metastatic neck lymph node, usually upper deep cervical, on presentation, and this indicates a poor prognosis but not necessarily incurability. A quarter of patients will die from distant metastases, most commonly of the lung.

Adenoid cystic carcinoma is particularly difficult to eradicate because of its ability to spread via the branches of the trigeminal and olfactory nerves along perineurium.

Malignant melanomas constitute 1% of sinonasal carcinomas and usually arise from the septum or lateral nasal wall, where the prognosis is a little better. There is no relationship between Clark's classification (penetration of specific skin layers) and prognosis in this region, although prognonis is associated with Breslow's classification (thickness of the lesion in mm). Frontoethmoidal and antral malignant melanoma have a much worse prognosis.

Olfactory neuroblastomas were undoubtedly under-reported until recently when immunocytochemical stains for this tumour became available. It arises from neural crest stem cells, the precursors of olfactory cells, and microscopically resembles other small cell malignancies such as high-grade lymphoma and anaplastic carcinoma. All ages are affected and urine vanillylmandelic acid (VMA) is not usually detectable. It always involves the cribriform plate so if resection is contemplated this must be via a craniofacial approach.

High-grade T-cell lymphoma (formerly lethal midline granuloma) – see Nasal polyps.

Clinical features

1. Nasal cavity tumours. Epistaxis, nasal obstruction and a mass visible on nasendoscopy.

2. Frontal sinus. Features are similar to frontal osteomas except the history is shorter and more rapidly progressive.

3. Ethmoidal. Epistaxis, nasal obstruction and, if the lamina papyracea is breached, proptosis, epiphora and diplopia. Nasendoscopy may reveal tumour extruding from the middle meatus.

4. Antral. Epistaxis, nasal obstruction, cheek swelling, headache if blocking the osteomeatal complex and atypical facial pain (suggesting involvement of the pterygopalatine fossa or the infraorbital nerve). Oroantral fistula, ill-fitting dentures, trismus and ethmoidal symptoms occur with advanced disease.

Investigations

A high-definition CT scan on both bone and soft-tissue windows is the ideal investigation to show soft-tissue and bone involvement. A T2 weighted or STIR sequence MRI scan may distinguish tumour from inflammation, retained secretions and fat, but bone does not generate a signal.

Treatment	There are three main surgical options:

There are three main surgical options:

(a) Lateral rhinotomy for tumour limited to the lateral nasal wall, nasal cavity and ethmoid. An upper limb extension will allow tumour extending to the frontoethmoidal region to be accessed.

(b) Total maxillectomy. For antral carcinoma.

(c) Craniofacial resection is indicated when the cribriform plate is involved or breached. In general, orbital exenteration is indicated only if tumour breaches periosteum to involve orbital fat, and this is unusual. Adjuvant radiotherapy may be indicated depending on tissue margins.

Prognosis by stage is difficult for reasons already outlined. Overall a 5-year survival of 40–50% would be reasonable.

Follow-up and aftercare

Ideally an orthodontist should take an impression of the maxillectomy cavity at operation in order to make a temporary obturator. Further review allows a fine tuning of the prosthesis to provide a light, comfortable, well-fitting and easily removable obturator. Those who have a lateral rhinotomy or craniofacial cavity often have excessive crusting in the early postoperative phase. Glycerine and glucose nose drops and regular douching with saline will minimize this. Only the surgeon should extract crusts from the nares of the craniofacial patient as these may be attached to a fascia lata or temporalis fascia graft overlying the anterior cranial fossa. Follow-up involves nasendoscopy to inspect the surgical cavity created or direct inspection of a maxillectomy cavity after obturator removal, laryngopharyngeal examination to exclude a second primary and neck examination to look for metastases. It should be monthly for the first post-operative year, bimonthly for the second, quarterly for the third and 6-monthly until 5 years post surgery. Some surgeons thereafter review annually for a further 5 years.

Further reading

Harrison DNF. Lateral rhinotomy: a neglected operation. *Annals of Otology, Rhinology and Laryngology,* 1977, **86**: 756–9.

Lund VJ, Harrison DFN. Craniofacial resection for tumors of the nasal cavity and paranasal sinuses. *American Journal of Surgery*, 1988; **156**: 187–90.

Lund VJ, Howard DJ, Lloyd GAS, Cheesman AD. Magnetic resonance imaging of paranasal sinus tumors for craniofacial resection. *Head and Neck Surgery*, 1989; **11**: 279–83.

Related topics of interest

Examination of the nose (p. 93)
Nasal polyps (p. 172)

SINUSITIS – COMPLICATIONS

In most cases sinusitis is uncomplicated and spread of infection beyond the walls of the sinus is uncommon. Complications may follow an acute infection, but are most frequent during an acute exacerbation of chronic sinusitis. They can be divided into:

- Orbital complications (orbital cellulitis and orbital abscess).
- Osteomyelitis (maxilla or frontal bone).
- Mucocele.
- Locoregional complications (pharyngitis, laryngitis, otitis media).
- Intracranial complications (meningitis, intracranial abscess, cavernous sinus thrombosis).

Orbital complications

Orbital cellulitis and abscess usually result from direct spread of pus from the ethmoid and frontal sinuses. It can also spread from thrombophlebitis of mucosal vessels in any of the sinuses.

Aching around the orbit is followed by oedema of the eyelids and later the conjunctiva. Cellulitis requires treatment with intravenous antibiotics and nasal decongestants to resolve the infection and limit further spread. The ethmoids are separated from the orbit by the thin lamina papyracea. An abscess results from direct spread from the ethmoids and collects between the lamina papyracea and the orbital periosteum. The eye will become proptosed and its movements progressively restricted. The biggest anxiety is the risk of blindness as a result of tension and septic necrosis of the optic nerve. Visual acuity and fields and the optic disc should be examined. A CT scan will confirm the collection and extent of the disease. Urgent surgical drainage is indicated. An incision is made in the superomedial aspect of the orbit. Elevation of the orbital periosteum usually reveals the pus under pressure. An external ethmoidectomy is performed and a drain inserted. Synchronous infection of the maxillary sinus is treated by inferior meatal antrostomy and intravenous antibiotics.

Osteomyelitis

This only occurs in diploic bone and thus only in the maxilla of children and the frontal sinus of adolescents and adults. The common organism is *Staphylococcus aureus*. Osteomyelitis of the maxilla is rare and usually only seen in Third World countries. It presents as a painful swelling of the cheek and lower eyelid. Treatment comprises intravenous antibiotics and debridement when necessary. Osteomyelitis of the frontal bone is more extensive and dangerous. There is a build-up of dull local pain with oedema of the forehead and the upper eyelids. A subperiosteal abscess of the forehead may form (Pott's puffy tumour). This is a life-threatening condition with a high risk of intracranial complications. Prompt treatment with high doses of intravenous antibiotics is required and surgical drainage of the frontal sinus with debridement necessary if pus has formed.

Mucocele

A mucocele may develop when the outlet from a sinus becomes permanently blocked. It occurs most commonly in the frontal sinus, but the ethmoid, maxillary and sphenoid sinuses can all be afflicted. There is an accumulation of sterile mucus which becomes increasingly viscous. The cyst gradually expands and exerts pressure on the sinus walls causing erosion. This leads to displacement of adjacent structures, especially the orbit. The main complaints are headache and swelling. These features can be dramatic if infection supervenes (pyocele). Diplopia and proptosis may result if the mucocele expands into the orbit. Radiographs will show enlargement of the sinus with thinning of the bone. CT scans will further delineate the extent of the disease if needed.

Treatment is surgical evacuation and drainage of the sinus. To approach the frontal sinus, the two options in common use are external fronto-ethmoidectomy (Howarth's operation) and the osteoplastic flap procedure (Macbeth's operation).

Locoregional complications

Regional complications occur as a result of infection and inflammation spreading through the rest of the upper aerodigestive tract mucosa. Mucopus from sinusitis is carried back through the nasal airway into the pharynx and may cause a pharyngitis. Invasion of the subepithelial lymphoid tissue will produce a granular pharyngitis with visible nodules as the lymphatic tissue hypertrophies. Further downward spread may lead to irritation of the vocal cords causing a laryngitis. Sinusitis is also implicated as a cause and complication of tonsillitis and otitis media.

Intracranial complications

The cavities of the frontal, ethmoidal and sphenoid sinuses are closely related to and separated by a thin wall of bone from the anterior cranial fossa. Infection may involve the brain and meninges from either direct spread or retrograde thrombophlebitis. Meningitis is the commonest complication, but encephalitis, intracranial abscess (extradural, subdural or cerebral) and cavernous sinus thrombosis may complicate sinus infections. The clinical features of meningitis are well known. A lumbar puncture may identify the causative organism, but it is essential to exclude raised intracranial pressure before this is done by looking for papilloedema.

Cavernous sinus thrombosis will cause a high fever, reduced conscious level and cerebral irritation. The eyes will proptose and an ophthalmoplegia of the cranial nerves which travel in the cavernous sinus will occur (III, IV, ophthalmic and maxillary branches of V and VI). An intracranial abscess may be more difficult to diagnose. The important point is that the ENT surgeon should always maintain a high index of suspicion for this and the other intracranial complications, particularly in sinusitis patients who become drowsy or show some neurological deficit. A CT scan with enhancement or MRI scan may assist in diagnosis. Intracranial complications should all be treated with high-dose intravenous antibiotics. An extradural or subdural abscess will require drainage by a neurosurgeon, together with drainage of the offending sinuses by an ENT surgeon.

Further reading

Pickard BH. The complications of sinusitis. In: Mackay IS, Bull TR (eds) *Scott-Brown's Otolaryngology*, Vol. 5, 5th edn. London: Butterworths, 1987; 203–11.

Related topics of interest

Acute sinusitis (p. 5)
Chronic sinusitis (p. 47)
Functional endoscopic sinus surgery (p. 119)

SNORING AND OBSTRUCTIVE SLEEP APNOEA

Definitions

- Snoring: a noise generated as a result of partial upper airway obstruction during sleep.
- Apnoea: a period of no airflow at the nose or mouth for at least 10 seconds.
- Apnoea index (AI): the number of periods of apnoea per hour.
- Hypopnoea: 50% or greater reduction in normal tidal volume.

Sleep apnoea syndrome can be diagnosed if there are more than 30 apnoeic episodes in 7 hours of sleep or if the apnoea index is more than 5. Sleep apnoea is classified as mild (AI = 5–20), moderate (AI = 20–40) or severe (AI > 40). Sleep apnoea can be obstructive, central or mixed.

In obstructive sleep apnoea (OSA) there is complete upper airway obstruction yet the patient continues to make respiratory efforts to overcome this. In central apnoea, respiratory effort, and consequently airflow, ceases for a period of time. Central apnoea is due to a defect of autonomic control of respiration in the medulla or peripheral chemoreceptors resulting in a failure of respiratory drive. It is a symptom of serious neurological disease and is not considered further here.

Pathophysiology

The noise of snoring is produced by vibration of the soft palate and pharyngeal walls caused by turbulent airflow and the Bernoulli effect from a partial obstruction. The obstruction occurs when the negative intraluminal pharyngeal pressure exceeds the ability of the dilators to hold the pharynx open. Any cause of airway narrowing from nares to glottis can contribute to increased airway resistance. Neuromuscular incoordination interfering with the reflex activity of the pharyngeal dilators associated with inspiration, increased compliance of pharyngeal tissues, the Venturi effect and the decreased muscle tone associated with sleep can all predispose to upper airway collapse.

This obstruction has three effects:

(a) Hypoxia, which can in turn lead to pulmonary and systemic hypertension, cor pulmonale and cardiac dysrhythmias.

(b) Increased negative intrathoracic pressures and increased cardiovascular strain.

(c) Arousal, in an effort to overcome the obstruction and consequent poor sleep quality.

As a consequence patients with severe OSA have a significantly increased mortality rate from cardiovascular disease.

Clinical features

Snoring and OSA in adults are more common with increasing age, in men, and in the obese and those with a high alcohol intake. Snoring occurs in 10% of men under 30 and 60% of men over 60, while OSA can be found in approximately 6% of men. In children it most commonly occurs around the age of 5 when lymphoid hyperplasia is at its greatest. Snoring can be immensely socially disruptive and may lead to marital difficulties. OSA often leads to daytime somnolence, morning headaches, personality change, intellectual deterioration, impotence and an increased risk of a road traffic accident.

Investigations

It is important to establish whether the patient has simple snoring or OSA, to exclude any exacerbating factors (drugs, endocrine disorders, anatomical) and to identify the site and level of obstruction. A thorough history and examination is needed; while taking the history it is essential to have the bed partner present.

1. General. Full blood count (FBC), thyroid function tests (TFT), chest radiograph, electrocardiogram (ECG) and blood gases.

2. To identify sleep apnoea. An overnight sleep study. Polysomnography is the gold standard and involves the recording of an electroencephalogram (EEG), electromyogram (EMG), ECG, airflow, abdominal and chest movements, oxygen saturation, and microphone recording of the snoring. Unfortunately, this is expensive in terms of time and equipment but is an ideal research tool. Less thorough sleep studies may be performed with overnight pulse oximetry.

3. Site of obstruction. To differentiate between palatal and tongue base or multisegmental obstruction, a variety of tests have been developed including cine CT, sleep nasendoscopy, lateral cephalometry and somnofluroscopy. Probably the most widely used test is the Muller manoeuvre. This involves positioning per nasally a flexible fibreoptic endoscope to the level of the tongue base with the patient in the sitting position and with the mouth closed. The patient inhales vigorously while the nares are occluded and the degree of hypopharyngeal collapse noted. The manoeuvre is then repeated with the endoscope positioned just above the soft palate. In this way the level of obstruction can be identified in up to 85% of cases.

Management

1. General. Patients without OSA require no specific treatment beyond the reassurance that there is no serious pathology. Weight loss and advice with regard to alcohol and other sedatives are often helpful.

2. Nasal obstruction. In patients with nasal obstruction, medical treatment of rhinitis, surgical correction of a septal deviation and the use of the 'Nozovent' device to splint open the nasal valve are all useful.

3. Pharyngeal. Where the level of obstruction is palatal, uvulopharyngopalatoplasty (UPPP) by excision or laser treatment to stiffen the soft palate results in a significant improvement in snoring. Continuous positive airway pressure (CPAP) may still be required to improve cor pulmonale. In OSA due to tongue base and multisegmental airway collapse, CPAP delivered via a nasal mask is extremely effective. An adequate nasal airway is required and compliance is often a problem.

4. Maxillofacial. Techniques to advance the mandible or hyoid and move the tongue base forward have been tried with some success.

5. In children. The condition is, in most cases, adequately dealt with by adenotonsillectomy as this is the usual site of obstruction.

Finally in severe OSA, when all other forms of treatment have failed, a tracheostomy can be life-saving.

Further reading

Douglas NJ. The sleep apnoea/hypopnoea syndrome and snoring. *British Medical Journal*, 1993; **306**: 1057–60.
Fairbanks DNF. Snoring: surgical versus non-surgical management. *Laryngoscope,* 1984; **94**: 1188–92.

Related topics of interest

SPEECH AUDIOMETRY

In many animals the sense of hearing is adapted for a specific purpose. In the human, the ear is specifically tuned to the speech frequencies (500–4000 Hz). The main function of the human ear is therefore the perception of speech. Indeed, most of the handicap of hearing loss is due to loss of the ability to perceive the spoken word. Speech audiometry provides a measure of this ability and any corresponding deficit. Voice tests can be considered as a very basic form of speech audiometry. However, in general, speech audiometry implies the formal qualitative assessment of a subject's perception of speech. It measures the actual disability produced by the hearing impairment. It is useful in a variety of contexts including:

(a) Assessment and diagnosis of peripheral and central hearing disorders.
(b) Prediction of the usefulness of a hearing aid.
(c) Evaluation of the benefit which might be obtained by an operation (pre- and postoperative assessment).
(d) Medicolegal assessment.

Materials

1. Instruments. Testing is performed in a soundproof room using a cassette player or microphone with the volume controlled from the audiometer which presents speech material to the subject via loudspeakers or headphones. Speech material presented by the tester using a microphone is prone to variation in both intensity and accent. Standardized, prepared speech material presented by cassette and controlled by the audiometer is much more preferable. The use of headphones, as opposed to the free-field situation with loudspeakers, allows each ear to be tested individually and allows the non-test ear to be masked.

2. Speech material. Phonemes are the building blocks of speech and represent the smallest unit of recognizable speech sound (e.g. ay, aw, ah, etc.). There are 49 phonemes in the English language. Speech material is chosen to provide a representative balance of phonemes and can be presented as words, sentences or synthetic sentences which have no meaning. A great number of lists of appropriate speech material have been developed by various agencies e.g. Medical Research Council, Institute of Hearing Research, Fry, Boothroyd and Manchester junior word lists and Bench, Koval and Bamford (BKB) sentences (University of Manchester).

Procedure

The subject is seated in a soundproof room and instructed in the test procedure. The recorded word lists are presented to the patient monaurally over headphones at various sound intensities. As speech audiometry is a suprathreshold test, masking of the non-test ear is required on all occasions. Masking sounds in speech audiometry are chosen to try and recreate an appropriate noise background such as speech, cocktail party and babble noise. Pink noise (equal energy for each octave over the hearing range) is often used when these are unavailable. The first presentation is usually at 20–30 dB greater than the pure-tone average for the frequencies 500, 1000 and 2000 Hz. Subsequent presentations are usually made at +10, +20, –10 and –20 dB from this level, although more may be required. The patient is asked to repeat the words as accurately as possible and the percentage of words or phonemes which are correctly repeated at each sound intensity (dB) is calculated and plotted on a graph.

The graphical display is compared with the calibration graph for that particular machine, which will have been obtained by testing otologically normal individuals on that machine, using the same tapes and test environment. The recorded data can then be used to formulate certain scores and the shape of the graph used to give information regarding the type of deafness.

Scoring

(a) The optimum discrimination score (ODS) is the subject's maximum score, no matter how loud the volume is turned up. It is a measure of optimal performance and should be 100% when normal.
(b) The speech reception threshold (SRT) is the sound intensity (dB) at which the subject can correctly repeat 50% of the presented words.
(c) The half-peak level (HPL) refers to the sound level (dB) at which the discrimination percentage is half the ODS.
(d) The half-peak level elevation (HPLE) refers to the difference between the pathological and normal HPL. This is the dB level at which the patient achieves half the ODS in comparison with the level at which normal individuals achieve 50%. This is considered to be the most valuable diagnostic score.

Shape of the graph

If the hearing is normal all the words will be understood if they are played loudly enough. The result is a sigmoid-shaped curve with a steep, near-vertical portion in the middle.

In patients with a conductive hearing loss all the words will be understood, but they must be played louder than for a normal subject. The curve is parallel to the normal but is shifted to the right (i.e. greater HPL) in proportion to the degree of hearing loss. The ODS is still 100% as discrimination is preserved.

In patients with a sensorineural hearing loss there is usually a loss of ability to discriminate speech, and consequently the ODS is often less than 100%. The gradient of the middle portion of the curve is often less and a plateau may be reached in which further increases in sound intensity do not improve discrimination. In severe cases 'roll over' may occur: beyond a certain point any further increase in sound intensity causes a reduction in the discrimination score. This type of curve is typical of a retrocochlear lesion.

Specific uses

1. Non-organic hearing loss. Speech audiometry can be used in the investigation of non-organic or feigned hearing loss. Two tests exist:

(a) Delayed speech feedback (DSF). The subject is asked to read text aloud. The speech is relayed to the test ear with a delay of 1–200 ms. If there is normal hearing in the test ear stammering and a raised voice are almost inevitable.

(b) Competition tests. The patient is asked to repeat speech material delivered to the good ear while competing speech material is introduced to the test ear. If the hearing is normal, stuttering is likely when the competing material is 40 dB louder than the test material.

2. Central function. Speech audiometry can also be used as a test of central auditory function. This can be done using a variety of techniques, including speech messages in competing noise, competing messages and overlapping messages in each ear, accelerated, interrupted and filtered speech. For further details on this the reader is referred to Keith and Pensak (1991).

Further reading

Ballantyne D. *Handbook of Audiological Techniques*. London: Butterworth-Heinemann, 1990.

Keith RW, Pensak ML,. Central auditory function. *Otolaryngologic Clinics of North America*, 1991; **24**(2): 371–9.

Related topics of interest

SPEECH THERAPY IN HEAD AND NECK SURGERY

The role of the speech therapist as a member of a multidisciplinary rehabilitation team working with patients undergoing head and neck surgery is threefold:
(a) The rehabilitation of voice following laryngectomy.
(b) Developing compensatory articulation strategies for patients who have had oral surgery.
(c) Assessment, advice and therapy of patients who have dysphagia following head and neck surgery.

Voice rehabilitation following laryngectomy

Preoperatively, the speech therapist should see the patient and relatives for assessment, information giving and support. An oral examination and communication profile are carried out. Factors such as speech rate, volume, articulation, posture, tension levels, hearing, motivation and communication needs can have a significant bearing on the prognosis for voice rehabilitation.

There are three options for alternative voice: the electrolarynx, oesophageal voice and surgical voice restoration (SVR) with a voice prosthesis.

The electrolarynx is useful as a temporary measure before oesophageal voice is functionally adequate or before placement of a voice prosthesis. It can be a long-term option when the pharyngo-oesophageal (PE) segment is not viable or when it is the patient's preference. The efficiency of the electrolarynx is dependent on accurate placement, clear articulation, appropriate phrasing and neck status – a hard, fibrotic postradiotherapy neck may not transmit the electronic signal into the oral cavity for articulation.

Both oesophageal voice and SVR require a viable PE segment or neoglottis. The segment is made up of the inferior constrictor including cricopharyngeus and the upper oesophagus. There must be adequate apposition of the oesophageal mucosa to form a functional PE segment, and the tonicity of the segment determines the quality of the voice achieved and the effort necessary to produce it.

The oesophageal speaker has to gain voluntary control of the PE segment in order to take air into the upper oesophagus. The air is then released, producing sound as it passes through the PE segment. It is then amplified by the resonating spaces and modified by the articulators in the normal way. There can be difficulties at any stage in this process. The patient has to learn to dissociate respiration from phonation, and the acquisition of a functional oesophageal voice can take months of intensive speech therapy.

Oesophageal voice lacks the duration, fluency, consistency and volume which can be achieved with a voice prosthesis using pulmonary air. In SVR, when the stoma is occluded, expired pulmonary air passes through the one-way silicone valve in the tracheo-oesophageal wall, setting the PE segment into vibration. Voice prostheses are of two main types: the non-indwelling type, e.g. Blom-Singer and Bivona, and the indwelling type, e.g. Provox and Groningen button. Indwelling valves have to be changed by a doctor, whereas non-indwelling valves can be changed and maintained by a speech therapist or by patients themselves. There are advantages and disadvantages to both of these.

Many centres now favour primary placement of the prosthesis during laryngectomy so that patients can leave the hospital with a voice. This means that much of the frustration, depression and strain on relationships caused by a lengthy period of postoperative aphonia can be avoided. When secondary placement is planned, the speech therapist or ENT surgeon carries out an air insufflation test (Taub and Bugner, 1973). A catheter is inserted via the nose to the level of the stoma and is connected to a housing, which is glued to the stoma, such that when the stoma is occluded pulmonary air is transmitted through the catheter to below the PE segment. The patient is asked to speak. The amount of air pressure needed to produce voice and the fluency and durability of the voice achieved are noted. This test can also be carried out before commencing oesophageal voice training as it provides information about the tonicity of the PE segment.

After valve placement speech therapy involves: training in maintaining the valve, achieving accurate occlusion of the stoma, breath/voice coordination, and modifying the speech rate and phrasing to maximize intelligibility. Laryngeal voice assessment is carried out at regular intervals, including objective measurement of:

- Duration, i.e. the number of syllables produced per breath or air charge.
- Maximum phonation time: how long the patient can sustain a vowel on one breath.
- Dynamic range.
- Availability of the voice, i.e. ease of initiation.
- Pitch (where instrumentation is available).

Intelligibility and communication skills can be rated subjectively by naive listeners or by the speech therapist, who also rates tension levels, fluency, articulation, rate, voice quality, etc. Ultimately the success of voice rehabilitation is a measure of patients' satisfaction with their communication: to what extent are they able to use their voice with confidence in all the situations enjoyed prior to the laryngectomy?

There is no doubt that the best possible voice results are obtained with a voice prosthesis, but these are not without complications and the patient remains dependent on the hospital for maintenance of voice. The available alternatives are not mutually exclusive, but individual ENT departments have to decide which is to be their method of choice and ensure that the other alternatives are available to patients if the first option is either contraindicated or unsuccessful.

Compensatory articulatory strategies following oral surgery

All patients should be seen preoperatively so that the therapist can obtain a sample (preferably taped) of the patient's speech. Postoperatively, once healing is complete, patients are assessed using phonetically balanced word lists to establish an objective measure of their intelligibility across all the phonemes of English. The speech therapist then works on improving excursion and control of available articulators and systematic exploration of potential compensatory articulations which will improve the patient's ability to make phonemic contrasts and hence improve intelligibility, e.g. the use of a uvula sound as a substitute for /k,g/ phonemes in a glossectomy patient. These compensations are then practised for integration into spontaneous speech.

Surgical dysphagia

The speech therapist should see any patient preoperatively when postoperative dysphagia is anticipated.

When healing is complete a bedside assessment of the swallow is carried out to identify the risk of aspiration. This includes:

- Evaluation of the range, rate and accuracy of the movement, and sensation in lips, tongue and palate.
- Sample swallows observing oral control, oral transit time, swallow initiation/delay, laryngeal elevation, evidence of penetration (substance entry into the airway above the vocal cords) and aspiration (before, during and after the reflex triggers).

Access to videofluoroscopy or modified barium swallow is essential with this patient group. It is useful not just to identify whether aspiration is taking place and why, but also to experiment with different consistencies, textures and volumes of contrast, to monitor the effect of altered head position on the safety of the swallow and to assess the efficacy of various techniques in improving airway protection.

When alternative feeding methods have been necessary, e.g. gastrostomy, the speech therapist continues to rehabilitate the swallow using exercises, airway protection techniques and thermal stimulation.

Follow-up and aftercare Follow-up as an outpatient or on a domiciliary basis should be available for as long as is necessary for this patient group. Most speech therapy departments organize a club for their laryngectomy patients aimed at providing information, support and social activities on a long-term basis. Members of the club also carry out pre- and postoperative visits and provide long-term support to new patients.

Eating and talking are not only essential but pleasurable activities, and it is important not to underestimate the trauma suffered by patients who have problems with either or both of these functions. The aim of speech therapy is to achieve maximum rehabilitation and, where preoperative functional levels are not achievable, to assist patients to compensate and adjust to their new set of circumstances.

Further reading

Groher ME, Laryngectomy. In: Edels Y (ed.). *Dysphagia – Diagnosis and Management*. London: Butterworths, 1984.

Logeman J. *The Evaluation and Treatment of Swallowing Disorders*. San Diego: College Hill Press, 1983.

Taub S, Bugner, LH. Air bypass voice prosthesis for vocal rehabilitation of laryngectomees. *American Journal of Surgery*, 1973; **125:** 748–56.

Related topics of interest

SPEECH THERAPY IN NON-MALIGNANT VOICE DISORDERS

The formation of the British Voice Association in the UK, incorporating laryngologists, speech therapists, voice teachers, singers, actors and phoneticians, has led to an increased interest in voice care and voice use.

Referral

All patients are referred for voice therapy from ENT clinics, with the exception of transexuals. The referral should include the following information: a description of the structure and function of the vocal cords, any significant ENT history and results of examinations of the ear, nose, pharynx and nasopharynx, any relevant medical history, and the occupation of the patient as, in most departments, professional voice users are prioritized for therapy.

An in-depth case history in the first session highlights factors which will have a bearing on therapy planning, e.g. the onset and course of the dysphonia, the patient's understanding and attitude to the problem, the patient's general health, any previous voice disorders and treatment, a profile of how the voice is used, and any predisposing factors, e.g. working conditions, relationship problems, mental illness, traumatic life events.

Conditions responding best to voice therapy are: early vocal nodules, chronic laryngitis, functional dysphonia, psychogenic aphonia, puberphonia, vocal cord palsy, Reinke's oedema, false cord phonation (dysphonia plica ventricularis), tensor weakness/bowing/incomplete adduction and globus sensation.

Conditions which do not respond well to voice therapy are: occult cysts, sulcus vocalis, recurrent papillomata, advanced cases of Reinke's oedema and hard fibrous nodules.

Assessment

Most speech therapy clinics employ a purely subjective description and assessment of dysphonia relying on the trained ear of the therapist. Assessment covers:

- Breathing pattern.
- Phonation: pitch/intonation/quality/glottal attack/loudness.
- Resonance.
- Articulation.
- Laryngeal and pharyngeal tension.
- Habits associated with voice production.
- A questionnaire concerning the patient's attitude to the

voice to be repeated following therapy to establish patient satisfaction with results.

Many centres now have joint ENT/speech therapy voice clinics, which are ideal for professional voice users. More time is allocated to each appointment, and using nasendoscopy and stroboscopy patients should be able to see their larynx on a TV monitor, have a clear understanding of the diagnosis and even try some therapy techniques on camera with clear visual feedback. This facility helps reduce anxiety and increases cooperation and motivation in therapy.

Some specialist clinics now have access to instrumentation such a PCLX laryngograph, which allow the dysphonia to be repeatedly analysed in terms of physical and acoustic parameters. Traditional assessment is supplemented with objective analysis of pitch, i.e. the mode frequency, the frequency range used and a percentage irregularity measure (a measure of the periodicity of vibration, which correlates with perceived hoarseness).

The laryngograph waveform gives quantitative and qualitative information about the closed phase of the vocal cord vibratory cycle. These objective measures can be used:

(a) To provide a baseline before therapy or surgery and to evaluate objectively improvement after therapy or surgery.

(b) As a therapy tool to provide instant visual feedback to the patient.

(c) For collection of data for comparative studies and for research and audit purposes.

Therapy

Following assessment the therapist attempts to elicit improvement in the voice quality by using various facilitation techniques, e.g. humming, yawning, shouting, growling, masking hearing, talking on inhalation, nasalizing, pushing, lip vibrating, etc. Experimenting in this way reveals further information about the disorder, helps plan therapy and gives some indication of the prognosis.

Objectives for therapy and the estimated number of sessions required are set and agreed with the patient. Examples of therapy aims may be to :

• Reduce excessive laryngeal and pharyngeal tension.
• Improve breath support and control.
• Eliminate abusive habits.
• Achieve easy natural phonation when there is maladaptive use of voice.

- Improve management of stress.
- Encourage certain lifestyle changes.
- Advise on vocal hygiene and economy.
- Teach voice projection techniques.
- Establish natural pitch.
- Shout without damaging the voice.
- Develop head/chest resonance.

Postoperative voice therapy is advisable in most conditions even if it is not suspected that vocal misuse/abuse was the cause of the problem. Organic changes to the vocal cords often lead to maladaptive patterns of voice use which may persist postoperatively.

Voice therapy with singers involves analysis of both the speaking and singing voice and generally a programme of therapy focusing on achieving an easy, natural voice without strain. When the healthiest possible voice has been achieved, the therapist may refer the patient to a singing teacher, whose role it is to develop technique and advise on singing style and material most suited to the voice. Up to three patients with a similar disorder, such as functional dysphonia in teachers, can be treated as a group to reduce cost and use time more efficiently.

The effective treatment of voice disorders requires sound scientific training and an understanding of the anatomical, physiological, acoustic and behavioural aspects of voice production combined with creativity and imagination in devising and implementing treatment programmes for individual patients.

Further reading

Arunson D. *Clinical Voice Disorders*. Stuttgart: Thieme Medical, 1990.
Fawcus M (ed.). *Voice Disorders and their Management*. London: Chapman & Hall, 1991.
Greene GM, Mathieson L. *The Voice and its Disorders*. London: Whurr , 1989.
Hiranu M. *Clinical Evaluations of Voice*. Berlin: Springer, 1981.

Related topic of interest

STRIDOR AND STERTOR

Definitions

- *Stridor* is noisy breathing caused by partial obstruction of the respiratory tract at or below the larynx.
- *Stertor* is noisy breathing caused by partial obstruction of the respiratory tract above the larynx.

Stridor

Aetiology

1. Congenital

Larynx:

Supraglottis	Laryngomalacia, web, saccular cyst, cystic hygroma.
Glottis	Web, vocal cord paralysis.
Subglottis	Web, stenosis, haemangioma.
Trachea and bronchi:	Web, stenosis, tracheomalacia, tracheo- and bronchogenic cyst, compression from vascular and other mediastinal tumours.

2. Acquired.

Trauma	Thermal and chemical, iatrogenic (intubation and surgical), blunt and sharp external.
Inflammatory	Acute laryngitis, acute laryngo-tracheobronchitis, diphtheria.
Foreign body	Laryngeal, tracheal, bronchial and external compression from an oesophageal foreign body.
Allergy	Angioneuroric oedema of the larynx or trachea.
	Extrinsic allergic alveolitis.
Neoplasia	Benign, e.g. laryngeal papillomatosis.
	Malignant, e.g. laryngeal or bronchial carcinoma.

Clinical features

Typically, supraglottic stridor is inspiratory, the negative inspiratory intralaryngeal pressure indrawing the supraglottic soft tissues, passive opening occurring on expiration. Tracheal and main bronchial airway obstruction causes stridor because of turbulence of air flowing through a narrow but rigid airway that does not collapse. It may be inspiratory or expiratory; but is usually biphasic. In the smaller bronchi and bronchioles obstruction accentuates the physiological construction occurring in expiration to cause an expiratory wheeze. A full history combined with examination of the nose, throat and neck, as in the stertorous subject, is indicated if circumstances permit. This should allow a confident or a working diagnosis to be made. Thereafter immediate treatment or appropriate investigations can be instituted.

Investigations

A lateral soft-tissue neck and chest radiograph or a CT scan of the larynx and lungs may be appropriate. A representative biopsy of any laryngeal or infralaryngeal mass may be indicated (see Related topics of interest).

Treatment

This depends on the diagnosis and the severity of symptoms (see Related topics of interest).

Stertor

Aetiology

Any condition restricting the nasal, nasopharyngeal or oropharyngeal airway.

1. Congenital (present at birth).

Nose	Choanal stenosis or atresia.
	External nasal deformity secondary to craniofacial abnormality.
	Dermoid, nasoalveolar, dentigerous and mucous cysts.
	Meningocele, encephalocele, meningo-encephalocele.
Nasopharynx	Craniofacial abnormality, especially Apert's syndrome and Crouzon's disease.
Oropharynx	Micrognathia secondary to a craniofacial abnormality, especially Treacher Collins syndrome.
	Macroglossia, most frequently in those with Down's syndrome.
	Lingual thyroid and thyroglossal cyst.

2. Acquired.

Trauma	Septal haematoma and secondary abscess.
	Nasal, septal and midfacial fracture.
Inflammatory	Infective acute and chronic rhinitis.
	Acute and chronic adenoiditis.
	Acute tonsillitis, especially secondary to infectious mononucleosis.

Parapharyngeal and retropharyngeal abscess.
Ludwig's angina.
Acute epiglottitis.
Wegener's granulomatosis.

Allergy   Allergic rhinitis.
                      Angio oedema of the floor of the mouth.
Neoplasia   Benign, e.g. simple nasal polyps, antrochoanal polyp, angiofibroma.
                      Malignant, e.g. oro- and nasopharyngeal squamous cell carcinoma, nasal T-cell lymphoma.

Clinical features   Stertor is usually inspiratory, but the accompanying features are diverse and depend on the cause. A full history should ascertain time of onset, symptom progression, aggravating and relieving factors, whether there is sleep apnoea, an intercurrent URTI or if trauma has occurred. Examination of the nose, throat (contraindicated in acute epiglottitis) and neck, pulse, temperature, respiratory rate and blood pressure may be necessary.

Investigations   A lateral soft-tissue neck radiograph or an MRI scan may be indicated to show the site of airway obstruction. In a child it is important to extend the neck to prevent the retropharyngeal soft tissue causing a pseudomass.

Treatment   Treatment depends on the cause, progression and severity of the stertor and on whether it is causing complications (see Related topics of interest).

Complications   Complications directly related to the airway obstruction include right ventricular failure and pulmonary hypertension (sleep apnoea), central respiratory arrest (in the first 3 months of life neonates are obligatory nasal breathers) and acute total airway obstruction.

Related topics of interest

SUDDEN HEARING LOSS

Sudden hearing loss is a significant subjective decline in the hearing acuity occurring either instantaneously or progressively over minutes or hours. Usually only one ear is affected. It can be classified into conductive and sensorineural causes.

Conductive causes

(a) External ear canal occlusion, e.g. from wax or a foreign body.
(b) Infection, e.g. otitis externa, acute otitis media or chronic otitis media.
(c) Ear trauma, from a direct blow, acoustic or barotrauma (see Related topics of interest).
(d) Iatrogenic.

Sensorineural

(a) Idiopathic.
(b) Iatrogenic.
(c) Serous and purulent labyrinthitis.
(d) Viral, e.g. measles and mumps virus.
(e) Cerebellopontine angle tumours, e.g. acoustic neuromas, cholesterol granulomas, congenital dermoids and meningiomas.
(f) Temporal bone fractures, in particular transverse fractures.
(g) Causes of perilymph fistula including round window rupture.
(h) Menière's *disease* (primary endolymphatic hydrops) and secondary endolymphatic hydrops (both of which may cause Menière's *syndrome*).
(i) Ototoxic drugs, in particular aminoglycoside antibiotics, non-steroidal anti-inflammatory drugs, beta-blockers, loop diuretics and chemotherapeutic drugs.
(j) Central causes, e.g. following a brainstem cerebrovascular accident.

Clinical features

In subjects with an identifiable cause of a sudden hearing loss the diagnosis is usually made from a thorough otological and neurological history, examination and relevant special investigations. Nearly all those with a sudden conductive hearing loss will have an definitive diagnosis made, but 60% of the sensorineural group will eventually be labelled as idiopathic, of which 60% will recover spontaneously.

Management

All patients with a sudden bilateral sensorineural hearing loss should be admitted to hospital for several reasons:

(a) Close monitoring of the hearing by pure tone and speech audiometry is possible and desirable in order to determine whether the hearing is stable, improving or declining. This will provide a prognosis and enable the patient's disability and handicap to be assessed.

(b) To obtain relevant special investigations. These include electric response audiometry, MRI imaging, viral titres (two sets 6 weeks apart), syphilis serology, a full blood count, fasting lipids, and thyroid and liver profiles in an effort to obtain a diagnosis.

(c) To provide rehabilitation by way of (i) counselling from a hearing therapist or (ii) a hearing aid and accessory aid provision (for example amplification of the TV, telephone bell, telephone receiver and door bell).

Treatment of the idiopathic group with vasodilators (e.g. betahistine), anticoagulants (e.g. heparin), blood viscosity-lowering substances (e.g. dextran 40), steroids, vitamins, inhalations of 5% CO_2 and 95% O_2, and antibiotics is empirical. It is generally agreed by those who advocate such treatment that it should commence as early as possible after the onset of the hearing loss and certainly within the first few days of symptoms. Most treatments report a response rate of 60%, about the same as those who spontaneously recover with no treatment.

Those with a sudden unilateral hearing loss will have less of a disability and handicap and do not require such urgent rehabilitation. As a general rule they do not require admission into hospital unless the aetiology (e.g. trauma, purulent labyrinthitis) dictates and they can be investigated as an outpatient.

Further reading

Byl FM. Sudden hearing loss: eight years experience and suggested prognostic table. *Laryngoscope*, 1984; **94**: 647–61.

Fisch U. Management of sudden deafness. *Otolaryngology and Head and Neck Surgery*, 1983; **91**: 3-8.

Kumar A, Maudelonde C, Maffee M. Unilateral sensorineural hearing loss: an analysis of 200 consecutive cases. *Laryngoscope*, 1986; **96**: 14-18.

Related topics of interest

Acoustic neuroma (p. 1)

Acute suppurative otitis media (p. 9)

Chronic suppurative otitis media (p. 51)

Labyrinthitis (p. 144)

Menière's disease (p. 169)

Otological aspects of head injury (p. 220)

Ototoxicity (p. 231)

Perilymph fistula (p. 244)

THYROID DISEASE – BENIGN

Benign thyroid disease can be analysed from three aspects: thyroid goitre, hypothyroidism and hyperthyroidism. Patients with thyroid goitre are the most important from a surgical standpoint as it is this group that is often referred to ENT surgeons by general practitioners for primary management. Hypo- and hyperthyroidism are not discussed further except when occurring with thyroid goitre. It should be recognized that hyperthyroidism may present without a goitre and require surgery either to determine the histology of a 'hot' nodule (rarely malignant) or because the disease is not controlled by medical management and the patient is deemed to be too young for radioiodine ablation.

Aetiology

1. *Physiological,* for example in puberty and pregnancy.

2. *Autoimmune.*
(a) Graves' disease. This is caused by thyroid-stimulating immunoglobulins (TSIs), IgG antibodies which bind to the thyroid-stimulating hormone (TSH) receptor to increase thyroid hormone production. TSI levels can now be quantified. TSI is usually associated with Graves' hyperthyroidism, although patients may be euthyroid or hypothyroid. It is associated with dysthyroid eye disease, which is caused by a specific antibody called exophthalmos-producing substance (EPS), that target retro-orbital tissue to cause oedema of fat and muscle. Graves' disease may also be associated with signs of vitiligo, pretibial myxoedema and autoimmune disorders such as pernicious anaemia.
(b) Hashimoto's thyroiditis. This is most common in late middle-aged women. Antibodies are directed against thyroglobulin and/or microsomal peroxidase. They cause lymphocyte infiltration, atrophy and regeneration of the thyroid, and ultimately a goitre. The gland is usually firm but rubbery. Initially patients are hyperthyroid but may become hypothyroid as the disease progresses. There is a high risk of developing thyroid lymphoma.

3. *Infection.*
(a) Acute. De Quervain's thyroiditis is secondary to an acute viral infection, often a flu-like illness, and associated with diffuse swelling and tenderness of the gland. There is usually a transient hyperthyroidism and a transient production of autoantibodies.
(b) Chronic. Riedel's thyroiditis is rare and associated with a woody hard, sometimes tender, irregular thyroid gland

which histologically shows marked fibrosis. This is thought by some to signify a fibrotic reaction to an underlying carcinoma or lymphoma.

4. Multinodular goitre and colloid goitre. The latter is occasionally associated with iodine deficiency, which is endemic in subjects living at high altitude, for example in the Alps or Himalayas. Those with a multinodular goitre are usually euthyroid. An ultrasound scan will confirm the most prominent nodule, and its benign nature is confirmed with a fine-needle aspiration.

5. Tumours.
(a) Benign. Thyroid adenoma. This is diagnosed from an ultrasound scan showing a solid nodule, a pentavalent technetium ($99mTc$) scan showing a non-functioning ('cold') nodule and fine-needle aspiration cytology confirming a benign thyroid adenoma.
(b) Malignant (see Related topic of interest).

6. Miscellaneous, for example sarcoidosis and tuberculosis.

Clinical features

Depending on the cause and duration of the goitre patients may be euthyroid, hyperthyroid or hypothyroid. A drug history is important because some are goitrogens, e.g. sulphonylureas. The goitre may produce discomfort on swallowing, dysphagia (implying oesophageal compression), or stridor (implying tracheal compression). It is important to confirm that the swelling moves with swallowing and to note its size, position and any retrosternal involvement. The latter is suspected from a manubrium that is dull to percussion. Examine the rest of the neck for nodes and perform indirect laryngoscopy to check the mobility of the vocal cords.

Investigations

A palpable, discrete mass within the thyroid gland should be subjected to a fine-needle aspiration for cytological examination. If there is diffuse involvement an ultrasound scan will distinguish solid from cystic nodules. If more than one nodule is present the largest should be targeted for fine-needle aspiration cytology. A technetium scan will distinguish a cold (10% malignant) from a hot (rarely malignant) nodule. It is thought unnecessary by many surgeons as both types will show up as a solid region on ultrasound and both types require fine-needle aspiration cytology for definitive histology.

Treatment	The indications for surgery are:
	(a) Suspected malignancy (see related topic of interest).
	(b)Cosmesis. The size of the goitre, although perhaps asymptomatic, is cosmetically unacceptable to the patient.
	(c) Tracheal compression. The longer the history of goitre and pressure symptoms, the greater the risk of a pressure-induced tracheomalacia.
Complications of thyroidectomy	As well as the hazards of any surgical operation there are specific potential complications of thyroidectomy.

1. Injury to related anatomical structures.
(a) Recurrent laryngeal nerve.
(b) Trachea.
(c) Pneumothorax.

2. Hormonal.
(a) Tetany (hypoparathyroidism secondary to parathyroid removal or bruising).
(b) Thyroid crisis (acute exacerbation of thyrotoxicosis).
(c) Myxoedema (secondary to extensive removal of thyroid tissue).
(d) Late recurrence of toxicity (inadequate removal of toxic gland).

3. Complications of the wound site.
(a) Haemorrhage. Immediate or early post-operative bleeding causing tracheal compression.
(b) Tracheomalacia.
(c) Wound infection.

Follow-up and aftercare	Those who have had a subtotal thyroidectomy for cosmesis or tracheal compression should be managed by their primary care physician to monitor thyroxine and TSH levels provided that satisfactory wound healing and vocal cord mobility have been confirmed. Serum corrected calcium levels should be routinely performed 24 hours postoperatively to ensure that there is no iatrogenic hypoparathyroidism.

Further reading

Drury PL. The thyroid axis. In: Kumar PJ, Clarke ML (eds). *Clinical Medicine,* 2nd edn. London: Baillière Tindall, 1990; 798–809.

Related topic of interest

Thyroid disease – malignant (p. 309)

THYROID DISEASE – MALIGNANT

Classification

1. Papillary, follicular and anaplastic carcinoma. From thyroid follicular epithelium.

2. Medullary carcinoma. From thyroid parafollicular cells.

3. Non-Hodgkin's lymphoma. From thyroid lymphoid tissue.

Aetiology

The only well-documented aetiological factor for those malignancies arising from thyroid follicular epithelium is exposure to ionizing radiation. This occurs in 1–7% of those exposed and develops 12–30 years after exposure. Subjects with a goitre secondary to a low iodine dietary intake may have an increased risk, perhaps related to chronically elevated TSH levels. Although 80% of medullary carcinomas are sporadic, the remainder occur as a component of either the autosomal dominant multiple endocrine neoplasia (MEN) IIA associated with phaeochromocytomas (10%) and parathyroid hyperplasia (60%) or MEN IIB (associated with mucosal neuromas, phaeochromocytomas and Marfan's syndrome).

Pathology

- The majority of papillary carcinomas also contain follicular components. They are unencapsulated with a high incidence of multifocal involvement. The peak incidence is in children and the 40–50 age group. Half of adults and 80% of children will have palpable cervical nodes at presentation, but only 10% have distant metastasis, usually to the lungs.
- Follicular carcinoma usually occurs in adults over 50 years, and two morphological subtypes are recognized. The first is encapsulated but has small areas of vascular or capsule invasion; the second shows frank invasion into the thyroid parenchyma with 20% showing lung or bone metastases but less than 10% metastases to the cervical nodes.
- Sporadic medullary carcinoma usually involves only a single lobe, but the familial variety is invariably bilobar. Most contain amyloid and 50% will have palpably involved cervical nodes, often with mediastinal involvement.
- Anaplastic carcinoma is very aggressive, spreads rapidly throughout the gland, invades locally and occurs in the elderly. It comprises swarms of small cells so must be distinguished from lymphoma, which has a good

prognosis. To this end, immunohistochemical staining for cytokeratin squamous cell marker, CD4 and CD8 lymphoid cell markers is required.

Clinical features

From the above it will be seen that patients present either with a diffuse or solitary thyroid nodule and/or a neck lump or symptoms of distant spread, especially to the lungs or bone. In addition, patients with medullary carcinoma may have symptoms ascribable to the MEN syndromes.

Investigations

Ultrasound and fine-needle aspiration cytology (FNAC) are the two most important investigations. Ultrasound will determine if a nodule is single or multiple. A gland showing multiple small cysts or nodules may simply be observed. If one is dominant, i.e. 1 cm, FNAC should be performed, if necessary under ultrasound guidance. A single cyst is not necessarily benign as many cancers appear cystic from haemorrhage into a nodule. An isotope scintiscan is often unnecessary as most nodules are cold whether benign or malignant, and even if hot will require an FNAC to exclude malignancy. Others argue an isotope scan will give a pointer towards prognosis. An ^{131}I isotope scan is recommended because ^{125}I is expensive and has a longer half life (^{131}I = 8 days, ^{125}I = 60 days). Pentavalent technetium (^{99m}Tc) is another isotope in common use. Although CT and MRI do not distinguish between benign and malignant nodules confined to the gland, they will provide an indication of the extent of local or cervical node invasion. Lymphoma must be referred to a medical oncologist for staging and further management.

Management

There are several scenarios for papillary and follicular carcinoma:

(a) When FNAC has given a histological diagnosis of follicular carcinoma, there are two choices: a total thyroidectomy with identification and preservation of one parathyroid gland or near-total thyroidectomy (in an effort to preserve a parathyroid gland) with radioiodine ablation of the thyroid remnant should histology show the invasive subtype. Total eradication of the thyroid is necessary with this subtype because of the high risk of distant metastases.

(b) When FNAC shows a papillary carcinoma, the options are similar to follicular carcinoma except if the cancer is small, when a thyroid lobectomy may suffice. Owing to its multifocal propensity there is a 7% chance of recurrence within 20 years if the latter option is chosen. This is difficult to detect by a radioiodine scintiscan or thyroglobulin assay because there is a residual lobe of functioning thyroid tissue. In these circumstances a thallium scintiscan is the investigation of choice. Recurrence can often be cured by further surgery, radioiodine, radiotherapy or a combination of these modalities, so many experts adopt this more conservative approach in children.

(c) Some patients will have had a thyroid lobectomy for a multinodular goitre or when FNAC of a discrete thyroid lump has suggested an adenoma. Should subsequent paraffin sections reveal a papillary cell or an encapsulated follicular carcinoma, the options are:

- To reoperate and perform one of the two options as in (a) above.
- To do nothing further except closely observe. With an encapsulated follicular carcinoma there is much less risk of subsequent distant metastases compared to the invasive type.
- To ablate the remaining thyroid lobe with ^{131}I and follow up as described below.

(d) Neck node metastasis occurring with a papillary or follicular carcinoma (previously and inappropriately named lateral aberrant thyroid if presentation was with a neck metastasis) requires a total thyroidectomy and either lumpectomy or a conservative neck dissection with a follow-up radioiodine scan at 6–12 weeks. If this shows residual disease ablative radioiodine therapy should be given as outlined below.

(e) If there is local invasion through the thyroid capsule to surrounding structures, then total thyroidectomy should be followed by ablative radioiodine and radiotherapy (Royal Marsden and Memorial Sloan-Kettering hospitals regimen).

(f) Distant metastases at presentation require a total thyroidectomy with a postoperative ^{131}I scan. If the metastases are iodine concentrating, ablative radioiodine therapy is indicated; if not, a curative regimen of radiotherapy is undertaken with a good chance of control for both papillary and follicular types.

- Medullary carcinoma requires a total thyroidectomy with resection of any palpable neck or mediastinal nodes. If calcitonin levels do not return to normal then postoperative radical radiotherapy is given to the involved region(s).

- Anaplastic carcinomas do not concentrate iodine and are nearly always unresectable because of local invasion. Radical radiotherapy may produce a short-term partial response. Although a total or partial response to chemotherapy has been reported (18% of patients in a Japanese study), these results have not been reproducible elsewhere.
- Lymphoma is treated according to stage with radiotherapy, chemotherapy or both.

Follow-up and aftercare

Normal thyroid tissue takes up iodine much more avidly than follicular and in particular papillary cancer cells. To detect or treat recurrence with radioiodine, all normal thyroid must first be resected or ablated. The dose of radioiodine is 5 mCi for scans and 200 mCi for ablation. Initial follow-up for follicular and papillary cell carcinoma comprises 6-monthly radioiodine scans to ensure eradication of all disease. If residual disease persists, another ablative dose of radioiodine is given and the patient rescanned after 6-months with further radioiodine given as necessary. Radiotherapy is indicated if there is any evidence of pulmonary fibrosis after multiple ablative doses or if suspected non-iodine-absorbing residual disease is confirmed with a thallium scintiscan

Replacement therapy is given postoperatively to suppress TSH because residual disease is usually TSH driven. Normal TSH levels are necessary, however, for normal thyroid and thyroid cancer cells to take up radioiodine when scanning or giving an ablative dose. T_3, because of its short half-life, is the ideal therapy as it need be stopped only 1 week before scanning to allow TSH levels to rise sufficiently. If a scan has confirmed that there is no residual disease, patients may be followed by monitoring thyroglobulin levels, which act as a marker of disease.

Medullary carcinomas are monitored by serial calcitonin levels. Progressively increasing levels suggest a recurrence but it is important to note that calcitonin levels may remain elevated in a successfully treated patient.

Further reading

Parsons JT, Stringer SP, Mancuso AA. Carcinoma of the thyroid, In: Million RR, Cassisi NG (eds). *Management of Head and Neck Cancer: A Multidisciplinary Approach*, 2nd edn. Philadelphia: JB Lippincott, 1994; 785–811.

Related topic of interest

TINNITUS

Definition

Tinnitus is the sensation of sound not brought about by simultaneously externally applied mechanoacoustic or electrical signals. This definition excludes vascular sounds and bruits.

Pathophysiology

The aetiology of tinnitus is not known. In developing an understanding of tinnitus mechanisms two points should be borne in mind: (a) there is a generated potential somewhere in the auditory system: (b) this signal will undergo extensive auditory processing before it is perceived as tinnitus. There are several hypotheses which attempt to explain the aetiology.

1. Altered auditory firing rate. There is some evidence that tinnitus is associated with an increase in the spontaneous firing rate of auditory nerve fibres. Other studies have shown a decrease in spontaneous firing rates, suggesting that tinnitus might result from reduced cochlear neural activity.

2. Cross talk. It has been postulated that mechanical (and perhaps other) insults to the cochlea, such as impulse noise or endolymphatic hydrops, may cause damage to the myelin insulation between axons in the peripheral auditory system, leading to 'cross-talk' between these structures and thus to phase locking of spontaneous neural activity, experienced subjectively as tinnitus.

3. Central processsing. The significance of emotions and a model which emphasizes the central auditory cortex in processing the tinnitus signal is now considered important.

Associated conditions

Almost every ear disease and cause of deafness can be associated with tinnitus, and the great majority of tinnitus sufferers have some measurable hearing loss. There is much evidence relating the prevalence and severity of tinnitus to the amount of hearing loss.

1. Local causes.

- Presbyacusis.
- Noise-induced hearing loss.
- Menière's disease.
- Otosclerosis.
- Acoustic neuroma.

2. General causes.

- Cardiovascular disease (hypertension, cardiac failure).
- Blood disease (anaemia, raised viscosity).
- Neurological (multiple sclerosis, neuropathy).
- Drug treatment (aspirin, quinine, ototoxic drugs).
- Alcohol abuse.
- Fever of any cause.

Clinical assessment

From the patient's history confirm that the patient is actually suffering with tinnitus and determine the character of the sound (intermittent or constant, pulsatile or non-pulsatile?). It is also important to establish how much trouble the patient is having because this will dictate whether treatment is necessary.

A full ENT examination should be performed to ensure the patient is not hearing transmitted sounds or does not have one of the potentially remedial causes of tinnitus. The ears should be examined under the microscope. Small movements of the tympanic membrane are sometimes visible (secondary to tensor tympani myoclonic contractions or abnormal patency of the Eustachian tube) and glomus jugulare tumours may be visualized. Auscultate the neck, head and ears with a stethoscope for bruits or myoclonus. The blood pressure and pulse should also be measured.

Investigations

1. In the absence of a clear diagnosis perform a full haematological screen to exclude anaemia, thyroid dysfunction, syphilis, dyslipidaemias and hypoglycaemia.

2. Audiometric investigations. It is usual to perform a pure tone audiogram, tinnitus pitch matching (tinnitus frequency match) with loudness balance (dB HL) and masking experiments (masking level) using audiometric white noise. Usually the pitch of the tinnitus is found to be at or around the frequency of the maximal hearing loss. The loudness is usually within 15 dB of the patient's pure tone threshold at the frequency of the pitch matching, and the tinnitus is usually masked at that frequency and at an intensity within 20 dB of that threshold. These measurements in no way indicate the intensity of the tinnitus which is apparent to the patient, as recruitment may be present and there is no reliable gauge of the severity of the noise as this is so subjective.

3. In patients with markedly asymmetrical tinnitus, it should be remembered that 10% of acoustic neuromas, present in this way. Brainstem electric response audiometry should be requested unless the hearing loss is more than 70 dB, when MRI scanning is required.

4. Pulsatile tinnitus may require angiography if a specific vascular lesion is suspected.

Management

1. Any underlying cause should be treated.

2. Hearing aids. These are only useful to those patients who have a 35 dB loss over the speech frequency range. If an appropriate aid with maximal gain at around the frequency of the tinnitus is fitted, the increased awareness of the background sound will make the tinnitus less apparent.

3. Maskers. These produce a controllable and more tonal masking sound which obliterates the sensation of the patient's own tinnitus. As there is adaptation to prolonged sound stimuli, the masker should be used for only short periods of less than 2 hours duration. A proportion of patients have residual inhibition of their tinnitus after a period of masking.

4. Combined hearing aid and masker unit.

5. A pillow radio or pillow speaker may help the patient get to sleep.

6. Many other treatments have been tried (i.e. lignocaine, magnetic stimulation, ultrasonic stimulation, iontophoresis, acupuncture, hypnotherapy, dietary supplements, electrical suppression), but success has been limited and adverse effects common.

Ideally management should be by a tinnitus clinic team, comprising a consultant otologist and one or more hearing therapists, scientists or audiology technicians. They should work in close liaison with a clinical psychologist and local self-help group to provide lay counselling and relaxation therapy.

Further reading

Coles RRA. Tinnitus and its management. *British Medical Bulletin*, 1987; **43**: 983–98.

Hazell JWP, Jastreboff PJ. Tinnitus I : Auditory mechanisms: a model for tinnitus and hearing impairment. *Journal of Otolaryngology*, 1990; **19**: 1–5.

Hazell JWP. Tinnitus II : Management of conditions associated with somatosounds. *Journal of Otolaryngology*, 1990; **19**: 6–10.

Hazell JWP. Tinnitus III : The practical management of sensorineural tinnitus. *Journal of Otolaryngology,* 1990; **19**: 11–17.

Related topics of interest

Evoked response audiometry (p. 85)
Hearing aids (p. 126)
Pure tone audiogram (p. 255)

TONSILLECTOMY

Indications for tonsillectomy

(a) Recurrent episodes of acute tonsillitis. (Surgeons differ in the definition of this. As a rule of thumb these episodes should last 5 days or more, five per year, for at least 2 years.)

(b) Previous episodes of peritonsillar abscess (quinsy).

(c) Suspected neoplasm (unilateral enlargement or ulceration).

(d) Part of another procedure (UVPP, access to glossopharyngeal nerve or styloid process).

(e) Gross enlargement causing airway obstruction (sleep apnoea syndrome).

Contraindications to tonsillectomy

These contraindications are not absolute, but surgery should be delayed until the particular problem is resolved. In some cases the decision to proceed with surgery should be reconsidered in the context of the potential problems.

(a) Recent episode of tonsillitis or upper respiratory tract infection (within 2 weeks).

(b) Bleeding disorder.

(c) Oral contraceptives.

(d) Cleft palate.

(e) During certain epidemics (e.g. polio).

Complications of tonsillectomy

1. Peroperative.

- Anaesthetic reaction.
- Haemorrhage.
- Damage to teeth.
- Trauma to the posterior pharyngeal wall (careless insertion of the tongue blade).
- Dislocation of the temporomandibular joint by overopening the mouth gag.

2. Immediate.

- Reactionary haemorrhage.
- Anaesthetic complications.

3. Early.

- Secondary haemorrhage.
- Haematoma and oedema of the uvula.
- Infection (may lead to secondary haemorrhage).
- Earache (referred pain or acute otitis media).

- Pulmonary complications (pneumonia and lung abscess are rare).
- Subacute bacterial endocarditis (if the patient has a cardiac defect).

4. Late.

- Scarring of the soft palate (limiting mobility and possibly affecting voice).
- Tonsillar remnants (which may be the site of recurrent acute infection).

The most significant complication is haemorrhage, which occurs in approximately 2% of cases. Most of the deaths associated with tonsillectomy are directly or indirectly associated with this complication.

It is essential to ensure adequate haemostasis at the end of the tonsillectomy procedure as blood in the airway at this time may cause laryngeal spasm or can occlude the airway. The postnasal space should always be checked for a blood clot (the so-called 'coroner's clot'). Patients are nursed in the reverse Trendelenburg position (head down) so that blood trickles out of the mouth rather than being swallowed or aspirated.

Reactionary (primary) haemorrhage by definition occurs up to 24 hours postoperatively, but the vast majority occur within the first 8 hours. It is one of the reasons why some surgeons are opposed to day case tonsillectomy. Continuing haemorrhage will result in hypovolaemia, and if not corrected circulatory failure (shock) will be the consequence. The signs of reactionary haemorrhage are obvious bleeding from the mouth, a gurgling sound in the throat on respiration, repeated swallowing, vomiting blood, a rising pulse rate and eventually a falling blood pressure and tachypnoea. Blood must be cross-matched and an intravenous infusion started. The tonsillar fossae should be inspected to identify a bleeding point. Any clot should be removed if possible and a gauze swab soaked in 1:1000 adrenaline applied to the fossa. If the bleeding continues, or there is any doubt, the patient should be prepared for a second anaesthetic and the bleeding point ligated under general anaesthesia. The second anaesthetic is hazardous and should only be administered by an experienced anaesthetist.

Secondary haemorrhage occurs some 5–10 days post tonsillectomy and is due to an infection of the fossae. The patient should be admitted to hospital for observation. A full blood count and cross-match should be performed. The infection and haemorrhage will usually settle after treatment with antibiotics (i.v. penicillin and metronidazole or erythromycin). It is unusual for such a patient to have to go back to theatre and when this is necessary the tonsillar fossae are found to be sloughy and friable and it is difficult to locate and ligate any specific bleeding point. It may be necessary to suture the faucial pillars together, or over Kaltostat or a gauze swab which is removed the next day.

Follow-up and aftercare No specific follow-up is required after a routine, uncomplicated tonsillectomy. Patients who have suffered a significant haemorrhage should be reviewed within 2 weeks to check their haemoglobin. Patients who have a tonsillectomy for reasons other than recurrent acute tonsillitis should be followed up appropriately to their problem.

Further reading

Hibbert J. Acute infection of the pharynx and tonsils. In: Stell PM (ed) *Scott-Brown's Otolaryngology*, Vol. 5, 5th edn. London: Butterworths, 1987; 76–98.
Hotaling AJ, Silva AB. Advances in adenotonsillar disease. *Current Opinion in Otolaryngology and Head and Neck Surgery,* 1993; **1:** 177–84.

Related topics of interest

Adenoids (p. 13)
Neck space infections (p. 186)
Snoring and obstructive sleep apnoea (p. 288)
Tonsillitis (p. 320)

TONSILLITIS

The tonsils are paired secondary lymphatic organs situated on the side of the oropharynx between the palatoglossal (anterior tonsil pillar) and palatopharyngeal folds (posterior tonsil pillar). They are part of Waldeyer's ring, a ring of lymphoid tissue consisting of the adenoids, the palatine tonsils and the lingual tonsils, which are embedded in the posterior third of the tongue. The ring as a whole is thought to have some protective function as a barrier against infection in the first few years of life. The tonsil is enclosed by a fibrous capsule, outside of which is a layer of areolar tissue. This separates the capsule from the pharyngobasilar fascia covering the superior constrictor muscle that forms the tonsil bed. The main blood supply of the tonsil is from the tonsillar branch of the facial artery.

Aetiology of acute tonsillitis

Although this is a common disease, its aetiology and pathogenesis are poorly understood. Acute tonsillitis is an infection which primarily affects the palatine tonsil. It is regarded as being distinctive from acute pharyngitis, which is most often felt to be a viral infection involving the lymphoid tissue on the posterior pharyngeal wall and may include the tonsil. Although the disease is seen in adults, it is most frequent in childhood, presumably because immunity to common childhood organisms has not been fully established. There is some doubt regarding the most common causative organisms in acute tonsillitis. It has been suggested that viruses (e.g. influenza, parainfluenza, adenoviruses, enteroviruses and rhinoviruses) may be responsible for tonsillitis in up to 50% of occasions. In many other cases it is felt that an initial viral tonsillitis may predispose to a superinfection by bacteria (β-haemolytic streptococcus, *Streptococcus pneumoniae*, *Haemophilus influenzae* and anaerobic organisms).

Clinical features

There may be a prodromal illness with pyrexia, malaise and headache for a day before the onset of the predominant symptom, which is a sore throat. Pain may radiate to the ears or may occur in the neck due to cervical lymphadenopathy. Swallowing may be painful (odynophagia) and the patient's voice may sound muffled. There may be trismus and dribbling. Some children may have abdominal pain and occasionally vomiting. The tonsils are found to be hyperaemic on examination with pus and debris in the crypts. There will be tender cervical lymphadenopathy, particularly the jugulodigastric nodes.

Differential diagnosis	Glandular fever, agranulocytosis, leukaemia and diphtheria must always be borne in mind. In general practice the clinical features usually make the diagnosis obvious without the need to resort to clinical investigations in the majority of cases. Cases that are referred to hospital are usually more severe, however, and it would be prudent to perform a Paul–Bunnell test, white cell count and a throat swab.
Management	Even though viruses are implicated as the pathogenic organisms in many cases, it is likely any patient who attends a medical practitioner with the clinical features of tonsillitis will be treated with antibiotics. Penicillin V is still the drug of choice, with erythromycin reserved for those patients allergic to penicillin. Ampicillin should never be used to treat acute tonsillitis in case the patient has infectious mononucleosis, when a generalized maculopapular rash may develop. The patient should have paracetamol for analgesia. Aspirin is contraindicated in children because of the risk of Reye's syndrome. Fluid replacement and bed rest are ancillary measures in the severe attack.
Complications of acute tonsillitis	*1. Local.*

- Severe swelling causing respiratory obstruction.
- Abscess formation: Peritonsillar (quinsy).
  Parapharyngeal.
  Retropharyngeal.
- Acute otitis media.
- Recurrent acute tonsillitis (chronic tonsillitis).

2. General.

- Septicaemia.
- Meningitis.
- Acute rheumatic fever.
- Acute glomerulonephritis.

Differential diagnosis of unilateral tonsil enlargement	(a) Asymmetry in a patient with recurrent bouts of acute tonsillitis. (b) Neoplasia (squamous cell carcinoma or lymphoma). (c) Apparent enlargement (peritonsillar abscess or parapharyngeal mass).
Differential diagnosis of ulceration of the tonsil	A working diagnosis can usually be determined from the history and clinical examination. Investigations include a full blood count, chest radiograph, serological tests and biopsy. Possible causes include:

1. Infection.

- Acute streptococcal tonsillitis.
- Diphtheria.
- Infectious mononucleosis.
- Vincent's angina.

2. Neoplasm.

- Squamous cell carcinoma.
- Lymphoma.
- Salivary gland tumours (adenoid cystic carcinoma or mucoepidermoid tumour).

3. Blood diseases.

- Agranulocytosis.
- Leukaemia.

4. Other causes.

- Aphthous ulceration.
- Behçet's syndrome.
- Acquired immunodeficiency syndrome (AIDS).

Further reading

Hibbert J. Acute infection of the pharynx and tonsils. In: Stell PM (ed) *Scott-Brown's Otolaryngology*, Vol. 5, 5th edn. London: Butterworths, 1987; 76–98.
Hotaling AJ, Silva AB. Advances in adenotonsillar disease. *Current Opinion in Otolaryngology and Head and Neck Surgery,* 1993; **1:** 177–84.

Related topics of interest

TRACHEOSTOMY

A tracheotomy is an operation to make an opening in the trachea, while a tracheostomy means converting this opening to a stoma on the skin surface. Tracheostomy should, whenever possible, be carried out as an elective procedure. Many disorders are now managed by endotracheal intubation, and this should always be carefully considered first, but the decision for tracheostomy should not be left until it is too late. Children especially can deteriorate very suddenly. There is an old adage that states 'the time to do a tracheostomy is when you first think about it'.

Indications

1. Airway obstruction. Advances in anaesthetics, including improved, less traumatizing types of endotracheal tubes, have reduced the number of potential tracheostomies. Upper airway obstruction is now the least common indication for tracheostomy.

- Congenital (subglottic stenosis, laryngeal web, laryngeal cysts).
- Trauma (foreign body, severe head and neck injury, swallowing corrosive, inhalation of irritants).
- Infection (acute epiglottitis, laryngotracheobronchitis, diphtheria, Ludwig's angina).
- Tumour (tongue, larynx, pharynx, trachea, thyroid).
- Vocal cord paralysis (thyroidectomy complication, bulbar palsy).

2. Protection of the tracheobronchial tree. This includes patients who need temporary protection of their airway (e.g. those patients undergoing head and neck surgery). Patients may benefit from a long-term tracheostomy if they suffer from any chronic condition (which are often neurological diseases) leading to inhalation of saliva, food, gastric contents or blood, or the stagnation of bronchial secretions. A cuffed tube will protect the airway from aspiration and allow easy access to the trachea for regular suction.

- Neurological diseases (polyneuritis, tetanus, myasthenia gravis, bulbar palsy, multiple sclerosis).
- Trauma (burns of the face and neck, multiple facial fractures).
- Coma (drug overdose, head injury, cerebrovascular accident).
- Head and neck surgery (oral or oropharyngeal resections, supraglottic laryngectomy).

3. Ventilatory insufficiency. Tracheostomy reduces upper respiratory dead space by about 70%, bypasses resistance to airflow in the nose, mouth and glottis, and allows the use of mechanically assisted respiration if necessary (intermittent positive-pressure ventilation).

- Pulmonary diseases (chronic bronchitis and emphysema, severe asthma, pneumonia).
- Neurological diseases (as above).
- Severe chest injury (flail chest).

Tracheostomy tubes

The selection of tracheostomy tube depends on the reason for the procedure and the postoperative requirements. A cuffed tube is preferred if the patient needs protection of the lower airway from aspiration or haemorrhage. Removable inner tubes facilitate cleaning and removal of crusted secretions while the outer tube maintains the airway. A fenestrated tube permits the passage of air upwards through the glottis, thereby allowing the patient to speak. Tube types can be divided into metal and synthetic.

1. Metal tubes. These usually consist of an obturator, an outer tube and an inner tube. They usually have an expiratory flap valve on the inner tube which allows phonation, but they do not have a cuff. Examples include the silver tubes of Chevalier Jackson and Negus. These are short and should only be used in patients with thin necks. The Durham tube has an adjustable flange so that it can be used in patients with either thin or very fat necks. The Koenig tube has a long flexible wire that can be used if there is a narrowing of the trachea. The Alder Hey tube is a typical example of a paediatric metal tube: both the inner and outer tubes are fenestrated and a valve is available to allow transglottic expiration and speech.

2. Synthetic tubes. Most of these are made from PVC, silicone or other synthetic plastics that are non-toxic. Examples include the Portex and Shiley tubes. These tubes can be connected to an anaesthetic connector or respirator. Nowadays they have low-pressure cuffs which can remain inflated for days, preventing aspiration and without causing pressure necrosis of the trachea. Paediatric synthetic tubes include the Franklin tube of Great Ormond Street, the Portex paediatric tube and the Shiley paediatric or neonatal tube. The Great Ormond Street tube and the Shiley are winged and sit comfortably in the infant's neck; the Portex is not winged but has square-ended flanges. None of the paediatric tubes have a cuff.

Postoperative management

1. Nursing care. Constant nursing attention is essential for at least the first 24 hours following the tracheostomy. The patient should be in a well-supported upright position; care must be taken in infants that the chin does not occlude the tracheostomy.

2. Suction. The patient will be unable to cough and clear secretions so suction should be applied regularly, by aseptic technique, to prevent a build-up of secretions in the trachea and bronchi. A sterile catheter is passed well down into each main bronchus in turn.

3. Humidification. Humidification of inspired air is essential to prevent drying of the airway, which encourages the formation of crusts and infection. Saline or sodium bicarbonate instillation into the trachea followed by immediate suction also helps to reduce the likelihood of such complications.

4. Apnoea. Some patients with chronic obstructive airways disease may develop apnoea following restoration of their airway. This is due to lowering of their Pco_2, with loss of stimulation of their respiratory centre. These patients need monitoring and the administration of carbon dioxide via a flowmeter through the tracheostomy if necessary.

5. Speech. A notebook or erasable pad should be provided for the patient to communicate. If the larynx is still functioning the patient can be shown how to speak by temporarily blocking the tube while exhaling. Patients with a permanent tracheostomy should if possible have a fenestrated tube with a speaking valve incorporated with the inner tube.

6. Swallowing. Some patients may experience problems, often because of the condition which necessitated the tracheostomy, but sometimes because of incoordination and the pressure of the tube's cuff. The tracheostomy tube may interfere with the normal mobility of the larynx during swallowing. Deflation of the cuff will sometimes help, but some patients may require a nasogastric tube.

7. Care of the tube. If there is an inner tube it should be taken out and cleaned whenever necessary; the outer tube must be held firmly while withdrawing the inner one. Replacement or cleaning of the outer tube is usually left for the first 5 days until a track has become established, then this should be done weekly or as required. If a cuffed tube has been used it should be inflated with the minimum amount of air that prevents an air leak, and it must have a low-pressure cuff to minimize the risk of tracheal stenosis. A spare tube of identical size and a tracheostomy dilator must always be available at the bedside in case a quick change is necessary. The first tube change is usually done about 48 hours after the tracheostomy and should always be performed by a doctor, preferably the surgeon who performed the procedure. Whenever the nursing staff perform subsequent tube changes it should be done when the whereabouts of a doctor is known in case of a problem.

8. Decannulation. The tracheostomy tube should be spigoted and removed as soon as is feasible. It should only be carried out when it is obvious that it is no longer required. The patient should be able to manage with the tube spigoted for a full 24-hour period, including a period of sleep. There may be difficulties in children who have had the tracheostomy for a long period of time, sometimes because of a psychological dependence on the tube. They also have a relatively smaller tracheal airway which may be partly blocked by granulation tissue, and surgical closure by excision of the scar tissue and the tracheocutaneous track may be required in some cases. After decannulation the patient should remain in hospital under observation for at least 2 days.

Complications

As with any operative procedure the complications of tracheostomy can be immediate (during the first 24 hours), intermediate (1–14 days) or late (>14 days). The following list can be a useful basis or plan for an examination answer.

1. Immediate.

- Anaesthetic complications.
- Damage to local structures (cricoid cartilage, recurrent laryngeal nerve, oesophagus, brachiocephalic vein).
- Cardiac arrest.
- Primary haemorrhage.

2. *Intermediate.*

- Dislodgement/displacement of the tube.
- Surgical emphysema.
- Pneumothorax.
- Obstruction of the tube or trachea (excessive crusting).
- Infection (perichondritis, wound infection, secondary haemorrhage).
- Tracheal necrosis (may lead to tracheal stenosis or tracheo-oesophageal fistula).

3. *Late.*

- Subglottic and tracheal stenosis.
- Decannulation difficulty.
- Tracheocutaneous fistula.
- Scar (hypertrophic or keloid).

Further reading

Bradley PJ. The obstructed airway. In: Stell PM (ed.). *Scott-Brown's Otolaryngology,* Vol. 5, 5th edn. London: Butterworths, 1987; 155–68.
Rogers JH. Tracheostomy and decannulation. In: Evans JNG (ed.) *Scott-Brown's Otolaryngology*, Vol. 6, 5th edn. London: Butterworths, 1987; 471–86.

Related topics of interest

TYMPANOPLASTY

Definition

Tympanoplasty is an operation to eradicate disease in the middle ear and to reconstruct the hearing mechanism with or without tympanic membrane grafting. Tympanoplasty may be combined with mastoid surgery (see Mastoidectomy, p. 165) when there is concomitant mastoid disease in patients with CSOM.

Myringoplasty is defined as an operation to repair or reconstruct the tympanic membrane. Strictly speaking it is not the same as a type 1 tympanoplasty because eradication of intercurrent middle-ear disease is not included in the definition. They are, however, often used synonomously.

Classification

Wullstein in 1953 described five tympanoplasty reconstruction techniques after eradication of middle-ear disease. A sixth was added by Garcia Ibanez in 1961.

1. Type 1. Reconstruction of the tympanic membrane when there is an intact and mobile ossicular chain.

2. Type 2. The malleus handle is absent. The tympanic membrane is reconstructed over the malleus remnant and the long process of the incus.

3. Type 3. The incus and malleus have been removed or eroded by disease. The tympanic membrane is reconstructed to lie on the stapes head to create a columella effect (myringostapediopexy). This is so called because in birds a single strut of bone, the columella, transmits sound from the tympanic membrane to the labyrinth.

4. Type 4. Only the stapes footplate remains. The footplate is exteriorized by leaving it exposed in the created mastoid cavity. The round window is acoustically separated from the oval window by reconstructing the tympanic membrane so that it's superior margin lies on the promontory below the oval window, creating a round window baffle.

5. Type 5. The stapes footplate is fixed and a fenestration of the lateral semicircular canal performed.

6. Type 6 or sono-inversion. There is an ossicular discontinuity. The round window niche is left uncovered and the tympanic membrane reconstructed so that its inferior edge lies on the promontory above the round window, thereby creating an oval window baffle.

In all of these procedures the aim is to aerate the middle ear by the Eustachian tube, but this is difficult to achieve because the repaired tympanic membrane often becomes atelectatic and adherent to the medial wall of the middle ear. In addition, it is evident that an intact ossicular chain is important to achieve a consistently good air–bone gap closure.

Ossicular chain reconstruction

Homograft tissue is now contraindicated because of the risk of Creutzfeldt–Jakob disease. Autograft reconstruction using cortical bone or remodelled incus is now usually preferred. An alternative is to use biodegradable porous hydroxyapatite tricalcium phosphate ceramics, which have been shown to be replaced at least in part by osteogenic cells and host connective tissue. There are several possible scenarios in reconstruction.

1. A stapes footplate remnant is present with or without the malleus. A myringostapediopexy or malleostapediopexy is performed using an autograft or ceramic total ossicular replacement prosthesis (TORP) to create the tympanic membrane or malleus-to-footplate assembly.

2. The stapes superstructure is intact with or without a malleus handle. An autograft malleus-to-stapes assembly or a ceramic partial ossicular replacement prosthesis (PORP) is used.

3. There is an incudostapedial discontinuity secondary to an absent lenticular process and/or stapes head. An incudostapediopexy using a cortical bone sliver as an incus-to-stapes assembly is the preferred method of reconstruction.

4. There is an incudostapedial discontinuity caused by an absent long process of the incus. A malleostapediopexy is performed after removing and refashioning the incus to create a malleus- to-stapes assembly.

To minimize extrusion of the ceramic implants most authorities recommend a sliver of autograft tragal cartilage is interposed between the tympanic membrane and prosthesis. Closure of the air–bone gap to within 20 dB has been reported in up to 80% of patients using ceramic PORPs and 50% of patients using TORPS. These results will probably decline in the long term.

Follow-up and aftercare   The ear canal dressing is removed after 7–14 days. Nasal decongestants may improve Eustachian tube function in the short term and help ensure aeration of the middle-ear cleft. Some authorities (e.g. Causse) advocate performing the Valsalva manoeuvre in the early postoperative period to achieve the same aim, although there is a theoretical risk of displacing the prosthesis. Exertion and flying should be avoided until healing is achieved at 4–6 weeks, although some otologists allow both in the first postoperative week. Swimming is contraindicated until healing, and diving may predispose to prosthesis displacement.

Further reading

Grote JJ. *Biomaterials in Otology*. Proceedings of the First International Symposium 1983. Leiden, The Netherlands: Martinus Nijhoff Publishers, 1983.
Montelaro JS, Horn KL. Techniques and materials in ossicular reconstruction. *Current Opinion in Otolaryngology and Head and Neck Surgery*. 1994; **2**: 382–7.
Wullstein H. Theory and practice of tympanoplasty. *Laryngoscope*, 1956; **66**: 1076–93.

Related topics of interest

Cholesteatoma (p. 43)
Chronic suppurative otitis media (p. 51)
Mastoidectomy (p. 165)

TYMPANOSCLEROSIS

Tympanosclerosis (also called chronic catarrhal otitis media) is an abnormal condition of the middle ear, characterized by calcareous deposits in the tympanic membrane, tympanic cavity and occasionally in the mastoid.

Aetiology

The exact cause remains in doubt, but it appears likely that there is an abnormal healing process in response to multiple acute or chronic inflammatory episodes. Another important aetiological factor is tissue trauma, which is substantiated by the frequent occurrence of tympanosclerosis after myringotomy with or without insertion of ventilation tubes; this may be due to intraepithelial haemorrhage.

Pathogenesis

Three stages are recognized. In the initial stage, inflammatory processes cause an exudate, the formation of granulation tissue and damage to collagen fibres. This phase is generally considered reversible. The second stage is the reparative phase, characterized by fibroblast invasion. This results in excessive collagen synthesis and hyalinization, as a result of which fibres become indistinct, fusing into a homogeneous mass. Most authorities now consider the process to be irreversible, and in the third and final stage calcification and occasionally ossification may occur. It has been well established that the pathological changes of tympanosclerosis are situated in the lamina propria, which is the connective tissue component of tympanic membrane and mucosa.

Clinical features

It has been suggested that the term myringosclerosis be used when the process is confined to the tympanic membrane and the term tympanosclerosis be exclusively reserved to describe sequelae of chronic otitis affecting the ossicular chain. Morphologically, however, no differentiation can be made between the two conditions. Furthermore, the occurrence of plaques in the tympanic membrane may indicate the presence of more extensive disease in the middle ear in patients with a history of chronic otitis.

1. Tympanic membrane. Tympanosclerosis that is restricted to the tympanic membrane is most commonly seen, usually following myringotomy and ventilation tube insertion. It may occur in all age groups. Otoscopically, deposits present as sharply demarcated areas of white opaque, chalk-like material. Plaques usually occur only in the pars tensa, mostly situated in the anterior or posterior segments, varying in size. The clinical importance of this calcification is dependent on its size. In most cases there is little if any effect on the patient's hearing, even with quite extensive plaques. However, with very large plaques and those that impinge across the annulus, measurable hearing loss may result (20–40 dB). The condition occurs in approximately 5% of children with otitis media with effusion who have had no previous surgery. There is, however, a natural tendency for resolution in this group.

2. Middle-ear. Middle-ear involvement is much less common, but when it occurs is usually accompanied by a perforation of the tympanic membrane (85–100%). Interestingly, these ears are often dry. The patients are usually over 30 years of age and have had a long history of ear problems. The condition tends to be most prevalent in the oval window niche, epitympanum and promontory. These patients often have a significant hearing loss, which is invariably due to fixation of the ossicular chain.

Investigation

The clinical appearance of tympanosclerosis in either the middle-ear cavity or tympanic membrane rarely presents any diagnostic difficulties although it may occasionally look like a cholesteatoma. Examination under a microscope will nearly always resolve the issue. In cases of tympanosclerosis the involved ear is usually dry with a large central perforation, whereas in an ear with cholesteatoma the perforation or retraction pocket is usually marginal and often there is malodorous otorrhoea. An audiogram to assess any degree of (conductive) hearing loss is always useful.

Management

Tympanic membrane tympanosclerosis with an intact drum rarely requires treatment. Occasionally removal of a plaque may be required during myringoplasty, for a coexistent perforation, to aid healing.

Conductive hearing loss caused by tympanosclerosis can be treated with either a hearing aid or surgery. A hearing aid is safe and effective; surgery is controversial. The choice of procedure depends on the extent of middle-ear involvement but may include stapedectomy and/or attic mobilization or clearance. Studies that show initial improvement in hearing also demonstrate a deterioration in hearing levels with time. Furthermore, it has been shown that a number of patients suffer a postoperative sensorineural hearing loss.

Follow-up and aftercare   This should be appropriate to the patient's surgery and any active otological pathology.

Further reading

Wielinga EWJ, Kerr AG. Tympanosclerosis (review). *Clinical Otolaryngology*, 1993, **18:** 341–9.

Related topics of interest

Cholesteatoma (p. 43)
Otitis media with effusion (p. 214)
Tympanoplasty (p. 328)

VERTIGO

Definition

Vertigo is the hallucination of movement. It is the cardinal symptom of disease of the vestibular system including its central connections.

The 'sense' of balance is very basic and phylogenetically predates sight and hearing. When this basic system goes wrong, the patient is left disabled. Sir Terence Cawthorne said that "labyrinthine disturbance may make one feel like the end of the world has arrived and I am told by sufferers from sea sickness that in the acutest phase of their distress they wish that it had". Remembering this enables us to understand the distress of these patients. It also, in combination with the very basic nature of the sense of balance, explains the many symptoms such as muzzy head, loss of memory and anxiety that are associated with vestibular disorders. These can therefore be explained as secondary effects from the vertigo and often remain after the vertigo has gone.

Anatomy and physiology

The vestibular sense organ consists of the three semicircular canals, the saccule and the utricle. These are membranous tubes within the dense temporal bone. The membranes are fluid filled and have cells with cilia which bend as the fluid moves relative to them. This excites or depresses the nerve cells and alters the tonic input into the brain. The semicircular canals are at right angles to each other and detect changes in angular acceleration. The utricle and saccule have otoconia embedded in a gel overlying the cilia and are positioned to detect linear acceleration.

The nerve impulses from the labyrinth go to the vestibular nuclei in the brain stem. Here they are integrated with two other inputs that enable us to balance. The two, other inputs are vision and proprioception, from the joints, skin and muscle receptors. The neck and ankles are the most important proprioceptive inputs. Approximately 70% of balance is due to visual input, 15% from proprioception and 15% from the vestibular system. The brain stem computerizes these three inputs and with the help of the cerebellum maintains the balance and co-ordination of the head and body.

Pathology and clinical syndromes

Non-vestibular disorders such as cardiovascular, metabolic, musculoskeletal or ocular disease may cause dizziness or a sense of light-headedness, though not usually vertigo.

Vestibular disorders are either central or peripheral. Central disease includes cerebrovascular disease, migraine, multiple sclerosis, brain tumours and very rarely vertebrobasilar insufficiency. The last hardly ever causes vertigo as a presenting symptom. Indeed, if the vertebral or basilar artery is constricted, dysarthria, visual phenomena, diplopia and weakness of one side of the body are usually the presenting signs. Cervical vertigo frequently occurs and is more likely to be due to disordered proprioceptive input from the neck. Iatrogenic vertigo caused by drugs (aminglycosides, diuretics, co-trimoxazole, metronidazole) is common due to either ototoxicity or a central effect. Non-organic dizziness and vertigo also exist and may be associated with hyperventilation. These causes aside, we are left with the peripheral causes of vertigo, of which there are three main symptom complexes.

- Benign positional vertigo commonly occurs after a head injury and is rotatory vertigo with a particular head movement. There are no other otological manifestations. It is diagnosed by the Hallpike manoeuvre.
- Menière's syndrome comprises paroxysmal fluctuating hearing loss, vertigo and tinnitus, each attack lasting many minutes or hours.
- Acute vestibular failure consists of marked vertigo for many hours or days often preceded by an upper respiratory tract infection.

Acoustic neuroma usually presents with a unilateral sensory hearing loss, but this is often accompanied by tinnitus and occasionally there is a non-specific dizziness. Middle-ear disease such as cholesteatoma can also cause vertigo, as can inner ear infections such as syphilis.

Clinical features

It is often difficult for patients to describe their sensations, and in taking a full and accurate history the feeling of vertigo must be differentiated from other types of dizziness such as fainting, light-headedness, claustrophobia, or some peripheral (musculoskeletal) dysequilibrium. A full description of the sensation should be obtained with reference to precipitating factors (e.g. neck movements), associated symptoms (e.g. deafness, tinnitus) and frequency and duration of the attacks. A previous history of trauma should be noted. Previous medical history, medication, and alcohol ingestion should also be considered in the context of possible causes or aggravation of the symptoms.

An otological and neurological examination is mandatory in all cases of vertigo. In particular middle-ear disease is looked for and nystagmus after finger following or after the Hallpike test. Gait assessment including Romberg's and Unterburger testing is important (see Vestibular function tests). A general medical examination may be required if the symptoms dictate.

The Hallpike manoeuvre

Positional nystagmus is best elicited by this positional test. The patient is positioned sitting on the edge of the bed and the procedure is explained. This explanation should include a reassurance to the patient that they will not be allowed to fall whatever happens. The patient is told to keep their eyes open and look straight ahead. The head is held firmly between the examiner's hands and turned 45° to the right or left. The patient is then rapidly laid backwards, with their head over the edge of the bed, 30° below the horizontal. The patient is asked if this provokes symptoms similar to those they have been describing and the eyes are observed for nystagmus. If neither occurs after 30 seconds then the patient is returned to the upright position and again asked if there is any vertigo and the eyes examined for nystagmus. If no symptoms or nystagmus are elicited the process is repeated but with the head to the other side.

Benign paroxysmal positional nystagmus elicited by the Hallpike manoeuvre usually has a latent period of 5–10 seconds before the onset of rotatory nystagmus, a fast component to the nystagmus directed towards the undermost ear, an associated vertigo which distresses the patient; and the nystagmus fatigues rapidly. This contrasts with nystagmus of central origin, which appears immediately, causes little or no vertigo and persists indefinitely if the head position is maintained. If there are no symptoms or nystagmus after the Hallpike manoeuvre, it is very unlikely that head positioning or neck extension has any role in the cause of the patient's vertigo.

Investigations

Vestibular testing consists of pure tone audiometry, evoked response audiometry, electronystagmography with caloric stimulation, optokinetic and positioning stimulation, and posturography (see Vestibular function tests). MRI with gadolinium enhancement is the radiological investigation of choice.

Management

1. Vestibular rehabilitation. This is now considered to be the mainstay of treatment in many vestibular disorders. The first step is to counsel the patient regarding their symptoms, to provide reassurance and to explain the importance of persisting with treatment. This is followed by a series of habituating exercises performed regularly to enable tolerance mechanisms to occur in the brain stem. It is known that structural changes occur to allow vestibular compensation such as a modification of the distribution and sensitivity of cholinergic synapses. These allow a new equilibrium situation to occur. With adequate counselling as many as 80% of patients with vestibular disorders will benefit from vestibular rehabilitation to encourage vestibular compensation. In addition to vestibular rehabilitation, patients may also benefit from spectacles to improve their visual acuity or a walking stick to aid peripheral balance function and to give them more confidence.

2. *Medical treatment.* This consists of lifestyle changes (e.g. less alcohol) and drugs. The latter are usually vestibular sedatives such as prochlorperazine or cinnarizine, histamine analogues such as betahistine, or antidepressants.

3. *Surgery.* This is usually used for episodic peripheral vertigo diagnosed as Meniere's syndrome and consists of endolymphatic sac shunting, vestibular neurectomy or labyrinthectomy. Occasionally it is used for benign positional vertigo when posterior semicircular canal obliteration or singular neurectomy is done.

Further reading

Wright A. Dizziness: *A Guide to Disorders of Balance.* London: Croom Helm, 1988.
Arenberg IK (ed.) *Dizziness and Balance Disorders.* Amsterdam: Kugler Publications, 1994.

Related topics of interest

Acoustic neuroma (p. 1)
Cholesteatoma (p. 43)
Chronic suppurative otitis media (p. 51)
Perilymph fistula (p. 244)
Vestibular function tests (p. 338)

VESTIBULAR FUNCTION TESTS

An individual maintains balance by coordinating sensory information provided by (1) the vestibular system, (2) the eyes and (3) the proprioceptors in the muscles of the limbs, trunk and neck. These sensory organs connect directly with the brain stem and the cerebellum and then with the cerebrum. The clinical correlate of this is that the assessment of any disorder of disequilibrium must be based on a multidisciplinary approach. A comprehensive history is essential, together with a complete general medical examination, with particular attention to the eyes, the ears, the central nervous system and the locomotor system.

Having established the need for a general medical approach to the problem of unsteadiness, it is necessary to identify the presence or absence of a vestibular component. Clinically, tests based on (a) the vestibulo-ocular reflex and (b) vestibulospinal reflexes can be performed.

Tests of the vestibulo-ocular reflex

Eye movements are generated in response to visual signals and vestibular activity. The central vestibulo-ocular and visuo-ocular pathways are intimately related, and both pathways share the common final pathway of the oculomotor neurone. If visually controlled eye movements are normal (e.g. saccades and the smooth pursuit system), derangement of the vestibulo-ocular reflex may correctly be ascribed to vestibular dysfunction. However, if visually controlled eye movements are abnormal, care must be taken in the interpretation of vestibulo-ocular responses.

Saccades	Saccades are rapid eye movements, which correct errors in the direction of gaze, and bring the desired object of fixation to the fovea in the shortest possible time. Central nervous system disease may cause abnormalities of latency, accuracy or velocity of saccades. Saccadic eye movements may be assessed by asking the patient to look back and forth between the examiner's index fingers, separated either horizontally or vertically.
Smooth pursuit	This system is responsible for maintaining gaze on a moving target, by comparing the eye velocity with that of the target velocity and producing a continuous match of eye and target position. It may be examined clinically by asking the patient to follow a pendulum swinging from side to side. Bilaterally impaired smooth pursuit is usually a non-specific abnormality observed in a fatigued patient or one who is on certain medication (alcohol, antidepressants, anticonvulsants or benzodiazepines). Unilateral impairment is a more reliable marker of central nervous system pathology.

Nystagmus

Nystagmus is an involuntary, rhythmical oscillation of the eyes away from the direction of gaze, followed by a return of the eyes to their original position. It can be either physiological or pathological.

Physiological nystagmus refers to nystagmus observed in normal subjects. It will be present in the majority of normal individuals if the irises of the eyes are deviated horizontally further than the punctum of the lacrimal sac: an important point to remember when testing for spontaneous nystagmus. Physiological nystagmus can also be induced by thermal (caloric) or rotational stimulation.

Pathological nystagmus may be congenital or acquired. Congenital nystagmus is present from birth. It is nearly always dependent on optic fixation and so disappears when this is removed by asking the patient to wear Frenzel's glasses. Acquired nystagmus is described as ocular, vestibular or central in origin.

1. Ocular nystagmus. This tends to be pendular. It is common in congenital blindness, but may occur without any defect of vision. Miner's nystagmus is a form of the ocular variety.

2. Vestibular nystagmus. This consists of a slow movement of the eyes in one direction followed by a quick return in the opposite direction. The slow component is produced by impulses from the vestibule. The fast component, or recovery movement, is a central correcting reflex. The direction of the nystagmus is named according to the direction of the fast component, e.g. a nystagmus whose quick component is to the right is called a nystagmus to the right. Nystagmus is most marked when the patient looks in the direction of the fast component and is lessened or abolished when looking in the direction of the slow component. Vestibular nystagmus can be spontaneous or positional.

(a) Spontaneous nystagmus can be elicited by asking the patient to follow a finger held 60 cm away to the left and then the right, and then up and down. Increasing degrees of severity of spontaneous nystagmus are recognized. First-degree nystagmus is present only when the eyes are deviated in the direction of the fast component. Second-degree nystagmus is present when the patient looks straight ahead. Third-degree nystagmus is still present when the patient looks in the direction of the slow component.

(b) Positional nystagmus is usually rotatory and accompanied by rotatory vertigo. Positional testing is described in detail elsewhere, see p. 334. Basically tests for positional nystagmus are done in the upright and supine positions with the head turned to either side. A nystagmus which is fatiguable and short-lasting is usually associated with a peripheral pathology (e.g. benign paroxysmal positional vertigo). A nystagmus which is not associated with vertigo and does not fatigue is more likely to be associated with a central lesion.

Specific tests based on the vestibulo-ocular reflex

1. Rotation tests. The nystagmus induced by acceleration and deceleration in a rotating chair is recorded. The test has the disadvantage of stimulating both labyrinths simultaneously. The test is also criticized because the stimulus is considered excessively violent, and it has found limited clinical application.

2. Caloric tests. In spite of improved imaging of the temporal bone and the advent of evoked response audiometry, this remains a popular investigation. It is also a popular topic in the Fellowship examination (see Caloric tests).

3. Electronystagmography (ENG). This technique is based upon the positive potential which exists between the cornea and retina. Electrodes are attached to the skin at each outer canthus close to the eyes. Changes in the corneoretinal potentials are recorded at the electrode sites as the eyes move from straight-ahead gaze. The changes in electric potential are used to follow nystagmus, and after amplification are recorded permanently on a moving paper strip. Full ENG testing includes a series of tests including different head positions, eyes open and closed, and caloric tests.

Test of the vestibulospinal reflex

Tests based on the vestibulo-ocular reflex are regarded as the most essential part of the investigation of the vestibular system. In contrast, tests of vestibulospinal function are commonly neglected in the evaluation of patients with balance dysfunction. Clinically vestibulospinal function is tested by examining stance and gait.

Romberg test	The Romberg test is used to assess a patient's ability to stand, feet together, arms by the side, with eyes open and then closed. The patient may fall towards the side of a recent peripheral vestibular lesion.
Unterburger test	This is performed by asking the patient to walk up and down on the spot for 30 seconds, with eyes closed and arms outstretched in front, with hands clasped together. Body rotation of more than 30°, or forward or backward displacement of more than 1 metre, is regarded as abnormal.
Gait testing	Gait is assessed by watching the patient walk normally with eyes open and then closed. A hemiplegic gait, cerebellar ataxic gait, Parkinsonian shuffle, or high stepping gait with loss of proprioception may become apparent. With eye closure some patients with uncompensated vestibular lesions will veer towards the affected side.
Specific tests based on the vestibulospinal reflex	Objective balance assessment has potential clinical use in the investigation of dizzy patients as a complement to existing tests. Posturography is the recording of postural sway. Several techniques have been used to evaluate such postural stability, but the most commonly used are force platforms. The data have enabled the effects of various sensory modalities upon balance to be identified, and some claim they allow various pathological conditions to be differentiated. A few of the more recent platforms have been used to rehabilitate patients with balance dysfunction by way of visual feedback. The high cost of many balance platforms has prohibited their use in both research and clinical practice.

Further reading

Luxon LM. Methods of examination – audiological and vestibular. In: Ludman H (ed.) *Mawson's Diseases of the Ear,* 5th edn. London: Edward Arnold, 1988; 153–89.
Schwaber MK. Vestibular function analysis. *Current Opinion in Otololaryngology and Head and Neck Surgery,* 1993; **1:** 35–9.

Related topics of interest

Caloric tests (p. 35)
Vertigo (p. 334)

VOCAL CORD PALSY

Anatomy

The roots of the vagus emerge from the pons and medulla to gain a trunk and exit the skull through the jugular foramen. The vagus gives two important branches for voice production: the superior and the recurrent laryngeal nerves. The superior laryngeal nerve branches into the external laryngeal nerve, supplying the cricothyroid muscle, a cord adductor, and the internal laryngeal nerve, which is sensory to the laryngeal mucosa above the vocal cords. The recurrent laryngeal nerve arises high in the chest on the right, looping around the subclavian artery to reach the tracheo-oesophageal groove, but on the left arises at the level of and looping around the aortic arch to reach the same groove. The nerve enters the larynx below the cricoid cartilage and the lateral origin of cricopharyngeus and so cannot be injured above this level. It supplies the remaining intrinsic laryngeal muscles and is sensory to mucosa below the cords.

Pathology

A vocal cord palsy may be unilateral or bilateral, and the movement the cords *cannot* initiate is described as an adductor or an abductor palsy. There are two theories describing the position of the vocal cord, neither of which is entirely satisfactory.

(a) Semon's law states that, for any lesion affecting the recurrent laryngeal nerve, the fibres supplying the adductors are more susceptible to injury. The cord should lie in a median position if this were true.

(b) The Wagner–Grossman theory proposes that, because the superior laryngeal nerve supplies the cord adductor cricothyroid, a low lesion of the recurrent laryngeal nerve will allow the vagus to exert an overall adductor effect on the vocal cord, but with a lesion affecting the origin or above of the superior laryngeal nerve the cord will lie in the cadaveric position. The fact that a cord palsy caused by a left apical bronchial carcinoma produces a median positioned cord somewhat discredits this theory.

A vocal cord palsy may arise from pathology of:

(1) The recurrent laryngeal nerve, e.g. iatrogenic, pressure damage or a neuropathy.

(2) The cricoarytenoid joint, e.g rheumatoid arthritis.

(3) The intrinsic muscles which move the vocal cord, e.g. a myopathy or infiltration by a malignancy.

Aetiology	(a) Malignant disease (30%), especially of the bronchus, oesophagus, thyroid and nasopharynx. (b) Iatrogenic (25%), especially thyroid and parathyroid, oesophageal, pharyngeal pouch and left lung surgery. (c) External trauma (15%), e.g. from road traffic or sporting accidents and stab or gunshot injury. (d) Idiopathic (15%), in which no cause is identified but which may be related to infection with a neurotropic virus. (e) Others (15%), e.g. neurological disorders, myopathies, Orton's syndrome and inflammatory disease.
Clinical feature	A breathy voice with a poor cough suggests an uncompensated adductor palsy. A voice which becomes weak or hoarse with use suggests an abductor palsy or a compensated adductor palsy. Stridor suggests a bilateral abductor palsy. Aspiration can occur with any palsy if the sensory supply to the larynx is compromised. Symptoms related to the cause may be present, such as haemoptysis or dysphagia.
Investigations	A chest radiograph, barium swallow and an MRI scan from the skull base to the aortic arch followed by a panendoscopy are necessary when no cause is obvious.
Management	*1. Unilateral abductor palsy.* In most cases no treatment is necessary because the normal cord compensates to produce a near-normal voice which tires with use. *2. Bilateral abductor palsy.* Many patients surprisingly are not stridulous unless they develop an upper respiratory tract infection. Others are stridulous and the treatment options are: an endoscopic laser cordectomy or arytenoidectomy or both, a permanent tracheostomy or a neuromuscular pedicle procedure using the ansa cervicalis and a strap muscle (described by Tucker). *3. Unilateral adductor palsy.* When the cause is idiopathic or there is a chance of spontaneous resolution, a wait of at least a year is necessary. Any improvement in voice will be at the expense of the airway, so judgement is required to achieve the optimum compromise. Treatment consists in a cord medialization procedure which comprises: • Injection of Teflon (available on a named-patient basis as it may cause granulation tissue formation) or a collagenase-resistant collagen (e.g GAX collagen), which

is injected just lateral to the vocalis muscle at two sites: just anterior to the vocal process and midway between this and the anterior commisure.

- An anterior thyroplasty (e.g. Isshiki), posterior thyroplasty (e.g. Woodman's operation) or a suture technique (e.g. Downie's arytenoidoplasty).

4. Bilateral adductor palsy. Most patients will aspirate and often the cause is a neurological or myopathic disorder so that medialization procedures do not usually help the cause. A permanent tracheostomy or even a laryngectomy as a last resort may be required.

Follow-up and aftercare
This is required:
(a) To exclude an occult carcinoma.
(b) To observe spontaneous resolution.
(c) To enable a stable situation to be reached with regard to the voice and airway.

Aftercare will be necessary for those patients requiring a tracheostomy.

Further reading

Tucker HM. Human laryngeal reinnervation. *Laryngoscope,* 1976; **86**: 769–79.
Woodson GE, Miller RH. The timing of surgical intervention in vocal cord paralysis. *Otolaryngology and Head and Neck Surgery*, 1981; **89**: 264–7.

Related topics of interest

Lasers in ENT (p. 161)
Stridor and stertor (p. 301)
Tracheostomy (p. 323)

INDEX

ALSO AVAILABLE FROM BIOS SCIENTIFIC PUBLISHERS LTD

Resuscitation: key data 2/e

M.J.A. Parr & T.M. Craft
respectively Bristol Royal Infirmary; and Royal United Hospital, Bath, UK

Updated to include all the latest treatment guidelines from the European
Resuscitation Council, the American College of Surgeons, and many others,
this second edition of Resuscitation: Key Data now provides an even more
comprehensive collection of essential data for the resuscitation of neonatal,
paediatric and adult patients. Treatment protocols for a broad range of
conditions are clearly presented as flowcharts and decision trees allowing
instant access to the key data in an emergency situation. Tabulated
information on Apgar and Glasgow coma scoring, the constituents of
intravenous fluids, antiarrhthmic drug doses and normal values for some of
the more common investigations. This book is an indispensable pocket
reference guide for all hospital doctors, nurses and paramedics.

"This book is definitely not one for gathering dust on the bookshelf, but would
be more at home in the white coat pocket where I have no doubt it will
become well thumbed." *J.Br.Assoc.Immediate Care* - "Don't just keep it in
your pocket. read it, use it and keep using it." Colin Robertson, Chairman of
the UK Resuscitation Council - "It should quickly become tatty in the hands
of those at the sharp end of medicine. It is a production of which the authors
can be justly proud." *Today's Anaesthetist*

Contents

Part 1 Adult resuscitation: Basic life support; Advanced life support; Cardiac;
Trauma; Burns; Anaphylaxis; Acute severe asthma; Hypothermia; Drug
overdose. Part 2 Paediatric resuscitation: Basic life support; Advanced life
support; Newborn; Infant and child; Trauma; Burns. Part 3 Normal
physiological values: Biochemistry; Haematology; Coagulation; Blood gases;
Conversion factors.

Of interest to:

All doctors, nurses, paramedics and practitioners trained in resuscitation.

Paperback; 112 pages; 1-85996-060-X; 1995

Key Topics in Accident & Emergency Medicine

P. Howarth & R. Evans
respectively Royal Cornwall Hospital, Truro, UK; and Cardiff Royal Infirmary, UK

Provides the key information on acute injuries and sudden illness which commonly present at Accident and Emergency Departments. The information is organised in a uniform manner with the focus on diagnosis and immediate management. The book is an ideal revision aid for postgraduate examinations, such as the FRCS examination in Accident and Emergency Medicine. It is also a valuable source of reference for anyone who deals with acute problems, including paramedics, general practitioners and nurses.

"Within a logical and attractive layout it covers 91 topics... All are relevant to everyday practice as well as being likely topics to be covered at some stage during the accident and emergency fellowship examination... readable and up-to-date... especially useful for candidates working for the fellowship examination." *BMJ*

Contents

100 key topics in current accident and emergency medicine presented in alphabetical order.

Of interest to:

Medical and nursing staff working in Emergency and Surgical Departments, particularly candidates for Fellowship or other postgraduate qualifications (such as the FRCS examination in Accident and Emergency Medicine). Also useful as a reference for paramedics; nurses and practitioners.

Paperback; 332 pages; 1-872748-67-8; 1994

Key Topics in Anaesthesia

T.M. Craft & P.M. Upton
respectively Bristol Royal Infirmary, UK; and Radcliffe Infirmary, Oxford, UK

Essential information on 100 major subjects pertinent to modern clinical practice in anaesthesia. The uniform, systematic structure of the text is designed to encourage a problem-based approach to clinical scenarios. An ideal revision aid for trainee anaesthetists and a useful reference source for qualified anaesthetists.

"I think this book is a winner. What about those to whom it is aimed? I have not yet found a member of our junior staff who, prior to taking the test [FRCA part III], has not already purchased a copy. May I also recommend it to their teachers?" *Today's Anaesthetist*

Contents

Each topic includes (wherever the subject allows): introduction; essential problems; anaesthetic management - assessment and premedication, conduct of anaesthesia, and postoperative care; further reading; and related topics of interest.

Of interest to:

Trainee anaesthetists studying for postgraduate examinations (e.g. FRCA Parts I and III, European Academy of Anaesthesiology examination, etc.); qualified anaesthetists, anaesthetic assistants, nurse anaesthetists and surgeons.

Paperback; 312 pages; 1-872748-90-2; 1992

ALSO AVAILABLE FROM BIOS SCIENTIFIC PUBLISHERS LTD

Key Topics in Paediatrics

A.E.M. Davies & A.L. Billson
respectively Bristol Royal Hospital for Sick Children, UK; and University of Nottingham, UK

Describes important issues in child health, and the identification and management of problems. The information is presented in a systematic format which makes the book ideal for revision purposes. The topic-orientated approach also ensures the book is a valuable source of reference.

Contents

100 key topics in current paediatrics presented in alphabetical order.

Of interest to:

Candidates studying for a postgraduate examination in paediatrics, such as the MRCP (Paed) Parts I and II or the Diploma of Child Health. Also useful as a reference source for all general practitioners, paediatricians, students and nurses.

Paperback; 348 pages; 1-872748-58-9; 1994

Key Topics in Obstetrics and Gynaecology

R.J. Slade, E. Laird & G. Beynon
respectively University Hospital of Wales, Cardiff, UK; Northampton General
Hospital, UK; and Queen Elizabeth II Hospital, Gateshead, UK

A compact, easy-to-read text for trainee obstetricians and gynaecologists.
This book provides information on 100 major topics regarded as essential
knowledge to pass a postgraduate examination. Wherever possible, the
information is presented in a uniform, systematic format to encourage a
problem-based approach to clinical scenarios. The book is an ideal revision
aid with each key topic designed to be read at an individual sitting.

"Whilst one hesitates to recommend such volumes as a basis for learning,
this particular publication will be found by many to be a useful guide to
preparation for examinations from final MB to the MRCOG." *Br.J.Obstetrics
& Gynaecology*

Contents

Of interest to:

Trainee obstetricians and gynaecologists studying for a postgraduate
examination, such as the MRCOG part II; also general practitioners and
medical students.

Paperback; 296 pages; 1-872748-07-4; 1993

ORDERING DETAILS

Main address for orders

BIOS Scientific Publishers Ltd
9 Newtec Place, Magdalen Road,
Oxford OX4 1RE, UK
Tel: (0)1865 726286
Fax: (0)1865 246823

Australia and New Zealand
DA Information Services
648 Whitehorse Road, Mitcham, Victoria 3132, Australia
Tel: (03) 873 4411
Fax: (03) 873 5679

India
Viva Books Private Ltd
4346/4C Ansari Road, New Delhi 110 002, India
Tel: 11 3283121
Fax: 11 3267224

Singapore and South East Asia
(Brunei, Hong Kong, Indonesia, Korea, Malaysia, the Philippines,
Singapore, Taiwan, and Thailand)
Toppan Company (S) PTE Ltd
38 Liu Fang Road, Jurong, Singapore 2262
Tel: (265) 6666
Fax: (261) 7875

USA and Canada
Books International Inc
PO Box 605, Herndon, VA 22070, USA
Tel: (703) 435 7064
Fax: (703) 689 0660

Payment can be made by cheque or credit card (Visa/Mastercard, quoting number and expiry date). Alternatively, a *pro forma* invoice can be sent.

Prepaid orders must include £2.50/US$5.00 to cover postage and packing for one item. Prepaid orders for two or more books are delivered postage free.